Contraception: Science and Practice

Contraception: Science and Practice

Edited by

Marcus Filshie, DM, FRCOG
Reader and Consultant, Department of Obstetrics and Gynaecology
University Hospital, Queen's Medical Centre, Nottingham

and

John Guillebaud, MA, FRCSE, FRCOG
Medical Director, Margaret Pyke Centre, Soho Square, London

Butterworth–Heinemann
London Boston Singapore Sydney Toronto Wellington

PART OF REED INTERNATIONAL P.L.C.

First published 1989
Reprinted 1990
Reprinted 1991

British Library Cataloguing in Publication Data

Contraception.
1. Contraception. For medicine
I. Filshie, Marcus II. Guillebaud, John
613.9′4
ISBN 0–7506–1186–3

Library of Congress Cataloging in Publication Data

Contraception: science and practice.
Includes bibliographies and index.
1. Contraception. I. Filshie, Marcus. II. Guillebaud, John.
[DNLM: 1. Contraception—methods. WP 630 C7616]
RG136.C5715 1989 613.9′4 88–26213
ISBN 0–7506–1186–3

Typeset by Latimer Trend & Company Ltd, Plymouth, UK
Printed and bound by Hartnolls Ltd, Bodmin, Cornwall

Preface

Much has been written on the subject of contraception, yet there remain two incontrovertible facts. The first is that the world's population is increasing by rather more than one million every five days. The continuing lack of priority given to tackling this growth in human numbers (by reducing it rather than merely attempting to accommodate to it) shows that neither politicians nor voters have yet appreciated its devasting implications for meeting human needs.

The second fact is the great extent of individual need even today. This was shown in developing countries by the World Fertility Survey. Numerous consumer surveys in developed countries have also demonstrated how deficient our current birth-control methods remain, despite much research, in terms both of perceived safety and of simplicity for users. Yet the methods are not nearly so bad as they are often made to appear by the media. Moreover, these methods could be so much better delivered by the caring professions to the ordinary couples of the world.

This book has been conceived as a guidebook both in facing the emergency threatened by the first fact, and in using the available methods better to meet the human needs implicit in the second.

The contributors are each world experts and innovators in their particular subject. They have been given free rein and have written with infectious enthusiasm as well as knowledge. The scene is set with a fascinating overview by Dr Malcolm Potts and Dr Bhiwandiwala. As a matter of policy the chapters have been only minimally edited, to preserve the stamp of each author's individuality. Therefore we believe the book reads more like an anthology or a proceedings than a treatise.

Although there is much 'science', the aim throughout has been to aid 'practice'. Much space has been given to the expanding subject of hormonal contraception. Despite the improvements in formulation and hence increased safety, 'the pill' and its cousins continue to be attacked by the popular press. The relevant chapters should help to put the subject into perspective.

The book is particularly intended for physicians engaged in teaching or research in birth-control techniques, although it will be a valuable reference book and resource for many others.

It has been a privilege to work with such an articulate and talented team of invited experts, from whom we have had great cooperation. We gratefully thank each one for his or her invaluable contribution. We also acknowledge the help of Mr John Harrison of Butterworths and of the many secretaries and production assistants whose labours (so often unsung) have turned our ideas into the finished product.

MARCUS FILSHIE
JOHN GUILLEBAUD

Contributors

P. Bhiwandiwala *MB, BS, MSPH*
University of North Carolina, Chapel Hill, North Carolina, USA

John Bonnar *MA, MB, ChB, FRCOG*
Professor of Obstetrics and Gynaecology, and Dean of the Faculty of Medicine, University of Dublin, Trinity College, Dublin, Eire

Walli Bounds *SCM*
Associate Research Fellow, University College London; Research Co-ordinator, Margaret Pyke Centre for Study and Training in Family Planning, Soho Square, London, UK

Peter Bowen-Simpkins *MA, MB, BChir, FRCOG*
Consultant Obstetrician and Gynaecologist, Singleton Hospital, Swansea, West Glamorgan, UK

Elizabeth B. Connell *MD*
Professor of Obstetrics and Gynecology, Emory University School of Medicine, Atlanta, Georgia, USA

James Drife *BSc, MD, ChB, FRCS (Ed), MRCOG*
Consultant and Senior Lecturer, University of Leicester, Department of Obstetrics and Gynaecology, Clinical Sciences Building, Leicester Royal Infirmary, Leicester, UK

Marcus Filshie *DM, FRCOG*
Reader/Consultant in Obstetrics and Gynaecology, University Hospital, Queen's Medical Centre, Nottingham, UK

Anna M. Flynn *MB, BCh, BAO NUI, FRCOG*
Senior Clinical Research Fellow, Department of Obstetrics and Gynaecology, Birmingham Maternity Hospital, Queen Elizabeth Medical Centre, Birmingham, UK

K. Fotherby *PhD*
Reader in Chemical Pathology, Royal Postgraduate Medical School, Hammersmith Hospital, London, UK

Ian S. Fraser *MD, BSc(Hons), MB, ChB, FRCOG, FRACOG*
Department of Obstetrics and Gynaecology, University of Sydney, New South Wales, Australia

Michael Gillmer *MA, MD, FRCOG*
Consultant Obstetrician and Gynaecologist, John Radcliffe Hospital, Oxford, UK

John Guillebaud *MA, FRCSE, FRCOG*
Medical Director, Margaret Pyke Centre for Study and Training in Family Planning, Soho Square, London, UK

W. F. Hendry *ChM, FRCS*
Consultant Genitourinary Surgeon, St Bartholomew's and Royal Marsden Hospitals, London, UK

S. L. Jeffcoate *MB, BChir, PhD, FRCPath*
National Institute for Biological Standards and Control, Hertfordshire, UK

A. Kubba *MB, ChB, MRCOG*
Deputy Medical Director, Margaret Pyke Centre for Study and Training in Family Planning, Soho Square, London, UK

M. Potts *MB, BChir, PhD*
President, Family Health International, Research Triangle Park, North Carolina, USA

Jacques-E. Rioux *MD, MPH*
Professor, Department of Obstetrics and Gynaecology and Director, Department of Gynaecology – Reproduction, Le Centre Hospitalier de l'Université Laval, Sainte-Foy, Quebec, Canada

G. Robinson *BSc, PhD, CBiol, MIBiol*
Senior Lecturer, Department of Pathology, University of Nottingham, Nottingham, UK

Howard J. Tatum *MD, PhD*
Professor, Department of Gynecology-Obstetrics, Emory University School of Medicine, Atlanta, Georgia, USA

Martin Vessey *MD, FRCP, FFCM, FRCGP*
Professor, Department of Community Medicine and General Practice, Gibson Laboratories Building, Radcliffe Infirmary, Oxford, UK

C. C. Welch *MB, ChB, MRCOG*
Consultant, Department of Obstetrics and Gynaecology, Basildon Hospital, Essex, UK

A. Yuzpe *MD, MSc, FRCS(C), FACOG, FACS*
Professor, Department of Obstetrics and Gynaecology, The University of Western Ontario, London, Ontario, Canada

Contents

Chapter 1

Birth control: a world view

M. Potts and P. Bhiwandiwala

Need

All non-seasonally breeding mammals have evolved mechanisms for the optimum spacing of pregnancies. The higher primates such as man and the chimpanzees are slow breeders, and on the average reproduce every 3–5 years. Throughout most of human evolution the total fertility rate (average number of children born during a fertile lifetime) was probably 5–6. The !Kung, who live in the Kalahari desert, have a population doubling time of approximately 300 years even though they use no 'modern' methods of birth control.

In hunting/food-gathering societies, as among the large primates, the pregnancy interval is determined by the suppression of ovulation during lactation. In the West we think of breast-feeding as an unimportant and unreliable method of family planning. However, a woman in, say, Bangladesh who is breast-feeding at one year is much more likely to be anovulatory than an American woman who also happens to breast-feed for one year. It appears that the suppression of ovulation is more complete and consistent when the child is exclusively dependent upon the mother's breastmilk, when (*a*) suckling is frequent (on average the !Kung suckle every 14 minutes), (*b*) when the child sleeps with the mother at night, and (*c*) when the mother has an adequate but not overgenerous diet and is physically active. Under these conditions ovulation can be suppressed for 30–40 months. For the !Kung, the average child-spacing interval is 44 months.

Epidemiological studies confirm that the human reproductive system has been finely tuned by evolution to produce an optimum interval between two pregnancies. Both infant and maternal mortality and morbidity rise when pregnancy intervals are reduced by abandoning traditional methods of breast-feeding.

Currently the human race is experiencing a second population explosion. The first occurred when hunter/gatherer societies moved into agricultural communities, beginning ten thousand or so years ago when there were probably 50 million people in the world. Fertility almost certainly rose due to minor changes in lactation and access to more food with less effort, but infant mortality remained high – or possibly even rose a little as population densities grew. Until the Industrial Revolution, most human populations grew slowly at about half a percent per year and a poor harvest or an outbreak of disease often caused a sudden rise in the death rate. Historical demographers, reconstituting families from church records, have shown that such jumps in the death rate were often limited to small geographical areas.

In industrialized nations during the nineteenth century the population grew at about 1% per annum. Improved transport, ameliorated localized food shortages, better sanitation, clean water, and a gradual growth in economic wealth all helped cut down infant mortality and led to some improvement in adult health. In England and Wales in 1771 there were less than 6.5 million people, whereas in 1871 there were more than 21.5 million. The birth rate during that interval probably fluctuated between about 36 and 40 per thousand, and the death rate fell marginally from 22 to perhaps 18 per thousand of the population. The growth in numbers in the Western industrialized nations was associated with emigration to North and South America, Africa, Australia, New Zealand and other colonies of the European powers.

When animals become crowded, the age of sexual maturity, infant mortality, and the interval between births all tend to rise. During the nineteenth- and twentieth-century population explosions, the age of the menarche has declined. The interval between pregnancies grew less with reduced intervals of breast-feeding, early weaning, and finally an increase in artificial feeding. While these changes were instrumental in the rise in fertility, the infant mortality rate also fell.

Since the Second World War, the population explosion has spread to the developing world. The changes that took place in the West have occurred much more rapidly in the Third World. Mortality has fallen due to improvements in political stability, the ability to meet local food shortages, improvements in sanitation, the vaccination of infants, the advent of antibiotics, and the partial control of malaria and other endemic diseases. Fertility has risen as bottle feeding has spread and as the age of the menarche has decreased slightly.

When a nuclear weapon explodes, 99.9% of the energy release occurs in the last seven generations of the 58 generations of nuclear fission before the core of the bomb is vaporized. The human population explosion takes decades rather than microseconds to occur, but as with a nuclear explosion, nearly all the consequences are concentrated in the last one or two doublings of the population. Whatever actions are taken, barring a global war on an unprecedented scale, human population will certainly double, may treble, and could even quadruple in the twenty-first century. Global population passed the two thousand million mark in the 1920s, reached four thousand million by 1975, five thousand million in 1987 and will certainly exceed six thousand million by the year 2000. The so-called 'low' projection of the United Nations is for 8.4 thousand million people by the year 2050, and the 'high' projection is 12.4 thousand million for that date. Which of these two numbers is achieved depends largely upon the vigour with which birth control initiatives are pursued in the 1990s.

More than half the population of the developing world is below the age of marriage, and even if those now born were to settle for only two children – which is certainly not going to happen – the distortion of the age pyramid that has occurred since the Second World War would ensure that populations continue to grow rapidly. Most of this growth will occur in the countries of Asia, where the population base is largest, although the highest absolute rates of population growth are being recorded in Africa.

In the world as a whole the percentage rate of growth in population has declined marginally in the last ten years, but so much demographic momentum has already been set up that the *absolute* annual increment in population continues to grow. To take a specific example, the population of Japan continues to increase by almost one million people a year, even though the total fertility rate is near to biological replacement – that is, each woman is currently expected to bear slightly more than two children in her fertile lifetime. For zero population growth to occur, which is the number of deaths equalling the number of births in the society, the population structure of the society must also be stable, as in Western Europe in the 1980s. Some countries have had less than replacement birth rates, and such an event always triggers political extremists to make wild statements about a 'birth dearth', although in reality population changes tend to be slow and to correct themselves. It is always easier to rise slowly to some sort of ceiling than to try to control an explosion.

The annual increment in the world's population is, by pure coincidence, approximately in step with the Western calendar year – 88 million more births than deaths in 1988 and 89 million more a year later. The population and the calendar year are marching in step towards a difficult and threatening future.

The world has accommodated significant population increases before: thus, some forecasting the future find comfort in the fact that the prices of raw materials tend to fall with increasing demand, and they also feel that these extra hands and brains will be available to solve problems. However, the unprecedented growth in population is making itself felt in relation to employment even before it impinges on food and natural resources. In order for agriculture to become more productive it must be more mechanized, and is thus likely to employ fewer rather than more people. The biggest migration in human history is taking place as hundreds of millions of people leave a traditional village way of life, which in many ways has changed little over the past 4000 years, to enter the exploding cities of the contemporary world with their multiplying problems. In the past 15 years nearly 600 million people, approximately the population of India, have become city dwellers for the first time. By the end of this century there will be another 1.5 thousand million, approximately equal to the total world population in 1900. In 1950 Brazil was 64% rural; in 1970, it was 56% urban.

It costs many thousands of dollars to create a new non-agricultural job in any part of the world. Between 1970 and 1985 the number of Asians of working age increased by 500 million. Unemployment, and with it political frustration and social instability, is bound to increase. Millions of people will live in squatter areas in the meanest of shacks on the poorest land, while governments pretend they do not exist or bulldoze down their fragile homes. Mexico City is probably destined to contain more than 30 million people by the year 2000. Such a concentration of human beings is unprecedented and its consequences difficult to predict.

The AIDS epidemic is reminding the world that *Homo sapiens* is not the omniscient species we believed ourselves to be. Most virologists believe the human immunodeficiency virus (HIV) has jumped from a primate host into the human population. It is a reasonable speculation that such a transition has probably occurred on a number of occasions in the past. The reason that the epidemic appeared in the 1970s and 1980s was that urbanization had provided the tinder where the spark of HIV infection could catch hold. In Africa the massive migration to cities and the breakdown of family life set up a situation where many men were having sufficient sexual partners to spread HIV infection rapidly. In the West, socially disadvantaged and largely unemployed urban groups joined the subculture of drug abusers and spread the disease through contaminated needles, while the specialized lifestyles of urban gay men in North America proved to be the flash point for homosexual transmission of the virus.

If uncontrolled, HIV infection may involve 100 million people by the turn of the century. If such a catastrophe occurs, it could lead to three times as many deaths from AIDS in the decade 2000–2010 than occurred during the Black Death in the fourteenth century, yet it would still only represent one year's global population growth for the end of the twentieth century: AIDS has the potential to kill vast numbers of people but not to reverse the population explosion.

In undeveloped countries fertility is high, most women are delivered by traditional birth attendants, and maternal mortality reaches appalling levels. Studies by Family Health International (FHI) show that some rural areas of Egypt and Indonesia have up to 77 times the maternal mortality rate of the US. It is likely that more women will die in childbirth between now and the end of the century than at any similar interval in human history. Whereas 85% of all births and 95% of all the infant mortality are in the developing world, an astonishing 99% of all maternal deaths occur in Third World countries, predominantly in rural areas outside the reach of medical services. More women die in one month in India from pregnancy, childbirth and illegal abortions than die in the whole of North America, Eastern or Western Europe and Scandinavia, Japan, Australia and New Zealand in *one year*. At a global level, maternal mortality is equivalent to crashing a jumbo jet full of parturient or aborting women every 5 hours, day after day.

Response

It took Great Britain more than a hundred years to bring its births and deaths into balance after the Industrial Revolution. Over most of this interval, contraceptives were of poor quality, the medical profession made little or no contribution to research or services, abortion was illegal, and voluntary sterilization was rarely used. Population was dependent upon do-it-yourself methods of family planning, such as *coitus interruptus* or corner-store and mail-order sales of relatively poor-quality condoms and spermicides. Illegal abortions were rampant, showing that desired family size was for a great many people smaller than what was being achieved.

All the countries in Asia except Burma and North Korea, and nearly all the countries of the developing world, now have a national commitment to family planning and the reduction of population growth. Governments are attempting to make services available to people. In the last 10–15 years a revolution in legislation has abrogated restrictive laws on contraception in most countries, with a few exceptions such as Madagascar. The majority of the population now lives in countries where abortion is legal, from Muslim Tunisia and Turkey to capitalist USA and Western Europe to Communist China and Cuba.

The World Fertility Survey conducted in the 1970s was the largest exercise in social science ever undertaken. It found a surprisingly strong desire for fertility control in nearly all societies. Almost without exception, desired family size is less than achieved family size. At present about half of all the women in the world who currently have three or more children do not wish to have any more. However, a gap remains between the stated desire to control fertility and actual practice. And even desired family size remains high when considered in the light of the world's demographic problems. Nevertheless the vigorous and realistic provision of services in the remaining years of this century may still permit mankind to control its numbers on a voluntary basis. The problem that faces those professionally involved in any aspect of fertility regulation, whether in rich or in poor countries, is to ensure that the services that we make available actually meet the perceived needs of the societies we have the privilege to serve.

In the developing world an instructive contrast can be drawn between the experiences of India and China in fertility regulation. In the last 15 years the birth rate in the Peoples' Republic of China has plummeted from 34 per thousand to 18 per thousand – a 47% reduction. Fundamental social changes have taken place, and unique concepts such as the one-child family have evolved. However, the two main lessons to come out of China are the dangers of delaying action in the face of population growth and the need to make the full range of fertility regulation services available.

The problem that faces China, which the leadership of the country now fully understands, is that for too long in the 1960s and 1970s population growth was either ignored or too little was done too late. It is a measure of the momentum of demographic change and the predominantly young population of developing countries that, if 70% or more of all Chinese couples now adopt the one-child family policy, the population of the nation will still *grow* by 200 million in the next 20 years. This means that a country the physical size of the United States will add almost as many people as now live in the United States to a base population of 1 thousand million. The imposition of the one-child family is unpopular, and has been accepted by the political leaders, the medical profession and the citizens of the country only because there is no viable alternative. Tragically, many women in China today find themselves having to abort a wanted pregnancy, often under considerable social pressure from their neighbours, because their parents a generation ago were not able to prevent *unwanted* pregnancies. It will be interesting to see if Nigeria, Brazil, Mexico, and other countries with rapidly growing populations learn from the errors of China.

The second lesson to be gained from China is that the successes that have been achieved have resulted from policies encouraging the widespread availability of the maximum number of methods – including voluntary sterilization through a variety of channels.

India started family planning earlier than China but has still not really come to grips with what needs to be, or can be, done. The Indian census estimate for 1981 (638 million) was considerably higher than had been hoped. The birth rate was 36 per thousand and the death rate 14.8 per thousand. India adds 13 million extra people to its population each year, and may well have the dubious honour of being the most populous nation in the world by the year 2000. Unlike China, India has concentrated on single-method solutions to her problems: first, the use of IUDs, and later, sterilization. Unlike the 'barefoot doctors' in China who play an important family planning role, the traditional practitioners who are their counterparts in India and who are found in every one of India's half-million villages, have been steadfastly excluded from the programme. There is no reason why they should not have been taught to handle pills and even injectables and simple surgical techniques. The Indian Government has never offered oral contraceptives on a significant scale: injectables, which would probably prove popular, have been rejected by the medical establishment.

The medical infrastructure in many developing countries is woefully weak. What doctors there are, are concentrated in the cities. Government workers often have considerable security, but are paid less than their colleagues in business so that motivation to provide quality services is often weak. Sick people, driven by pain or fear, will usually seek out some form of health care. However, in the case of family planning, especially when it is a novelty within society, people are easily deterred from seeking advice. Geographical or social distance can appear as insurmountable barriers even to individuals who wish to limit their family size.

Services

Non-formal services

Much of the analysis of family planning services has been limited to formal government programmes. This is a mistake, both because it overlooks the important role played by informal, non-governmental services and because it makes it more difficult to overcome possible cultural barriers to the acceptance of modern methods of contraception. It also focuses too much attention on the mechanics of birth control and too little on other variables.

Lactation is nature's contraceptive. In much of the world the traditional patterns of breast-feeding avert more pregnancies than modern methods of contraception. In Bangladesh, women not using contraceptives have their babies approximately 30 months apart, because most breast-feed for two years or more. In the early 1970s it was estimated that 35 million couple years of protection was provided by breast-feeding, but only 27 million after the family planning programmes were established. The situation may have changed in some places; however, in sub-Saharan Africa breast-feeding still remains 10–40 times as demographically significant as the adoption of modern methods of contraception.

It is difficult to counsel the individual lactating woman on when to start an artificial method of contraception. Research in Mexico and Thailand suggests that if women breast-feed at least ten times a day, they are unlikely to ovulate. More research is needed in this field, as is an appreciation of the fact that the advantages and disadvantages of artificial contraceptives vary when they are offered to a lactating, as opposed to a menstruating, woman.

An IUD can be safely inserted immediately postpartum, but if insertion is delayed for a day, then perforation rates will rise. Combined oral contraceptives may have an adverse effect on the quantity of milk produced and the duration of breast-feeding, although not all the available data point in this direction. However, injectable contraceptives such as Depo-Provera (medroxyprogesterone) or the progestogen-only pills have no effect on the quantity and quality of milk yield or content and in some cases may even increase it.

In many ways the most important traditional method of fertility regulation is induced abortion. Almost every historical society and certainly every contemporary society has developed some means of terminating pregnancy. It is always difficult to measure induced abortion accurately when it is illegal, but there is reasonable circumstantial evidence, from a number of different sources, that illegal abortion rates were high in the nineteenth century in most industrialized countries and were a major element in the uniquely low fertility achieved during the years of the Depression in Europe and in the United States. Experience in the reversal of previously liberal patterns of abortion legislation, as in Romania, shows that the law is not a significant determinant in the total number of abortions taking place. Socioeconomic pressures, urbanization, and the opportunity for women to work outside the home outweigh such variables as legislation or religious teachings.

In Europe and the Americas, the Middle East and the Indian subcontinent, mechanical methods of illegal abortion, such as the passage of a urinary catheter or the use of a twig or leaf stem were, or are, common. In the Orient, massage abortion is performed, often by the traditional birth attendant. A survey in Thailand suggests that a quarter-million illegal massage abortions were performed in the villages of that country alone. Many countries have widespread availability and sale of abortifacient drugs. Some of these such as ergot, quinine, and lead-based compounds, may work but present considerable danger to the mother, or to the fetus if pregnancy continues.

Others are probably ineffective but continue to be sold in situations where exploitation is easy.

In Europe, arguments for liberalizing abortion laws were largely based on the hard case: the woman who has been raped or is carrying a congenitally defective fetus; or on the grounds of expediency: that abortions will happen anyhow, and the health of women will be improved and the burden on the health services reduced if the operation is performed under hygienic conditions. In the United States, abortion was legalized on grounds of the right to privacy, and a major philosophical battle continues to rage around the respective rights of the woman and of the embryo or fetus.

Some of the lowest birth rates in history occurred in Eastern Europe in the 1950s and were achieved largely by a combination of *coitus interruptus* and induced abortion. Amongst older couples in the Orient, *coitus reservatus* may be relatively common. Do-it-yourself methods of contraception, including alternative patterns of sexual congress, are numerically important in many countries. Even in Britain, the use of *coitus interruptus* and condoms exceeded that of pills and IUDs until well into the 1960s. In Uttar Pradesh (Northern India), *coitus interruptus* was found to be used by 42% of a sample of doctors. Those who work in family planning programmes are often unrealistically critical of this method; they forget that they see only those couples who have problems with it and not those who are relatively successful. The 1949 Royal Commission on Population in the United Kingdom found no difference between users of appliances and users of non-appliance methods as regards the average number of children. The Indianapolis study found no difference in failure rates between diaphragm users and those adopting *coitus interruptus*. In Sri Lanka, of all the people using contraceptives, one-half are using traditional methods, roughly divided between *coitus interruptus* and some form of periodic abstinence. Both methods have the advantages of costing nothing, and requiring no resupply – and a couple cannot forget them when they go away for the weekend!

Unfortunately even less is known about the effectiveness of periodic abstinence when used on a large scale than about *coitus interruptus*. It would seem a reasonable guess that widespread use of *coitus interruptus*, although in an irregular and inaccurate way, does make an overall difference within a society. High degrees of effectiveness can be obtained with certain methods of periodic abstinence, such as the mucus method and symptothermal techniques, but these are only used by very small numbers of individuals. It is a challenge to see if knowledge and insight into periodic abstinence can be systematically improved on a large scale.

The private sector

The over-the-counter sale of contraceptives and their private prescription by physicians are significant channels of service in many countries. They account for the majority of artificial contraception in North America, and even with the availability of family planning through the British National Health Service, a significant number of people still choose to go to fee-for-service clinics.

Some of the most cost-effective programmes in the developing world have been associated with an intelligent cooperation between the private and public sector, as for example in Korea and Taiwan. The concept of social marketing, or commercial retail sales, has been demonstrated to be highly acceptable, open to rapid implementation, cost-effective, and to have a relatively low socioreligious profile. Yet it has been adopted by relatively few countries. The most successful programme was launched by Population Services International in Bangladesh in 1975 and now extends protection to 1.3 million couples. It is responsible for selling 7 million condoms, 150 thousand cycles of pills, and 300 thousand foaming tablets per month. In addition, the same marketing system is now selling safe delivery kits to enhance the care that traditional birth attendants can give to women in labour. Social marketing programmes have also been initiated in Jamaica, Honduras and Colombia. However, they must be multiplied rapidly in many countries if the world is to deal with the massive health and social problems associated with rapid population growth.

Happily, many Third World countries are making economic progress and some, particularly on the Pacific rim, have made spectacular strides. Revealingly, those countries with the greatest economic growth over the last three decades have also been those with the most vigorous and effective family planning programmes, such as Korea, Taiwan, Singapore, and to a lesser but still substantial extent, Thailand. As communities become richer, they can and should pay for more and more of their own family planning services. The need for subsidy is likely to disappear, first in relation to the reversible methods of contraception such as condoms or oral contraceptives; it is likely to remain longest in relation to voluntary sterilization; this latter is financially a 'good buy' as it provides many years of protection against unintended pregnancy, but involves more up-front money, which individuals in many developing countries cannot afford.

The government sector

Governments can subsidize family planning through commercial retail sales, but it is also self-evident that direct involvement in services is necessary and will remain necessary until well into the twenty-first century. Unfortunately, government effort has often been put into inappropriate aspects of family planning. On the whole, most countries have launched their family planning services with the government provision of IUDs and/or oral contraceptives rather than providing sterilization services or making injectable contraceptives available on a large scale. One of the outcomes of the controversy which always surrounds early involvement in family planning is that it is often politically most acceptable to begin to make available the least controversial, but also least effective, methods of birth control through the most expensive channels, namely using the medical profession and health services rather than retail-market outlets.

Another result of the political pressures opposing the provision of straightforward birth control services has been the policy adopted by some countries and international agencies for so-called integrated family planning programmes. It is argued that family planning must be presented as part of the maternal and child health services or it will not be culturally acceptable to the community. In practice, there is little or no evidence for this view, which remains controversial; and the pursuit of such a policy often means that family planning is only offered as a token service, as in Kenya, or is easily pushed into the background by the imperatives of providing curative services, as so often occurs in India. These attitudes, combined with the overall weakness of the medical infrastructure in many developing countries, have emasculated some national family planning services.

The solution to the problem is more straightforward than commonly recognized. It should be self-evident that family planning must be an intrinsic part of any maternal and child health (MCH) service but it would be wrong to suggest that such services should be the exclusive outlet for contraception. Indeed, women often need contraception before their first child and long after their last one is beyond infancy. In addition, MCH services automatically exclude male methods of contraception which often need to be made more, rather than less, visible, particularly in male-dominated societies, such as many Islamic countries. Family planning must be recognized not only as an essential element of primary health care but also as often the first element that can be made available in remote areas. One of the advantages of family planning is that it requires no diagnostic skill; it is the result of a mature decision by an adult couple, rather than the identification of a disease. Therefore, community providers do not need the higher level of training required for other aspects of primary health care. In addition, family planning is a non-seasonal need that, when provided, can produce results that are visible to the community in a relatively short time.

Mechai Viravaidya in Thailand has pioneered the policy of fertility-related development. He has demonstrated that village volunteers can provide contraceptive services after only one day's training; however, they do need continuing supervision and further training. It is an added motivation if they can get some financial return from the methods they provide. In Thailand, a network of 16 000 volunteers has been built up and has become the basis of other aspects of health care, such as parasite control, and a channel by which needed agricultural technologies can be introduced. In its fully developed form, fertility-related development leads to providing better markets for rural products and a systematic attempt to cut down on the exploitation by middlemen which is common in Third World countries, often removing more from the rural economy than is received in foreign aid or government development grants.

In short, family planning policies must recognize the impact of fertility control on health, as well as recognizing the many variables such as family income and educational opportunities that impact on family size. In Dacca, Bangladesh, contraception and other efforts to raise the status of women have been happily combined.

Investment and policy

During the 1990s, the number of fertile-age couples will increase by over 30%. If contraceptive prevalence is to continue to rise in developing countries to meet the median UN population projection for the twenty-first century, then the number of couples using contraception, at a minimum, must double. If the Soviet Union and eastern Europe are to escape from the family planning dark ages in which they find themselves, then there must also be a vast increase in contraceptive use in these nations.

The vigour and realism with which family planning is pursued in the 1990s will, to a considerable extent, determine the final stable population of the planet. The demand for family planning is strong and a global target of doubling the number of individuals using contraception in the 1990s is not unrealistic. Given the resources, it may even be possible for the world to reach the lower UN population projection for the next century.

Currently less than \$2 bn a year goes into the subsidy of family planning services for those who are too poor to afford the contraceptives and sterilizations they desire. If the above goals are to be met, then a minimum of \$2.5–3 bn a year will be required by the end of the decade. These costs do not include the infrastructure costs, training and censuses. With the intelligent application of scientific technology – and a great deal of luck – the world might just bring ten billion to some semblance of wealth without exceeding its biological limits and irreversibly destroying the human environment. With fourteen or fifteen billion people in the second half of the twenty-first century, we would almost certainly irreversibly damage huge areas of the planetary biosphere.

Currently all the industrialized nations of the world give slightly more than the equivalent of the cost of one B-2 bomber to international family planning each year.

The handful of developing countries where the number of medical personnel equal or outnumber military personnel is so short that it can be listed in toto: Canada, Venezuela, Britain, Scandinavia, Switzerland, Austria, Japan, Australia, Ghana and South Africa. By contrast, in a number of countries, such as Pakistan, Nepal, Israel and Ethiopia, soldiers outnumber health workers ten to one.

The investment in reproductive research and contraceptive development is even more inadequate than that for contraceptive services. Currently, the US spends only slightly over 10 cents per capita per year of federal money on contraceptive research and development. The US is now in the paradoxical position that it may exit the twentieth century with fewer contraceptive choices than were available in 1900. In 1986, all the commonly used intrauterine devices were removed from the US market by problems of product liability, and when they are marketed again, it is likely that a plastic and copper device costing less than one dollar to make will have to be sold for over $100 in order to cover the risks of litigation. One multi-million dollar award has already been given against a commonly used spermicide, even though the scientific basis of the complaint was exceptionally weak and has subsequently been refuted by additional epidemiological research. The anti-progesterone, RU–486, is unlikely to ever be marketed in the USA because of its abortifacient effects. Safe, simple, potentially reversible methods of female sterilization are unlikely to be used in the USA because of the abnormally high fear of patient suits should unintended pregnancy ever occur.

The failure of the Western World to develop adequate methods of contraception or effective services in the years 1850 to 1950, and the still halting and uncertain assistance which industrialized nations provide to less privileged countries, combine to place the world our children will inhabit in very real jeopardy.

Conclusion

Currently available methods of contraception are not as good as they would have been if an appropriate amount of investment had been put into this important area of medical research. Nevertheless, the need for family planning around the world is great and growing, and human fertility has been successfully controlled in a number of very different societies and against a variety of socioeconomic backgrounds, using the somewhat clumsy and limited methods we have available.

Ethically and legally the need for human fertility regulation has been almost totally misunderstood. Theologians of all religions have tended to focus on the drama of human copulation and to have lost sight of those lifelong cycles of human fertility which actually determine the welfare of women and children. Once society accepted the technology of artificial formulae, glass feeding bottles and rubber nipples to feed newborn infants, it had no alternative but to accept contraception and rubber condoms to restore the balance of nature and the natural spacing of pregnancies which evolution had given our species. The choice facing Western policy makers at the present time is either to increase vastly the resources going into research and services using reversible methods of contraception, or to settle for the present cumbersome compromise where inadequate methods have to be backed up with abortion and sterilization. There is no way that five thousand million people are going to muddle by and reach their fertility goals merely through the availability of natural family planning, pills and condoms; neither will the fragile biosphere of our planet survive the growth in human numbers unless countries, both rich and poor, understand the choices that face them and act on those choices quickly.

Chapter 2

Metabolic effects of combined oral contraceptives

Michael D. G. Gillmer

It is now more than 25 years since oral contraceptives became available for general clinical use. During this time our state of knowledge about their metabolic effects, and in particular our understanding of the relationship between metabolic and side-effects, both beneficial and adverse, has progressed from a state of profound ignorance to one of relative ignorance. In view of the fact that oral contraceptive steroids have been more widely studied than almost any other drugs, this may seem to be an unduly pessimistic statement. It is, however, sadly true that we remain uncertain of the significance of many of the metabolic effects that have been observed when these potent drugs are administered to healthy young women. I have in preparing this chapter endeavoured to highlight not only what is known about the metabolic effects of the pill, but also to stress the areas that require further research.

Historical overview

The most important clinical effect of the combined oral contraceptive pill is inhibition of ovulation. The term 'combined' relates to the combination of two synthetic sex hormones, oestrogens and progestogens. Although it had been demonstrated in the mid-thirties that progesterone administration caused inhibition of ovulation in rats and rabbits [1], the technique could not be applied in women for two reasons. Firstly the naturally occurring compounds were extremely scarce because their only available source was the ovaries of animals such as the sow, and secondly when given by mouth they had remarkably little effect. Russell Marker, an enigmatic American chemist overcame the first problem by synthesizing kilogram quantities of steroid from the Mexican yam in the early 1940s. Marker was co-founder of a small pharmaceutical company incorporated in Mexico City in 1944. Carl Djerassi later modified testosterone to produce norethisterone (norethindrone), the first orally active progestogen, and the US patent for this compound was filed by Syntex SA on 12 November 1952. Although the patent for the second orally active compound norethynodrel was not filed until nearly a year later by G. D. Searle on 31 August 1953, the patent for norethynodrel was issued in November 1955, five months earlier than that of norethisterone. Searle had a strong research and trials capability as well as full production, packaging, marketing and advertising facilities. As a result Searle introduced Enovid, their preparation for clinical use, in the USA in June 1960, nearly three years ahead of Syntex, who licensed their progestogen to Ortho who introduced it in the USA in January 1963 under the name Orthonovum [2, 3]. Later the same year Syntex marketed Norinyl.

There followed a succession of compounds derived from norethisterone, including norethisterone acetate, ethynodiol diacetate and lynoestrenol, and also progestogens derived from progesterone, of which the first was megestrol acetate patented by Searle in 1959. Norgestrel, developed by Wyeth and patented in 1964, was the first progestogen to be manufactured by total chemical synthesis. It was subsequently licensed to Schering AG, who separated the racemic mixture into an inactive structural isomer l-norgestrel and the active d-norgestrel – more usually known as dextronorgestrel and levonorgestrel respectively, because of the optical isomerism that each displays.

The idea of using progestogens for contraception is attributed to Gregory Pincus, a Searle consultant [4]. The first trials were conducted in Puerto Rico because of the country's high birth rate and to avoid moral censure in the USA.

Norethynodrel 10 mg daily for 21 days, followed by a 'pill free' week was used in these pioneering studies. This proved spectacularly successful in inhibiting ovulation and inducing 'withdrawal bleeds'. It was then discovered that the oestrogen mestranol was present as a contaminant, which accounted for 1.5% of the preparation in use. When the mestranol was removed, cycle control deteriorated and some pregnancies occurred. It was therefore decided to reintroduce the mestranol in the amount present as a contaminant, viz. 150 μg. The 'combined' pill was born – a product of serendipity. It was, however, some years before it was realized that the artificial hormones that this preparation contained were present in much higher doses than subsequently proved to be necessary or advisable.

Pharmacology

Ethinyloestradiol, which is now used more or less exclusively as the oestrogen in combined oral contraceptive preparations, was first marketed by Parke-Davis in 1964. Although the micronized form of the naturally occurring oestrogen 17-beta-oestradiol is orally active, the addition of an ethinyl group at C–17 greatly enhances the oral activity of this compound (Figure 2.1). There has for many years been controversy about the relative biological activity (potency) of ethinyloestradiol and mestranol (the 3-methyl ether derivative of ethinyloestradiol). This has been resolved by studies demonstrating that mestranol is demethylated to varying extents (50%–100%) at C–3 to form ethinyloestradiol and that this variable conversion entails some loss of activity [5, 6]. Although lower peak levels of ethinyloestradiol are observed after the administration of equal doses of mestranol and ethinyloestradiol, it is unknown whether or not this is beneficial. It has similarly been shown that norethisterone derivatives such as ethynodiol diacetate (Figure 2.2) are pro-drugs rapidly converted to norethisterone [7–9].

All synthetic progestogens are derivatives of either 17-alpha-hydroxyprogesterone or 19-nortestosterone. The 17-alpha-hydroxyprogesterone derivatives are also known as pregnanes and are characterized by the presence between the A and B rings of a methyl group which greatly reduces the androgenic effects. The 19-nortestosterone derivatives lack this methyl (C–19) substituent at C–10 and also have in the 17-alpha position an ethinyl group, which delays hepatic inactivation – as in norethisterone (Figure 2.3). They can be subdivided into oestranes and gonanes. The distinguishing feature of the gonanes is the additional presence of a methyl group at position 18, and

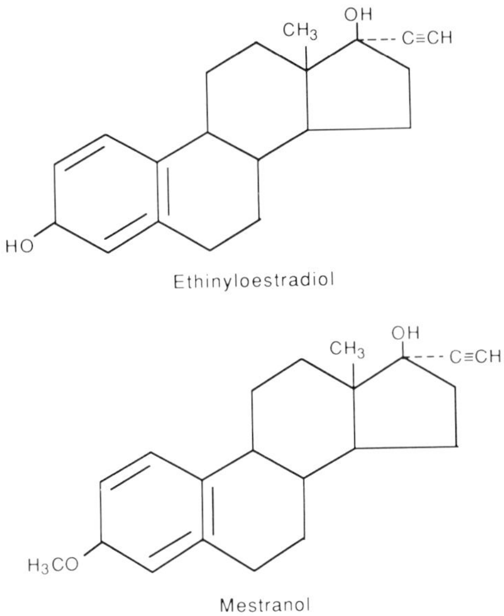

Figure 2.1 Structure of ethinyloestradiol and mestranol

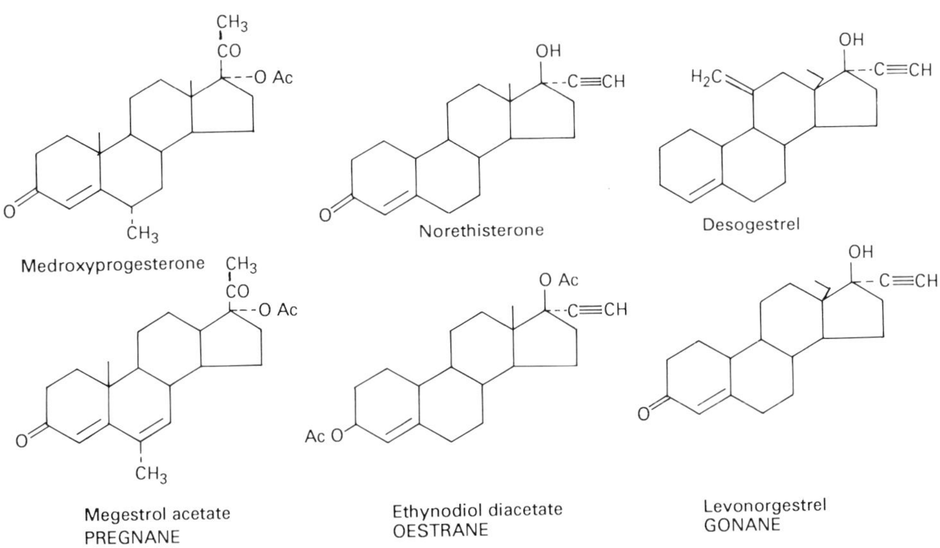

Figure 2.2 Structure of pregnane, oestrane and gonane progestogens

this increases progestogenic activity (Figure 2.2). The gonanes include levonorgestrel and the so-called third-generation progestogens, desogestrel, gestodene and norgestimate (Figure 2.4).

Although levonorgestrel is biologically active and is not converted to norethisterone, the two compounds are closely related structurally (Figure 2.2). Recent studies by Bergink and Kloosterboer [10] have demonstrated three important sites for

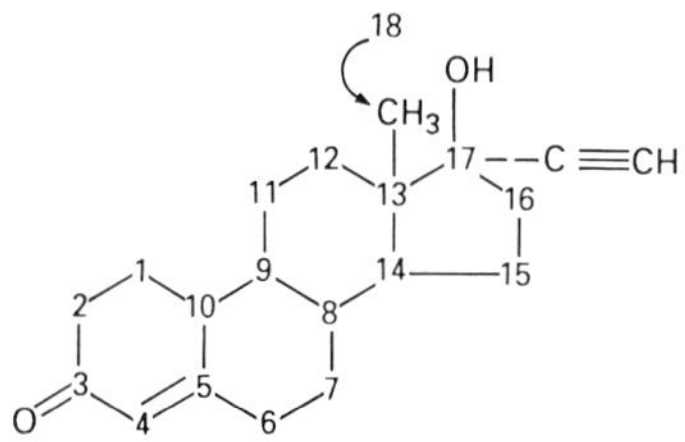

Norethisterone

Figure 2.3 Norethisterone: numbered rings

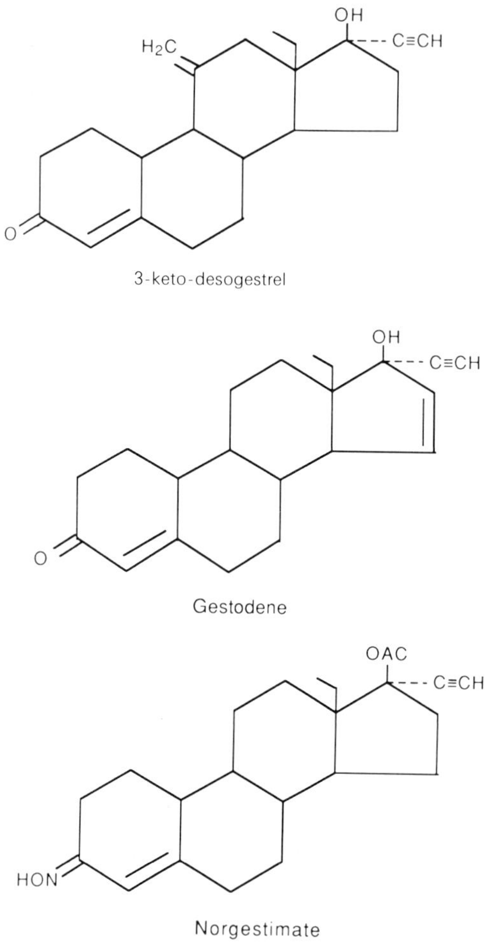

Figure 2.4 'Third-generation' progestogens

substitutions to the norethisterone molecule, all of which enhance binding to the progesterone receptor. These are the methyl group at C–18, a methylene group at C–11 and a double bond at C–15. The presence or absence of these substituents (which remain intact throughout the processes of metabolism) creates the eight possible compounds shown in Table 2.1.

Only four of these progestogens have names and are currently used in oral

Table 2.1 Norethisterone derivatives. (From Bergink and Kloosterboer [10] by permission)

Compound	*18-methyl*	*11-methylene*	*delta-15*
Norethisterone	−	−	−
Levonorgestrel	+	−	−
$11 = CH_2$-NET	−	+	−
delta-15-NET	−	−	+
3-keto-desogestrel	+	+	−
Gestodene	+	−	+
delta-15,$11 = CH_2$-NET	−	+	+
delta-15,$11 = CH_2$, 18-CH_3-NET	+	+	+

Table 2.2 Relative receptor affinities of norethisterone and its derivatives for the human progesterone and androgen receptor in intact MCF-7 cells. (After Bergink and Kloosterboer [10])

Compound	*RBA* for progesterone receptor*	*RBA* for androgen receptor*	*Selectivity ratio*
Norethisterone	1	1.0	1.0
Levonorgestrel	6	2.5	2.4
$11 = CH_2$-NET	7	1.2	5.8
delta-15-NET	3	0.7	4.3
3-keto-desogestrel	9	1.2	7.5
Gestodene	15	2.2	6.8
delta-15,$11 = CH_2$-NET	10	0.3	33.3
delta-15,$11 = CH_2$, 18-CH_3-NET	9	0.3	30.0

*RBA: relative binding affinity

contraceptives: norethisterone, levonorgestrel, 3-ketodesgestrel (the active metabolite of the Organon progestogen desogestrel) and gestodene (developed by Schering AG). All have, however, been synthesized and their relative binding to the progesterone and androgen receptors of intact MCF–7 cells has been studied [10]. Although binding to the *progesterone* receptor is enhanced by all three substituents, *androgen* receptor binding is enhanced solely by the 18-methyl substitution, is inhibited by the 11-methylene substitution, and is unaffected by the insertion of a double bond at delta-15. Analyses of the selectivity ratio – which is the ratio of the relative binding affinity (RBA) for the progesterone receptor to the RBA for the androgen receptor – show major differences (Table 2.2). Norethisterone has the lowest selectivity, levonorgestrel is more selective, but 3-keto-desogestrel and gestodene have a highly selective binding affinity for the progesterone receptor [10a]. Two of the so far unnamed compounds in Table 2.2 display higher selectivity than any of the remaining six. It is interesting to speculate that either or both may prove to be the progestogens of the future.

Norgestimate, developed by Ortho in the USA, is another third generation progestogen now becoming available for clinical use. In common with gestodene and 3-keto-desogestrel, norgestimate (Figure 2.4) has an 18-methyl substitution, but lacks both the double bond between C–15 and C–16 seen in gestodene, and the C–11 methylene group of 3-keto-desogestrel. It is, however, unique in possessing an oxime group at C–3 and an acetate group at C–17. These two substituents are split off during the processes of metabolism. It is still uncertain how much of the progestogenic activity of this steroid is due to norgestimate itself and how much to its metabolites. The pharmacological profile reveals antiovulatory activity with virtually no androgenic response or oestrogenic activity according to Hahn et al. [11].

Pharmacokinetics and metabolism of hormonal contraceptives

Ethinyloestradiol is absorbed totally from the gastrointestinal tract and peak concentrations are observed in plasma within 1–2 hours of oral ingestion. Rapid conversion to the conjugate ethinyloestradiol sulphate occurs in the bowel wall, and although some ethinyloestradiol may exist free in plasma most of the hormone and its sulphate are bound to albumin [12]. Any ethinyloestradiol escaping gut-wall conjugation is available for both hepatic conjugation and first-phase metabolism, viz. oxidation, reduction or hydrolysis [13]. The sulphate and glucuronide conjugates and those arising from first-phase metabolism are excreted in bile and can subsequently undergo hydrolysis by the bacterial flora of the colon to produce ethinyloestradiol, which is reabsorbed, creating an 'enterohepatic' circulation. Wide interindividual variations exist, and the bioavailability of ethinyloestradiol after oral administration, as judged by the area under the plasma concentration time curve, varies tenfold [6, 12, 14]. This may be due in part to the varying degrees of bacterial deconjugation of the ethinyloestradiol glucuronide excreted in bile and subsequent reabsorption of free ethinyloestradiol by the gut that are observed in different women. The clinical relevance of these observations is uncertain, but a tenable hypothesis derived from the variability in plasma concentrations of ethinyloestradiol and all progestogens studied to date is that the highest levels may be causally associated with greater metabolic changes and clinical side-effects. Insufficient studies have been done to check this hypothesis, but Ahluwalia et al. [15] showed significantly higher plasma levels of ethinyloestradiol in hypertensive combined-pill users as compared with a comparison group who were normotensive pill-takers. The implications are discussed in Chapter 5. The mean half-time of elimination of ethinyloestradiol reported by Back et al. [16] was 6.5 ± SD 2.9 hours, but wide interindividual variation has been demonstrated by Fotherby [12] with values of 5–16 hours in 67.5% women, less than 5 hours in 8.8%, and up to 30 hours in the remainder. The half-time of elimination, estimated in patients with an ileostomy (to minimize the effect of the enterohepatic circulation) was 6.7 ± SD 2.2 hours [17].

Norethisterone is fully absorbed from the gut but its bioavailability is reduced to approximately 65% as a result of first-pass metabolism in the gut wall and liver. Urinary metabolites reflect subsequent reduction of the A ring and conjugation to sulphate and glucuronide [12, 13]. Absorption is slower than that observed with ethinyloestradiol. Peak plasma concentrations occur in most women within 1–4 hours, but times in excess of 5 hours were observed in nearly a quarter of subjects studied by Fotherby [12]. Elimination half-times of between 8 and 12 hours have been reported by Grimmer and Orme [13], and a mean of 8–9 hours by Shi et al. [18].

Orally administered levonorgestrel is absorbed totally and is not subject to any significant first-pass effect through the gut and liver, resulting in almost 100% bioavailability [19]. Over 25 urinary metabolites have been identified, most of which are apparently of minor importance, although hydroxylation at C–2 and reduction at C–3 and C–5 are considered to be quantitatively significant [20]. According to Goldzieher and Chenault [19] it also has a longer elimination half-life than norethisterone (mean 11.4 hours), possibly due to the ethyl group at C–13 [8]. Plasma concentrations display a near tenfold variation between individuals comparable to that observed with norethisterone and ethinyloestradiol [21].

Desogestrel is rapidly converted to the active metabolite 3-keto-desogestrel during the first liver passage and has a bioavailability of 76% [21a,b]. It is inactivated by A-ring reduction and conjugation [22].

A review of the pharmacological profile of gestodene has been published [23]. It is rapidly absorbed after oral administration, with a mean elimination half-time of approximately 10 hours.

Peak norgestimate concentrations are observed within 2 hours of oral ingestion, reflecting rapid absorption. The half-life of radioactivity due to carbon-14 labelling of norgestimate has been reported as approximately 60 hours [24], but this result cannot readily be compared with the elimination half-lives determined by serial radioimmunoassays. Norgestimate appears to be extensively metabolized following oral administration. This includes hydrolysis of the oxime and actate moieties, A-ring reduction, polyhydroxylation, and conjugation, a pattern of metabolism similar to that observed for the other synthetic progestogens in man. Five major metabolites, including norgestrel, have been characterized in urine [25].

Oestrogen and progestogen activity

Some actions of oestrogens are listed in Table 2.3 and those of progestogens in Table 2.4 (adapted from Hawkins and Elder [26]).

The relative 'potency' of the progestogens used in oral contraceptives is a source of considerable controversy. It is now generally accepted that in order to establish the relative potency of two drugs, certain fundamental requirements must be met. To quote from Goldzieher [27], 'The potency of a drug is determined by the location of the dose/response curve along the dose axis; the relative potency of two drugs is the ratio of doses that have equivalent effect when the dose/response curves are parallel'. In addition, the species, target organ or tissue, route of administration and bioavailability must all be specified, and the sample size must be sufficient to ensure precision. Of the many potential end-points for assessing progestogen potency, those relating to menstrual effects have received most clinical attention. The acceptability of the combined pill rests on the predictability of the withdrawal bleed which the individual woman experiences. The earliest attempt to assess the bioactivity of combined oral contraceptives was therefore aimed at assessing the endometrial effect of these oestrogen–progestogen combinations, using the so-called 'delay of menses' test.

Swyer [28] demonstrated two basic flaws in most early reports on progestogen

Table 2.3 Some actions of oestrogens

The systemic actions of oestrogens include:
Nitrogen, calcium and phosphorus retention
Promotion of skeletal growth and epiphyseal closure
An increase in connective-tissue water
An increase in the pelvic blood supply
Stimulation of uterine growth
An increase in cervical mucus
Maturation of vaginal epithelium
Development of the breast ducts, lobules and areolae
An increase in the pelvic musculature

Table 2.4 Some actions of progestogens

The systemic actions of progestogens include:
An overall catabolic effect
Elevation of basal body temperature
A hypnotic action
Diminution of pituitary gonadotrophin secretion
An endometrial decidual response
A mild natriuretic and diuretic effect
Reduction and thickening of cervical mucus
Stimulation of primary alveolar growth in the breasts

potency. Firstly, that the potency of progestogens cannot be assessed in isolation; these products are of necessity combined with oestrogens and the interaction between the oestrogen and progestogen concerned will profoundly influence the resulting assessment of progestogen bioactivity. Secondly, the nature of the interaction – synergistic or antagonistic – will depend not only on the target organ under study but also the relative dose of oestrogen and progestogen under test. Amidst all this confusion two things are clear. The relative bioactivity of two progestogenic compounds established for a particular oestrogen–progestogen combination should never be extrapolated from one species to another or from one end-organ to another. In addition, it is clear from the data presently available that there are no truly reliable studies of any particular oestrogen–progestogen combination on any target organ in women, with the possible exception of the endometrium [29, 30]. The clinician must therefore be prepared to question the reliability and validity of any potency estimates which are presented.

Venous thromboembolism

Shortly after their introduction, oral contraceptives were shown to cause a number of changes in haemostatic function which at least on theoretical grounds could be expected to increase the risk of thrombosis. Case reports in the early 1960s of venous thromboembolism in women taking oral contraceptives [31] were followed later in the decade by epidemiological data which confirmed these suspicions and suggested a link between the oestrogen content of the pill and the incidence of venous thromboembolic disease [32]. The validity of these findings has, however, been questioned because of the frequent uncertainty of the clinical diagnosis in this condition, the inadequate *in vitro* methodology used for assessing blood coagulation, and the absence of a specific association between any of the measured changes in coagulation function and venous thromboembolism in any individual. These issues have been comprehensively reviewed by Mammen [33].

Three main components participate in the process of haemostasis, viz. the vessel wall, the platelets, and the coagulation system. Abnormalities have been observed in each of these components in women using combined oral contraceptives.

Studies of the vessel wall [34] have revealed endothelial proliferation in some women. These rare lesions are, however, not specific for oral contraceptive use, and as they can only be determined in biopsy specimens they are of no predictive value in determining which patients will develop venous thrombosis.

Platelet interaction with the vessel wall involves prostaglandin derivatives. Prostacyclin is the most powerful inhibitor of platelets known and is also a potent vasodilator. The platelet membrane produces thromboxane A_2, a powerful platelet aggregator and vasoconstrictor. The interplay between these prostacyclin derivatives controls platelet adhesiveness, and may therefore be important in thrombin formation. Studies of platelets and endothelium in users of combined oral contraceptives have, however, produced contradictory data. This is probably due in part to the poor reproducibility of the methods currently available to assess these mechanisms. As there is no clear evidence at the present time that platelet changes measured *in vitro* are predictive of thromboembolism *in vivo*, the variable changes observed in oral contraceptive users to date are of dubious practical relevance [33].

The coagulation system has been more fully investigated than any other aspect of the haemostatic mechanism in women using combined oral contraceptives. Several clotting factors have been shown to increase in women taking oestrogen-containing oral contraceptives, including fibrinogen, prothrombin and Factors VII, IX, X, and XII [33]. In addition, the concentration of antithrombin III, the most important of the natural anticoagulants, has been shown consistently to be decreased. These observations, together with the epidemiological reports in the late 1960s of a positive correlation between the incidence of venous thromboembolism and the oestrogen content of combined oral contraceptives would seem to indicate a causal association.

This argument has been cautiously maintained by Meade [35], who observed a positive relationship between Factor VII concentrations and the oestrogen content of combined oral contraceptives. Mammen [33] and Beller and Ebert [36] have, however, questioned these assumptions, pointing out that while a reduction in clotting factors is a cause of haemorrhagic diatheses, the clotting factors are already present in excess in blood and that increases, both innate and acquired, have not been shown to be associated with thrombosis. Although congenital or acquired reductions in antithrombin III concentrations are associated with a tendency to thrombosis, there is no certainty that the changes observed in women using combined oral contraceptives are the cause of venous or arterial thrombosis. Indeed, Mammen [33] has suggested that the increase in $alpha_2$ macroglobulin, another natural 'anticoagulant' which has been found in some studies [37, 38], may compensate for decreased antithrombin levels and inhibit thrombin formation during clotting.

Congenital deficiency of protein C, a vitamin-K-dependent coagulation inhibitor [39], has recently been shown to be associated with thromboembolic disease [40]. Studies of women taking combined oral contraceptives have, however, shown either an increase [41, 42] or no change in this protein [43]. The differences between these studies may have been due to differences in laboratory methodology or the preparations used.

Compensatory changes have also been observed in the fibrinolytic system in users of combined oral contraceptives, in particular an increase in circulating plasminogen concentrations and decreased antiplasmin activity. This appears, however, to be balanced by a reduction in the level of tissue plasminogen activators [44].

The complexity of these interactions, the difficulties that arise when extrapolating from *in vitro* studies to *in vivo* events, and the controversy concerning methodology all conspire to confuse rather than to clarify the issues.

A further complication so far given little consideration is the interaction between the oestrogen and differing progestogen components of combined oral contraceptive preparations. This has been highlighted by Bonnar and Sabra [45]. Their studies, which compared products of different oestrogen and progestogen content, led them to conclude that the progestogen content and type modified the oestrogenic effects on the coagulation system. In particular, the oestrogen-induced fall in antithrombin III appeared to vary depending on the progestogen under study. These differences may, however, have been due to the balance of oestrogen–progestogen effects rather than to a specific progestogen, as the doses of each compound studied were not identical.

In conclusion, although specific changes in the coagulation system can be identified in women using combined oral contraceptives (and some of these appear to be related to the oestrogen dose, probably modified by the progestogen type and content), none of the changes observed has proved predictive of thromboembolic disease. Recent epidemiological evidence suggests that the reduced oestrogen doses used in the 1970s have been associated with a lessening of the incidence of thromboembolic disease [46]. Kierkegaard [47] has suggested that this study, which depended on adverse drug reaction reports, is unreliable because of biased reporting. Current research is, however, aimed at finding oestrogen–progestogen combinations that produce minimal changes in the haemostatic system. It therefore seems reasonable to anticipate some genuine reduction in the incidence of thrombotic complications of oral contraceptives, with modern formulations containing low doses of both oestrogen and progestogen [45, 48–50].

Carbohydrate metabolism

Although it has been known for more than a century that pregnancy produces a diabetogenic stress [51], at the time that combined oral contraceptives were first used it was not apparent that this was hormonally induced. Since the late 1960s oestrogens and progestogens alone and in varying combinations have been the subject of intense study. These investigations were initially stimulated by the advent of radioimmunoassays for the pancreatic hormones insulin and glucagon, which play a central role in carbohydrate homeostasis. Early studies demonstrated that oral contraceptives, like pregnancy, caused mild impairment of glucose tolerance and an increase in circulating metabolites such as pyruvate, despite enhanced insulin secretion and an apparently paradoxical fall in plasma glucose [52].

Subsequent studies in animals and man have, however, demonstrated that oestrogens alone do not have any significant effect on glucose tolerance or insulin secretion, but that the effects observed in pregnancy can be reproduced by progestogen treatment. Small doses of oestrane progestogen (i.e. norethisterone, Figures 2.2, 2.3) and those 19-nor-progestogens converted to norethisterone) as used in progestogen-only pills do not appear to affect glucose tolerance, but have been reported to increase the insulin response to an oral glucose load [53, 54]. The data relating to gonane progestogens (i.e. those 19-nor-progestogens with an ethyl group at C–13) are less clear. Spellacy et al. [55, 56] reported both an impairment of glucose tolerance and an increase in insulin secretion of women taking 75 μg of norgestrel without oestrogen for 18 months. A significant increase in the weight of the women studied was also observed during this time, and their altered carbohydrate metabolism may simply have been due to insulin resistance consequent upon an increased adipose mass.

The mechanism of action of combined oestrogen–progestogen oral contraceptives on carbohydrate metabolism has been investigated by Wynn's group [57]. They demonstrated a marked suppressive effect on the glucagon-secreting pancreatic alpha cells of ovariectomized rats treated with 17-beta-oestradiol alone. This was associated with an enhanced insulin: glucagon molar ratio in the portal blood and an increase in activity of hepatic lipogenic enzymes (acetyl CoA carboxylase), and inhibition of the gluconeogenic rate-limiting enzyme phosphoenolpyruvate carboxykinase. The characteristic fall in fasting plasma glucose during pregnancy and in women treated with combined oral contraceptives, therefore, appears to be due to reduced hepatic glucose output consequent upon an oestrogen-induced change in insulin:glucagon ratio, causing inhibition of hepatic gluconeogenesis. Progesterone administration on the other hand produced an increase in the portal-vein insulin concentration and did not affect the portal-vein insulin:glucagon ratio.

Wynn's group have also performed the most extensive clinical investigation of combined oral contraceptives containing different doses of oestrogens and progestogens. They have shown that high doses of oestrogen plus oestrane progestogen produce deterioration in glucose tolerance and suppressed insulin levels. Glucose tolerance was most markedly impaired by pills of high oestrogen dose containing high doses of oestrane progestogen. Insulin values were, however, only modestly increased by these preparations whereas those containing lower doses of oestrogen and either oestrane or gonane progestogens produced much smaller changes in glucose tolerance with relatively greater increases in insulin secretion after an oral glucose load [54].

A clear dose-dependent effect of oestrane and gonane progestogens on insulin secretion has been demonstrated in these and other studies [53, 58]. An oestrogen dose-dependent effect has also been demonstrated by Wynn and co-workers [59]. Preparations containing the same dose of oestrane progestogen but different doses of oestrogen produce degrees of glucose intolerance which are directly related to the oestrogen content. Wynn has suggested that the oestrogen suppresses insulin secretion, allowing the progestogenic effect to become dominant at lower oestrogen doses. He has also postulated that the insulin:glucose ratio is influenced by the progestogen under study and that gonane progestogens produce more marked hyperinsulinism than oestrane progestogens when combined with oestrogens in similar doses [54]. These data are, however, open to criticism because of the varying oestrogen doses in the preparations used by the groups of women studied. Pregnane progestogens do not appear to affect glucose tolerance or insulin metabolism.

Recent studies of low-oestrogen and progestogen preparations show that these produce very minor effects on insulin secretion and little or no change in glucose tolerance. This is a clear example of the clinical benefits that have resulted from modifications of formulation stimulated by biochemical investigations of the metabolic effects of the pill [50, 58, 60, 61, 61a].

Although combined oral contraceptives may produce significant glucose intolerance in susceptible individuals, this is rare. Insulin-dependent diabetics should, however, be warned of the possible need for increased insulin doses to maintain optimal diabetic control.

Lipid metabolism

Current interest in the effects of combined oral contraceptives on lipid metabolism stems from two sets of epidemiological data. Firstly, the recognition of an increased risk of ischaemic heart disease in women using these preparations [62, 63] (See Chapter 3 for review) and secondly the association between high blood lipid concentrations and the risk of atherosclerotic heart disease in several large population studies [64].

Total plasma cholesterol was the first lipid measurement found to have predictive power for coronary heart disease, and much publicity has been given to dietary means of lowering blood cholesterol exemplified by the recent National Institutes of Health

Consensus Opinion [65]. In the last decade it has become apparent, however, that several aspects of lipoprotein metabolism are relevant to atherogenesis, in particular as evidenced by low-density and high-density lipoproteins.

Lipids are insoluble in water. They are transported in blood in micellar complexes consisting of phospholipids and carrier apoproteins that form a hydrophilic membrane around the hydrophobic triglyceride and cholesterol esters. The four main subclasses of lipoproteins can be subdivided by their density, electrophoretic mobility, size, or apoprotein constituents (Table 2.5) [66].

The values for the contents of the various lipoprotein fractions shown in the table are approximate. Each is heterogeneous and contains a number of different apoprotein constituents and varying proportions of lipids, which change as the lipoproteins fulfil their physiological functions. The lipoproteins arise from the liver and intestine. Chylomicrons arise from fat absorption and are cleaved of triglyceride by lipoprotein lipase. Very-low-density lipoproteins (VLDL) are secreted by the liver and intestine; cleavage of triglyceride from this fraction forms intermediate density lipoproteins (IDL). IDLs lose more triglyceride due to the action of hepatic lipase, and with the loss of apoprotein C and E are converted to low-density-lipoproteins (LDL), containing mainly apoprotein B (apo-B). This fraction carries approximately 70% of plasma cholesterol. It is metabolized in part by the liver, but is also taken up peripherally by tissues with LDL receptors for apo-B. The cholesterol ester is hydrolysed within the cell and inhibits cholesterol and LDL receptor synthesis by the cell, thus controlling further LDL uptake.

HDL apoproteins are synthesized in the small intestine and liver and secreted into the circulation. They appear to 'take up' cholesterol from cell membranes. This is then esterified by lecithin-cholesterol transferase (LCAT) and enters the core of the 'nascent' HDL apoprotein envelope, and is in part taken up by the liver and excreted. HDL exists in subfractions of which the most important are HDL_2 and HDL_3. Free exchange of phospholipids, cholesterol, and apo-C occurs between HDL and VLDL. HDL_3 takes up cholesterol and in the process becomes converted to HDL_2, which is less dense. HDL_2 in turn may be converted to VLDL as described above. There is a reciprocal relationship between plasma HDL cholesterol and VLDL triglyceride concentrations, and a positive relationship between HDL cholesterol and lipoprotein lipase activity.

This complex interchange between the lipoprotein fractions explains their heterogeneity and the overlap between the various fractions with regard to particle size,

Table 2.5 Characteristics of the lipoproteins

	Chylomicrons	*VLDL*	*LDL*	*HDL*
Density (g/ml)	0.95	0.95–1.006	1.019–1.063	1.063–1.21
Electrophoretic mobility	Origin	Pre-beta	Beta	Alpha
Lipid content (% total mass)	98	90	75	48
Cholesterol	3	18	47	18
Triglyceride	90	55	7	5
Phospholipid	5	17	21	25
Protein (%)	1–2	10	25	50
Apoproteins				
Major	C (90%)	C, B	B (74%)	A–I (46%) A–II (23%)
Minor	A, B, E,	E	C–III, E	C, E

density and lipid–protein content. These complex dynamic interrelations are depicted in a simple graphic form in the adjacent Figure 2.5. For more detailed descriptions the reader is referred to Krauss [67] and Fotherby [68].

The association between high lipid concentrations and an increased risk of cardiovascular disease reported in epidemiological studies [64] is supported by a number of other observations, including premature cardiovascular disease associated with genetic disorders of lipid metabolism, experimental atherogenesis in animals fed a high-cholesterol diet, and the higher cholesterol concentrations measured in populations with higher incidences of ischaemic heart disease.

Low-density lipoprotein cholesterol accounts for approximately 70% of serum cholesterol, and a positive association has been demonstrated between LDL-C and the risk of myocardial infarction. In women, HDL cholesterol accounts for approximately 25%–30% of serum cholesterol, and displays a negative association with ischaemic heart disease risk which is independent of and stronger than that displayed by LDL cholesterol. It has also been suggested that HDL_2–C (the more variable component of HDL–C) is a more sensitive indicator of coronary atherogenic risk, and measurement of the changes in the concentration of individual apoproteins has also been suggested. Neither of these techniques is, however, in widespread use. In practice the ratios of LDL:HDL cholesterol or total cholesterol:HDL cholesterol appear to provide the most easily measured and sensitive indicators of atherogenic risk.

HDL and LDL cholesterol are influenced by many factors [64] including age, sex, diet, obesity, exercise, alcohol, smoking, drug therapy, and certain disease states. LDL cholesterol concentrations are lower in premenopausal women but higher in postmenopausal women than in men. HDL–C and HDL_2–C concentrations are higher in women than men but HDL_3–C concentrations are higher in men. There is a slight increase in HDL–C with age in women but not in men. Genetic factors are also important and there is a strong correlation between levels in related family members. High-carbohydrate diets decrease HDL–C concentrations, while a high-cholesterol diet increases HDL–C with an increase in the ratio of HDL_3 to HDL_2. HDL–C is decreased in obese subjects, due mainly to reduced HDL_2. Alcohol increases HDL (probably HDL_2 [68]) and triglyceride concentrations. Smoking also increases triglyceride concentrations but, in contrast to alcohol, it lowers HDL–C. Exercise increases HDL–C (mainly HDL_2) and decreases LDL–C levels. Poorly controlled maturity-onset diabetes and hyperthyroidism are associated with reduced HDL–C

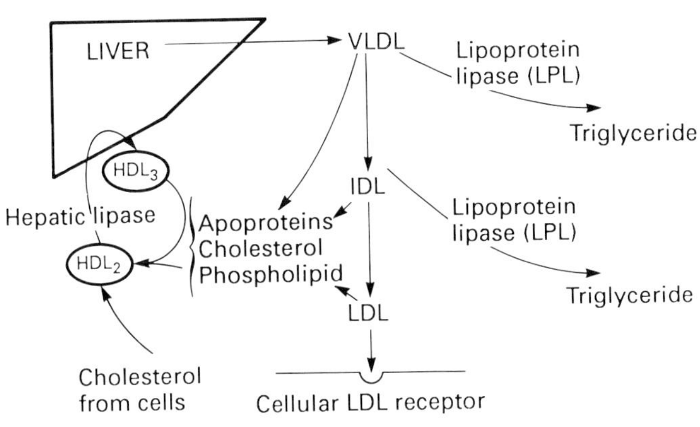

Figure 2.5 Simplified lipoprotein metabolic pathways. (After Tikkanen and Nikkila [74])

concentrations, while hypothyroidism is associated with increased levels of HDL–C (especially HDL_2) and increased LDL–C. Drugs such as clofibrate and nicotinic acid raise HDL–C and have been used to treat hyperlipidaemic states. Phenytoin, barbiturates, and other drugs which induce hepatic microsomal enzymes also increase HDL–C, while the sulphonylureas and beta-blockers lower it.

It is against this complex background that the influence of synthetic sex steroids on lipid and lipoprotein metabolism must be considered. These are summarized in Table 2.6.

The most extensively studied effects of oestrogens in women are their ability to reduce LDL cholesterol and increase HDL cholesterol, altering the LDL:HDL cholesterol ratio in a direction associated in population studies with a decreased atherogenic risk. It is, however, important to be aware that a truly beneficial association cannot yet be extrapolated to users of combined oral contraceptives. Preliminary data from the Lipid Research Clinics Program Follow-up Study [69] have shown that deaths from cardiovascular disease over a five-year period of observation were reduced by approximately two-thirds in postmenopausal women taking unapposed oestrogens, and that this was indeed associated with higher HDL–cholesterol concentrations in the oestrogen group.

The combined oral contraceptive pill was developed as a medication that would achieve a state of pseudopregnancy. It would thus be expected to alter maternal lipid metabolism in a manner similar to that of fetoplacental oestrogens and progesterone. The effect of pregnancy on lipid and lipoprotein metabolism may therefore be used as a reference point against which to assess the effects of the pill. Pregnancy is associated with a twofold increase in total triglyceride and a 25% increase in total cholesterol [70, 71]. There are also increases in LDL and HDL cholesterol with no real change in the HDL:LDL cholesterol ratio [72].

Soon after their introduction, combined pills were found to cause elevated triglyceride concentrations, believed by some authorities to be a risk factor in cardiovascular disease [73, 73a]. Extensive studies [74] have demonstrated that oestrogens and certain progestogens have opposite effects on triglyceride levels. Pregnane progestogens, i.e. those derived from progesterone (e.g. megestrol acetate and chlormadinone acetate) have no effect on triglyceride concentrations. First- and second-generation progestogens derived from 19-nor-testosterone, viz. the norethisterone derivatives and levonorgestrel (so-called oestrane and gonane progestogens, respectively) may, however, antagonize the effects of endogenous and exogenous oestrogens on lipid and lipoprotein metabolism, particularly when administered in high doses.

These pharmacodynamic effects may for simplicity be viewed as antioestrogenic or

Table 2.6 Effects of oestrogen and progestogens (pre-'third generation') on plasma lipids and lipoproteins in normal women (from LaRosa [138] by permission)

	Oestrogens	*Progestogens*
Total cholesterol	No change or sl. ↑	No change or sl. ↓
Total triglyceride	Increase	Decrease
VLDL cholesterol	Increase	Decrease
LDL cholesterol	Decrease	Increase
HDL cholesterol	Increase	Decrease
HDL_2 cholesterol	Increase	Decrease
HDL_3 cholesterol	No change	No change

androgenic in nature. When these progestogens are administered in relatively high doses without oestrogen they cause a reduction in serum triglyceride and VLDL levels. The newer third-generation progestogens (desogestrel, gestodene and norgestimate) do not appear to have any significant antioestrogenic/androgenic actions *in vivo*, and their effect on triglyceride and VLDL concentrations in combination with low doses of ethinyloestradiol appears to be essentially neutral [75]. The overall effect of combined preparations containing progestogens with antioestrogenic/androgenic actions, e.g. levonorgestrel and norethisterone, depends on dose and the relative amounts of oestrogen that they contain [76]. The mechanism of the hypertriglyceridaemia observed with oestrogen therapy appears to be an increased production of apoprotein B. The mechanism of the triglyceride-lowering action of progestogens is unclear, but may be due to enhanced removal of triglyceride [74].

Oestrogens reduce LDL cholesterol concentrations by increasing the binding and uptake of LDL particles by the liver. Progestogens in combination with oestrogen, on the other hand, tend to produce a variable increase in LDL cholesterol levels. This is a dose-related 'androgenic' effect observed with high doses of levonorgestrel and the progestogens metabolized to norethisterone. It does not appear to occur with low-dose formulations containing the newer (third-generation) progestogens.

Knopp and co-workers [77] have shown an elevated triglyceride:cholesterol ratio in LDL particles with most of the combined oral contraceptives they studied. In addition, oestrogen increases the amount of protein in LDL [73]. These changes result from the production of triglyceride-enriched small LDL particles during ester exchange between VLDL and LDL.

Synthetic and natural oestrogens increase HDL cholesterol levels [68]. Conversely, progestogens with antioestrogenic/androgenic actions lower HDL cholesterol. The mechanism by which these changes occur is, however, only partly understood. Tikkanen [74] has reported that oestrogen suppresses hepatic lipase activity and increases the levels of cholesterol, triglycerides and phospholipids in HDL_2 without altering HDL_3. Levonorgestrel alone or in combination with oestrogens, on the contrary, increases hepatic lipase activity and decreases HDL_2 cholesterol. This effect was not observed with medroxyprogesterone acetate or desogestrel. Sex hormones may also regulate HDL levels by influencing the synthesis of HDL apoproteins, and a dual mechanism has been proposed [74].

Progestogen-only preparations containing norethisterone or norgestrel have been reported by Wynn and Niththyananthan [78] to be associated with lower HDL_2/LDL cholesterol concentrations. These effects were not confirmed in our own studies (Ball et al. Unpublished observations).

Although innumerable studies of combined oral contraceptives on lipid and lipoprotein metabolism have been published, it is impossible to achieve a meaningful comparative overview of all of them, in part because of variations in laboratory methodology, but also because of differences in patient selection, preparations used, etc. It is, however, clear that whereas the high oestrogen/progestogen preparations of the sixties caused significant changes in both total triglyceride and cholesterol and most of the lipoprotein subfractions, those of the seventies were essentially progestogen dominant. They were thus associated with much smaller changes in total triglyceride and cholesterol, but caused significant alterations in the lipoprotein fractions, especially a reduction in HDL cholesterol and an increase in LDL cholesterol, with a potentially 'atherogenic shift' in the profile of these lipoproteins. It is important to realize that no prospective study has demonstrated either an increase or a decrease in the risk of cardiovascular or in particular myocardial disease to be associated with sex-hormone-induced changes in lipid metabolism.

In addition it is necessary to remember that our understanding of the effect of combined oral contraceptives on lipid metabolism remains very superficial, depending as it does on isolated measurements of the plasma concentrations of lipoproteins which are involved in complex dynamic interactions. As yet no information is available on the effect of combined pills on the turnover rates of the lipoproteins, nor is it clear whether the subtle changes in lipid or fatty-acid composition observed in some studies have any practical relevance.

Furthermore, although many studies have shown significant changes in total lipid and lipoprotein concentrations of women using combined oral contraceptives these changes are usually within the normal range and are seldom as great as those observed in pregnant women. The aim of the pharmaceutical industry during the 1980s has been to develop 'balanced preparations' which have a near neutral effect on lipid metabolism. On current evidence, low-dose preparations that contain the so-called third-generation progestogens (desogestrel, gestodene and norgestimate) have the least apparently adverse effects on lipid metabolism, and from this point of view are a logical clinical choice for the next decade.

Oral contraception and sex-hormone-binding globulin (SHBG)

The possible adverse effects of combined oral contraceptives on lipid metabolism have largely been attributed to the potential 'androgenicity' of the progestogens that they contain [79]. Great interest has therefore been expressed in the effect of the pill on sex-hormone-binding globulin, a hepatic carrier protein that binds androgens and progestogens. As with many carrier proteins (e.g. thyroid-binding globulin (TBG), cortisol-binding globulin (CBG), and ceruloplasmin), coagulation factors, and lipid apoproteins, hepatic production of SHBG is stimulated by endogenous and synthetic oestrogens. The resulting increase in the plasma SHBG concentrations can, however, be suppressed by androgens and some progestogens. A similar effect is seen with TBG but not with CBG or ceruloplasmin [80, 81]. These effects are important, as an increase in SHBG levels reduces the free testosterone fraction, thus also reducing androgenic effect, while a fall in the SHBG level causes an increase in free testosterone and an enhanced clinical androgenic effect.

The progestogens currently in use display widely differing binding affinities for SHBG, and this is of practical relevance as it influences the availability of free steroid and hence the biological effect of the compound. Norethisterone binds to SHBG with less affinity than endogenous androgens and oestrogens [81] while levonorgestrel displays a binding affinity for SHBG between that of oestradiol and testosterone. 3-keto-desogestrel (the active metabolite of desogestrel) binds to SHBG with less affinity than levonorgestrel [82]. The binding of these progestogens to CBG appears to be negligible [81, 82]. Progestogen treatment alone in high dosage has been shown to reduce SHBG. Whether this is due to inhibition of endogenous oestrogen production or a direct hepatocyte-blocking effect is not clear [83].

Progestogens in combination with ethinyloestradiol suppress the oestrogen-induced increase in SHBG concentrations to varying degrees depending on the particular progestogen and dose used [76]. Thus, ethinyloestradiol 50 μg in combination with 1 mg of norethisterone acetate causes an approximately twofold increase in SHBG, but when 3 mg norethisterone acetate is combined with the same dose of oestrogen there is no change in SHBG [81]. Differences in the antioestrogenic effect of desogestrel and levonorgestrel on SHBG have been the subject of several studies [82].

Thus, while combinations of levonorgestrel and desogestrel (each 150 µg) and ethinyloestradiol (30 µg) both produce a twofold increase in CBG concentrations, levonorgestrel inhibits the two- to threefold increase in SHBG seen with the desogestrel/ethinyloestradiol preparation. This was associated with significantly lower total and, in particular, free testosterone measurements in the desogestrel group. In contrast to the 150/30 monophasic levonorgestrel preparations, those containing relatively more oestrogenic triphasic combinations of ethinyloestradiol and levonorgestrel produce a twofold increase in CBG *and* SHBG. Similar SHBG increases have been reported with the new monophasic gestodene and norgestimate combinations with ethinyloestradiol [61] and also the gestodene triphasic preparations [72, 75].

In practice, these low-dose preparations and those containing desogestrel are particularly suitable for women with a tendency to acne [82, 84].

Oral contraception and hypertension

Blood pressure appears to increase slightly in most women taking combined oral contraceptive preparations and although few experience a rise that justifies the diagnosis of hypertension, marked elevation can occur [85]. This increase in blood pressure may contribute to the known cardiovascular risk even though the rise observed may not fulfil the diagnostic criteria for hypertension. The extensive literature on the pill and hypertension and in particular the role of the renin–angiotensin system has been comprehensively reviewed by Roberts [86] (Figure 2.6).

An oestrogen-induced increase in the plasma renin substrate of 3–5-fold has been reported in women using the pill, but there was no difference in the rise observed in women who became hypertensive or those who remained normotensive [87–89]. An associated increase in plasma renin activity (PRA) has been reported; this appears to return towards normal with long-term use. No difference in PRA has been found in women who become hypertensive or remain normotensive.

Synthetic progestogens have mineralocorticoid activity and expand the plasma

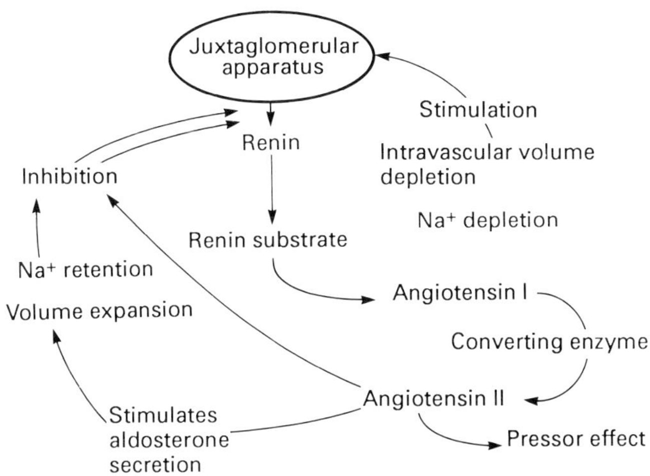

Figure 2.6 Components of the renin–angiotensin system. (After Roberts [86])

volume, with subsequent suppression of renin release [90]. The result of these interactions depends on the dose of oestrogen and progestogen and on the duration of use.

Angiotensin II has been found to be elevated in patients using oral contraceptives, but again no difference has been observed in hypertensive or normotensive pill users [91–93]. Whether real differences in the renin–angiotensin–aldosterone system do exist but are masked by measurement problems cannot be determined at present. The presence of high blood concentrations of synthetic oestrogen may well be a crucial determinant but the work of Ahluwalia et al. [15] needs to be confirmed for modern low-dose combined oral contraceptive formulations containing less than 50 μg of ethinyloestradiol.

A link between progestogen content of oestrogen-containing pills and hypertension has been demonstrated in epidemiological studies [62], but no particular progestogen has been implicated. This finding was not, however, confirmed by Meade et al. [94]. Oral progestogen-only preparations have not been shown to cause hypertension [95, 96]. Elevation of blood pressure has, however, been observed in association with depot injections of medroxyprogesterone acetate by Hall et al. [95], but not with norethisterone oenanthate by Wilson et al. [96].

Cardiac output and plasma volume increases have been reported in women taking 75–100 μg of mestranol [97]. Studies with 50 μg of mestranol did not, however, reveal any changes [98].

Studies of other aetiological factors including oestrogen effects on the sympathetic nervous system and prostaglandin pathways have failed to identify the cause of blood pressure changes in women using oral contraceptives.

In practice, pills containing low doses of oestrogen and progestogen should always be prescribed, as these are least likely to cause blood-pressure changes. All women using oral contraceptives should have their blood pressure checked at regular intervals.

Gallstones and combined oral contraceptives

Although obesity is the most important risk factor for gallstones, oral contraceptives increase the risk of the condition in certain predisposed women [84, 99, 100]. In otherwise normal women using combined oral contraceptives, Bennion and co-workers [101] have shown an enhanced biliary cholesterol secretion that is independent of any change in bile acid or bile phospholipid output. Thornton and colleagues [102] observed a direct relationship between bile cholesterol saturation and plasma HDL cholesterol concentrations. Bennion's group did not, however, identify any link between plasma HDL cholesterol and biliary cholesterol secretion, or between bile acid secretion and VLDL triglycerides. They concluded that contraceptive steroids alter the relationship between bile acid and cholesterol secretion rates so that more cholesterol is secreted at any given level of bile acid secretion, explaining the increased incidence of cholesterol cholelithiasis among users of oral contraceptives. See also page 47.

Oral contraceptives, vitamins, and minerals

Although the effects of oral contraceptives on carbohydrate, lipid, and protein metabolism have been well documented, the information available on the effects of the pill on vitamin metabolism is, by comparison, limited and on the whole conflicting. The available literature has been extensively reviewed [103–105].

As in pregnancy, decreased concentrations of the water-soluble vitamins B_2, B_6, B_{12}, C, and folic acid have been reported in users of the pill. One may speculate that this may be due in part to impaired intestinal absorption, but plasma volume expansion leading to haemodilution may also be a factor. The fat-soluble vitamins A and K are increased in pill users and this probably reflects the increases in circulating lipids that occur with these preparations.

Vitamin A (retinol)

Gal and associates [106] were the first to report increased plasma levels of vitamin A. As high doses of this vitamin are known to cause fetal malformations in laboratory animals, the authors expressed concern that the effect might be observed in women who conceived shortly after stopping the pill. Their anxiety has thus far proved to be without foundation. Increases in serum retinol-binding proteins and decreases in plasma carotene levels and liver content of vitamin A have been reported and it has been suggested that oral contraceptives may affect mobilization and redistribution of tissue vitamin A.

Vitamin B_6

Pyridoxine is absorbed in the upper intestine and converted to pyridoxal phosphate, the coenzyme form which acts as a catalyst in the formation of niacin from tryptophan. Low availability of pyridoxine disrupts this process and causes accumulation of intermediary metabolites, e.g. xanthurenic acid. Pyridoxine has been extensively studied in women using oral contraception because of the apparent link between disturbances in some pyridoxine-dependent enzyme systems and symptoms of depression [107]. Treatment with pyridoxine (40 mg daily) in a double-blind crossover study effectively improved the depression. Although most women taking combined oral contraceptives can be shown to have reduced pyridoxal phosphate levels, this does not appear to have a demonstrable effect, and in the vast majority vitamin supplementation is not considered necessary.

Vitamin B_2 (riboflavin)

Measurement in long-term pill users of erythrocyte glutathione reductase, a red-cell enzyme used as an index of riboflavin nutrition, has suggested a deficiency which is not of dietary origin [108]. The reason for this is uncertain and the apparent deficiency does not appear to have any clinical effect.

Folic acid and vitamin B_{12}

Reduced serum folate concentrations have been reported in women using oral contraceptives [109]. The absorption of polyglutamates, the major food source containing folic acid, is reduced in oral contraceptive users, but monoglutamate absorption is normal. As polyglutamic folate must be enzymatically deconjugated in the small intestine before absorption can occur, it has been suggested that the process may be affected by the synthetic sex steroids [110]. These changes are not observed during pregnancy, which suggests that synthetic oestrogens and progestogens act differently from the naturally occurring hormones.

Vitamin B_{12} concentrations have been reported to be reduced in the serum but not in the erythrocytes of oral contraceptive users [111–114]. The reason for this is uncertain, but a number of possible causes have been suggested, including malabsorption and increased renal excretion. It has also been postulated that the production of transcobalamin 1, a glycoprotein involved in plasma vitamin B_{12} transport, may be inherited [115]. These observations do not, however, appear to have any clinical relevance.

Vitamin C (ascorbic acid)

Women using oral contraceptives have been shown to have reduced vitamin C concentrations in plasma, leucocytes [116], and urine [117]. The clinical significance and cause of this is, however, uncertain. Ceruloplasmin, a copper-containing protein which is elevated by oestrogens, has ascorbic acid oxidase activity *in vitro* and it has therefore been suggested that this carrier protein may be the cause of the lower concentrations of the vitamin observed in the plasma and tissues of these women [103]. Alternative explanations include lower levels of reducing agents such as glutathione [118], impaired vitamin absorption, and altered tissue distribution [119].

Vitamin E (alpha-tocopherol)

Little or no change in the plasma concentrations of vitamin E has been observed in users of oral contraceptives [120]. Renaud and co-workers [121] have, however, observed platelet 'hyperactivity' associated with a reduced Vitamin E concentrations in long-term users of combined oral contraceptives. These changes were corrected by treatment with 200 mg vitamin E daily for two months.

Vitamin K

Because of the increase in the circulating concentrations of vitamin-K-dependent clotting factors observed in oral contraceptive users, it has been suggested that vitamin K requirements of women on the pill are reduced [104]. This is, however, of doubtful clinical relevance.

Oral contraception and minerals

Serum iron, total iron-binding capacity (TIBC), and transferrin are all increased in women using oral contraceptives [122–124]. This appears to be due to a combination of reduced menstrual iron loss, enhanced iron absorption, and an oestrogen-induced increase in carrier protein concentration. The resulting highly significant reduction in anaemia in women using the pill is one of the useful health benefits of this method of contraception.

Serum copper concentrations are also increased in women taking oral contraceptives [125], an effect that appears to be largely due to an oestrogen-induced increase in ceruloplasmin [124]. Although a reduced dietary requirement for this mineral has been postulated [105], the metabolic significance of these findings is unknown.

Serum zinc concentrations have been shown to be reduced in women using oral contraceptives [126, 127]. Several theories have been proposed to account for this, including decreased absorption, increased urinary excretion, redistribution to erythrocytes or a decrease in serum albumin, a major carrier of zinc [128]. This finding is again of unknown clinical relevance.

Drug interactions with oral contraceptive steroids

In the 1960s failure of combined oral contraceptive preparations was attributed to patient non-compliance. However, in 1971 Reimers and Jezek [129] reported an increased incidence of 'intermenstrual' bleeding in users of contraceptive steroids who were also taking antituberculous drugs; their analysis revealed that this was due to the antibiotic rifampicin. Subsequent studies have confirmed these findings and implicated anticonvulsant drugs and antibiotics in contraceptive failure [130].

Rifampicin

Rifampicin has been shown to be a potent inducer of hepatic microsomal enzymes. Bolt and co-workers [131] demonstrated a fourfold increase in the hydroxylation of ethinyloestradiol in the livers of patients treated with this drug. Back and colleagues [132] have also shown that circulating norethisterone concentrations are nearly halved in women taking preparations containing this progestogen. It is, however, uncertain whether rifampicin affects the gut wall in addition to the hepatic metabolism of these drugs.

Anticonvulsant drugs

A large number of pregnancy failures have been reported in women taking anticonvulsant drugs and oral contraceptives concurrently. The drugs implicated, which are all inducers of hepatic microsomal enzymes, include phenytoin, phenobarbitone, methylphenobarbitone, primidone, carbamazepine and ethosuximide [16]. There is, however, considerable interindividual variation and while some women display marked falls in plasma ethinyloestradiol concentrations after starting treatment with these drugs, others show no change. SHBG capacity has also been noted to increase during phenobarbitone therapy, which reduces the free concentration of progestogen in plasma (*vide supra*).

Reduction over the years in the oestrogen content of combined oral contraceptive preparations from 50 μg or greater to as little as 20 or 30 μg has led to an increased awareness of these interactions. In clinical practice it may be necessary to increase the daily dose of steroid to as much as 100 μg to prevent breakthrough bleeding and maintain contraceptive efficacy.

Griseofulvin

Griseofulvin is also a potent inducer of hepatic enzyme activity. Intermenstrual bleeding and amenorrhoea have been reported in 20 women treated with this preparation. Two pregnancies were also observed, but these occurred in patients who were taking sulphonamides and so cannot be attributed solely to griseofulvin with certainty [133].

Other antibiotics

An increased incidence of breakthrough bleeding and contraceptive failure have also been observed in women for whom antibiotics have been prescribed. The first reports concerned ampicillin, but chloramphenicol, sulphonamides, and nitrofurantoin have also been implicated [134]. These antibiotics alter the gut flora and thus interfere with the enterohepatic circulation of ethinyloestradiol [135], reducing the concentrations in some women. There does, however, appear to be considerable variation between individuals, and Friedman and co-workers [136] were unable to demonstrate any significant effect when women taking a 50-μg ethinyloestradiol preparation were treated with ampicillin. These findings were confirmed by Back and colleagues [137], who also failed to show any effect with erythromycin, tetracycline or co-trimoxazole. Indeed, treatment with co-trimoxazole was, if anything, associated with enhanced contraceptive effects, possibly due to inhibition of the metabolism of ethinyloestradiol by the sulphonamide component of this preparation.

Vitamin C

The effects of oral contraceptives can also be enhanced by vitamin C. This is due to competition between the vitamin and ethinyloestradiol for sulphate conjugation in the gut wall. Plasma concentrations of ethinyloestradiol increase by approximately 50% in women receiving 1 g of vitamin C a day [16].

Other drugs

Any drug which has enzyme-inducing properties may reduce the efficacy of the oral contraceptive steroids. Large lists of such compounds have been produced, but drugs have often been cautiously included on theoretical grounds and these lists are seldom of practical value. See chapter 5 for clinical guidelines (page 80–82).

Conclusion

Despite nearly three decades of clinical experience with the combined oral contraceptive pill, many questions remain unanswered. Although changes in dosage and the development of new progestogens over the last 25 years have undoubtedly been beneficial, they have also made it more difficult to evaluate the epidemiological and metabolic effects of these preparations. It seems unlikely that the oestrogen component of the pill will alter in the near future. A plethora of studies will, however, appear during the course of the next decade as the third-generation progestogens are more widely used. Whether these will in time be replaced by a fourth generation remains to be seen.

References

1. HABERLANDT, L. Die hormonale Sterilisierung des weiblichen organismus. *Thesis*, Fischer, Jena, Germany (1931)
2. PIOTROW, P. T. and LEE, C. M. Oral contraceptives. *Population Reports*, Series A, No. 1 (1974)
3. DJERASSI, C. *The Politics of Contraception* W. W. Norton and Co., New York, pp. 227 (1979)
4. VAUGHAN, P. *The Pill on Trial*. Weidenfeld and Nicholson, London (1970)

5. WARREN, R. J. and FOTHERBY, K. Plasma levels of ethinyloestradiol after administration of ethinyloestradiol or mestranol to human subjects. *Journal of Endocrinology*, **59,** 369 (1973)

6. GOLDZIEHER, J. W., DOZIER, T. S. and DE LA PENA, A. Plasma levels and pharmacokinetics of ethynyl estrogens in various populations. I. Ethynylestradiol and II. Mestranol. *Contraception*, **21,** 1 (1980)

7. FOTHERBY, K. Metabolism of synthetic steroids by animals and man. *Acta Endocrinologica (Copenhagen)* [Suppl.], **185,** 119 (1974)

8. DE LIA J. E. and EMERY, M. G. Clinical pharmacology and common minor side effects of oral contraceptives. *Clinical Obstetrics and Gynecology*, **24,** 879 (1981)

9. VOSE, C. W., BUTLER, J. K., WILLIAMS, B. M. *et al.* Bioavailability and pharmacokinetics of norethisterone in women after oral doses of ethynodiol diacetate. *Contraception*, **19,** 119 (1979)

10. BERGINK, E. W. and KLOOSTERBOER, H. J. Structural requirements for optimal receptor binding of contraceptive progestogens. *Advances in Contraception*, **1,** 256 (1985)

10a. REKERS. H. New generation of monophasic oral contraceptives. In: *Contraception Into the Next Decade* (ed. Keller P. J.), Parthenon, Carnforth, pp. 13–24 (1988)

11. HAHN, D. W., ALLEN, G. O. and MCGUIRE, J. L. The pharmacological profile of norgestimate, a new orally active progestin. *Contraception*, **16,** 541 (1977)

12. FOTHERBY, K. Variability of pharmacokinetic parameters for contraceptive steroids. *Journal of Steroid Biochemistry*, **19,** 817 (1983)

13. GRIMMER, S. F. M. and ORME M. L'E. The basic pharmacology, pharmacokinetics and drug interactions of hormonal contraceptives. *British Journal of Family Planning*, **12,** 38 (1986)

14. STADEL, B. V., STERNTHAL, P. M., SCHLESSELMAN, J. J. *et al.* Variation of ethinylestradiol blood levels among healthy women using oral contraceptives. *Fertility and Sterility*, **33,** 257 (1980)

15. AHLUWALIA, B. S., CURRY, C. L., CROCKER C. L. and VERMA, P. S. Evidence of higher ethynylestradiol blood levels in human hypertensive oral contraceptive users. *Fertility and Sterility*, **28,** 627 (1977)

16. BACK, D. J., BRECKENRIDGE, A. M. and ORME, M. L'E. Drug interactions with oral contraceptive steroids. *IPPF Medical Bulletin*, **17,** 1 (1983)

17. GRIMMER, S. F. M., BACK, D. J., ORME, M. L'E. *et al.* The bioavailability of ethinylestradiol and levonorgestrel in patients with an ileostomy. *Contraception*, **33,** 51 (1986)

18. SHI, Y-E., HE, C-H., GU, J. and FOTHERBY, K. Pharmacokinetics of norethisterone in humans. *Contraception*, **35,** 465 (1987)

19. GOLDZIEHER, J. W. and CHENAULT, C. B. Low dose oral contraceptive steroids: Implications of first-pass effect. Presented at the ACOG meeting, Las Vegas, Nevada (1987)

20. SISENWINE, S. F., KIMMEL, H. B., LIU, A. L. and RUELIUS, H. W. Excretion and stereoselective biotransformation of dl-, d-, and l-norgestrel in women. *Drug Metabolism and Disposition*, **3,** 180 (1975)

21. BACK, D. J., BRECKENRIDGE, A. M., ORME, M. L'E. and ROWE, P. Clinical pharmacology of oral contraceptive steroids: drug interactions. *Journal of Obstetrics and Gynaecology*, **1**, 126 (1980)

21a. HASENACK, H. G., BOSCH, M. G. and KARR, K. Serum levels of 3-keto-desogestrel after oral administration of desogestrel and 3-keto-desogestrel. *Contraception*, **33,** 591 (1986)

21b. BLACK, D. J., GRIMMER, S. F., SHENOY, N. and ORME, M. L'E. Plasma concentrations of 3-keto-desogestrel after oral administration of desogestrel and intravenous administration of 3-keto-desogestrel. *Contraception*, **35,** 619 (1987)

22. PINKERTON, S. M. Does the choice of progestogen in a combined oral contraceptive matter? The case for selectivity. *Drugs of Today*, **19,** 569 (1983)

23. SPONA, J. and HUBER, J. Pharmacological and endocrine profiles of gestodene. *International Journal of Fertility*, **32** [Suppl.], 6 (1987)

24. WEINTRAUB, H. S., ABRAMS, L. S., PATRICK, J. E. and MCGUIRE, J. L. Disposition of norgestimate in the presence and absence of ethinyl estradiol after oral administration to humans. *Journal of Pharmaceutical Sciences*, **67,** 1406 (1978)

25. ALTON, K. B., HETYEI, C. S. and PATRICK, J. E. Biotransformation of norgestimate in women. *Contraception*, **29,** 19 (1984)

26. HAWKINS, D. F. and ELDER, M. D. The clinical pharmacology of oestrogens and progestogens. In *Human Fertility Control: Theory and Practice*, Butterworths, London (1979)

27. GOLDZIEHER, J. W. Use and misuse of the term potency with respect to oral contraceptives, *Journal of Reproductive Medicine*, **31** [Suppl. 6], 553 (1986)

28. SWYER, G. I. M. Development of potency tests. *Journal of Obstetrics and Gynaecology*, **4**, S110 (1984)
29. GILLMER, M. D. G. Progestogen potency in oral contraceptive pills. *American Journal of Obstetrics and Gynecology*, **157**, 1048 (1987)
30. RUNNEBAUM, B. and RABE, T. B. New progestogens in oral contraceptives. *American Journal of Obstetrics and Gynecology*, **157**, 1059 (1987)
31. JORDAN, W. M. Pulmonary embolism. *Lancet*, **2**, 1146 (1961)
32. INMAN, W. H. W., VESSEY, M. P., WESTERHOLM, B. and ENGELUND, A. Thrombo-embolic disease and the steroidal content of oral contraceptives. A report to the Committee on Safety of drugs. *British Medical Journal*, **2**, 203 (1970)
33. MAMMEN, E. F. Oral contraceptives and blood coagulation: A critical review. *American Journal of Obstetrics and Gynecology*, **142**, 781 (1982)
34. IREY, N. S., MANION, W. C. and TAYLOR, H. B. Vascular lesions in women taking oral contraceptives. *Archives of Pathology*, **89**, 1 (1970)
35. MEADE, T. W. Oral contraceptives, clotting factors and thrombosis. *American Journal of Obstetrics and Gynecology*, **142**, 758 (1982)
36. BELLER, F. K. and EBERT, C. Effects of oral contraceptives on blood coagulation. *Obstetrical and Gynecological Survey*, **40**, 425 (1985)
37. CHANDRA, R. K. Serum levels of IgG and alpha-macroglobulin and incidence of cryofibrinogenaemia in women taking oral contraceptives. *Journal of Reproduction and Fertility*, **28**, 463 (1972)
38. ALKJAERSIG, N., FLETCHER, A. and BURSTEIN. R. Association between oral contraceptive use and thromboembolism: A new approach to its investigation based on plasma fibrinogen chromatography. *American Journal of Obstetrics and Gynecology*, **122**, 199 (1975)
39. STENFLO, J. A new vitamin K-dependent protein: purification from bovine plasma and preliminary characterisation. *Journal of Biological Chemistry*, **251**, 355 (1976)
40. GRIFFIN, J. H. *et al.* Deficiency of protein C in congenital thrombotic disease. *Journal of Clinical Investigation*, **68**, 1370 (1981)
41. GONZALEZ, R. *et al.* Protein C levels in late pregnancy, post-partum and in women on oral contraceptives. *Journal of Laboratory and Clinical Medicine*, **96**, 762 (1985)
42. MEADE, T. W. *et al.* Effects of oral contraceptives and obesity on protein C antigen. *Thrombosis and Haemostasis*, **53**, 198 (1985)
43. COHEN, H., MACKIE, I. J., WALSHE, K. *et al.* A comparison of the effects of two triphasic oral contraceptives on haemostasis. *British Journal of Haematology*. In press (1988)
44. MEADE, T. W., CHAKRABARTI, R., HAINES, A. P. *et al.* Characteristics affecting fibrinolytic activity and plasma fibrinogen concentrations. *British Medical Journal*, **1**, 153 (1979)
45. BONNAR, J. and SABRA, A. M. Oral contraceptives and blood coagulation. *Journal of Reproductive Medicine*, **31**, [Suppl. 6], 551 (1986)
46. BOTTIGER, L. E., BORMAN, G., EKLUND, G. and WESTERHOLM, B. Oral contraceptives and thromboembolic disease: effects of lowering the oestrogen content. *Lancet*, **1**, 1097 (1980)
47. KIERKEGAARD. A. Deep vein thrombosis and the estrogen content in oral contraceptives – an epidemiological analysis. *Contraception*, **31**, 29 (1984)
48. NOTELOVITZ, M., KITCHENS, C., COONE, L. *et al.* Low dose oral contraceptive usage and coagulation. *American Journal of Obstetrics and Gynecology*, **141**, 71 (1981)
49. BONNAR, J., DALY, L. and CARROLL, E. Blood coagulation with a combination pill containing gestodene and ethinyl oestradiol. *International Journal of Fertility* [Suppl.], 21 (1987)
50. RABE, T., RUNNEBAUM, B., KOHLMEIER, T. *et al.* Clinical and metabolic effects of gestodene and levonorgestrel. *International Journal of Fertility* [Suppl.], 29 (1987)
51. DUNCAN, J. M. On puerperal diabetes. *Transactions of the London Obstetric Society for the Year 1882*, **24**, 256 (1883)
52. WYNN, V. and DOAR, J. W. H. Some effects of oral contraceptives on carbohydrate metabolism. *Lancet*, **2**, 715 (1966)
53. SPELLACY, W. N., BUHI, W. C. and BIRK, S. A. Effects of norethindrone on carbohydrate and lipid metabolism. *Obstetrics and Gynecology*, **46**, 560 (1975)
54. WYNN, V., ADAMS, P. W., GODSLAND, I. *et al.* Comparison of effects of different combined oral contraceptive formulations on carbohydrate and lipid metabolism. *Lancet*, **1**, 1045 (1979)

55. SPELLACY, W. N., BUHI, W. C. and BIRK, S. A. The effects of norgestrel on carbohydrate and lipid metabolism over one year. *American Journal of Obstetrics and Gynecology*, **125,** 984 (1976)
56. SPELLACY, W. N., BUHI, W. C. and BIRK, S. A. Prospective studies of carbohydrate metabolism in 'normal' women using norgestrel for eighteen months. *Fertility and Sterility*, **35,** 167 (1981)
57. MANDOUR, T., KISSEBAH, A. H. and WYNN, V. Mechanism of oestrogen and progesterone effects on lipid and carbohydrate metabolism: alteration in the insulin:glucagon molar ratio and hepatic enzyme activity. *European Journal of Clinical Investigation*, **7,** 181 (1977)
58. SPELLACY, W. N., BUHI, W. C., BIRK, S. A. and VAN ARNARN, J. B. Carbohydrate metabolism studies in women using Brevicon, a low-estrogen type of oral contraceptive for one year. *American Journal of Obstetrics and Gynecology*, **142,** 105 (1982)
59. WYNN, V. The effects of low dose contraceptive formulations on carbohydrate metabolism. *British Journal of Family Planning*, **11,** 18 (1985)
60. SPELLACY, W. N., BIRK, S. A., BUGGIE, J. and BUHI, W. C. Prospective carbohydrate metabolism studies in women using a low estrogen oral contraceptive for one year. *Journal of Reproductive Medicine*, **26,** 295 (1981)
61. FOTHERBY, K., TRAYNER, I., LONGHORNE, P. N. *et al.* Metabolic investigations with Femodene–an oral contraceptive containing gestodene and ethinylestradiol. *Contraception*, **35,** 323 (1987)
61a. VAN DER VANGE, N., KLOOSTERBOER, H. J. and HASPELS, A. A. Effect of seven low-dose combined oral contraceptive preparations on carbohydrate metabolism. *American Journal of Obstetrics and Gynecology*, **156,** 918 (1987)
62. ROYAL COLLEGE OF GENERAL PRACTITIONERS' ORAL CONTRACEPTION STUDY. Mortality among oral contraceptive users. *Lancet*, **2,** 727 (1977)
63. ROYAL COLLEGE OF GENERAL PRACTITIONERS' ORAL CONTRACEPTION STUDY. Further analyses of mortality in oral contraceptive users. *Lancet*, **1,** 541 (1981)
64. LEWIS, B. The lipoproteins: predictors, protectors and pathogenesis. *British Medicical Journal* , **287,** 1161 (1983)
65. N.I.H. CONSENSUS DEVELOPMENT CONFERENCE. Lowering blood cholesterol to prevent heart disease. *Journal of the American Medical Association*, **253,** 2080 (1985)
66. FOTHERBY, K. Effect of oral contraceptives on serum lipids and cardiovascular disease. *British Journal of Family Planning*, **11,** 86 (1985)
67. KRAUSS, R. M. Effects of progestational agents on serum lipids and lipoproteins. *Journal of Reproductive Medicine*, **27,** 503 (1982)
68. FOTHERBY, K. Oral contraceptives, lipids and cardiovascular disease. *Contraception*, **31,** 367 (1985)
69. BUSH, T. L., COWAN, L. D., BARRETT-CONNOR, E. *et al.* Estrogen use and cardiovascular mortality. *The Lipid Research Clinics Follow-up Study*. Abstract 183. Winnipeg, Manitoba, Canada, Society of Epidemiologic Research (1983)
70. HYTTEN, F. E. Nutrition. In *Clinical Physiology in Obstetrics* (ed. Hytten, F. E. and Chamberlain, G.), Blackwell Scientific Publications, Oxford, pp. 163 (1980)
71. GILLMER, M. D. G. The relevance of potency tests. *Journal of Obstetrics and Gynaecology*, **4,** S128 (1984)
72. BALL, M., GILLMER, M. D. G., ASHWELL, E. *et al.* Which pill? The effect of various modern preparations on lipoprotein and glucose metabolism. *British Journal of Family Planning*, **14**, in press (1989)
73. AURELL, CRAMER, K. and RYBO, G. Serum lipids and lipoproteins during long-term administration of an oral contraceptive. *Lancet*, **1,** 291 (1966)
73a. WYNN, V., DOAR, J. W. H. and MILLS, G. L. Some effects of oral contraceptives on serum lipid and lipoprotein levels. *Lancet*, **2,** 720 (1966)
74. TIKKANEN, M. J. and NIKKILA, E. A. Oral contraceptives and lipoprotein metabolism. *Journal of Reproductive Medicine*, **31** [Suppl. 9], 898 (1986)
75. LEPOT, M. R. and GASPARD, U. J. Metabolic effects of two low-dose triphasic oral contraceptives containing ethinyl estradiol and levonorgestrel or gestodene. *International Journal of Fertility* [Suppl.], 15 (1987)
76. FOTHERBY, K. A metabolic assessment of different oral contraceptives. *Journal of Obstetrics and Gynaecology*, **3** [Suppl. 2], S77 (1983)
77. KNOPP, R. H., WALDEN, C. E., WAHL, P. W. *et al.* Oral contraceptive effects on lipoprotein triglyceride and cholesterol. *Journal of Clinical Endocrinology and Metabolism*, **53,** 1123 (1981)

78. WYNN, V. and NITHTHYANANTHAN, R. The effect of progestins in combined oral contraceptives on serum lipids. *American Journal of Obstetrics and Gynecology*, **142,** 766 (1982)
79. KUUSI, T., NIKKILA, E. A., TIKKANEN, M. J. and SIPINEN, S. Effects of two progestins with different androgenic properties on hepatic endothelial lipase and high density lipoprotein. *Atherosclerosis*, **54,** 251 (1985)
80. EL MAKHZANGY, M. N., WYNN, V. and LAWRENCE, D. M. Sex hormone binding globulin capacity as an index of oestrogenicity or androgenicity in women on oral contraceptive steroids. *Clinical Endocrinology*, **10,** 39 (1979)
81. BOWLES, S. M. and MILLS, R. J. Sex hormone binding globulin: effect of synthetic steroids on the assay and effect of oral contraceptives. *Annals of Clinical Biochemistry*, **18,** 226 (1981)
82. HAMMOND, G. L., LANGLEY, M. S., ROBINSON, P. A. *et al.* Serum steroid binding protein concentrations, distribution of progestogens, and bioavailability of testosterone during treatment with contraceptives containing desogestrel or levonorgestrel. *Fertility and Sterility*, **42,** 44 (1984)
83. CULLBERG, G. and MATTSSON, L. A. Androgenic, oestrogenic and antioestrogenic effects of desogestrel and lynestrenol alone: effects on serum proteins, sex hormones and vaginal cytology. In *Proceedings of the XIIth World Congress of Fertility and Sterility* (ed. Harrison, R. F., Bonnar, J. and Thompson, W.), MTP Press, Lancaster, 623 (1984)
84. PALATSI, R., HIRVENSALO, E., LIUKKO, P. *et al.* Serum total and unbound testosterone and sex hormone binding globulin (SHBG) in female acne patients treated with two different oral contraceptives. *Acta Dermato-Venereologica (Stockholm)*, **64,** 517 (1984)
85. ROYAL COLLEGE OF GENERAL PRACTITIONERS. Oral contraceptives and health: an interim report from the oral contraception study of the Royal College of General Practitioners. Pitman Medical, London (1974)
86. ROBERTS, J. M. Oestrogens and hypertension. *Clinical Endocrinology and Metabolism*, **10,** 489 (1981)
87. SARUTA, T., SAADE, G. A. and KAPLAN, N. M. A possible mechanism for hypertension induced by oral contraceptives. *Archives of Internal Medicine*, **126,** 621 (1970)
88. BECKERHOFF, R., LEUTSCHER, J. A., BECKERHOFF, I. and NOKES, G. W. Effects of oral contraceptives on the renin–angiotensin system and on blood pressure of normal young women. *Johns Hopkins Medical Journal*, **132,** 80 (1972)
89. BECKERHOFF, R., LEUTSCHER, J. A., WILKINSON, R. *et al.* Plasma renin concentration, activity, and substrate in hypertension induced by oral contraceptives. *Journal of Clinical Endocrinology*, **34,** 1067 (1972)
90. OELKERS, W., SCHONESHOFER, M. and BLUMEL, A. Effects of progesterone and four synthetic progestogens on sodium balance and the renin–aldosterone system in man. *Journal of Clinical Endocrinology and Metabolism*, **39,** 882 (1974)
91. KATZ, F. H. and BECK, P. Plasma renin activity, renin substrate and aldosterone during treatment with various oral contraceptives. *Journal of Clinical Endocrinology and Metabolism*, **39,** 1001 (1974)
92. CRANE, M. G. and HARRIS, J. J. Estrogens and hypertension: effect of discontinuing estrogens on blood pressure, exchangeable sodium, and the renin–aldosterone system. *American Journal of the Medical Sciences*, **276,** 33 (1978)
93. OGIHARA, T., HATA, T., MARUYAMA, A. *et al.* Effects of angiotensin II antagonist, (Sarcosine 1, Isoleucine 8) angiotensin II, on blood pressure, plasma renin activity and plasma aldosterone concentration in hypertensive and normotensive subjects taking oral contraceptives. *Endocrinologia Japonica*, **26,** 591 (1979)
94. MEADE, T. W., GREENBERG, G. and THOMPSON, S. G. Progestogens and cardiovascular reactions associated with oral contraceptives and a comparison of the safety of 50- and 30-microgram oestrogen preparations. *British Medical Journal*, **280,** 1157 (1980)
95. HALL, W. D., DOUGLAS, M. B., BLUMENSTEIN, B. A. and HATCHER, R. A. Blood pressure and oral progestational agents. *American Journal of Obstetrics and Gynecology*, **136,** 344 (1980)
96. WILSON, E. S. B., CRUICKSHANK, J., MCMASTER, M. and WEIR, R. J. A prospective controlled study of the effect on blood pressure of contraceptive preparations containing different types and dosages of progestogen. *British Journal of Obstetrics and Gynaecology*, **91,** 1254 (1984)
97. WALTERS, W. A. W. and LIM, Y. L. Haemodynamic changes in women taking oral contraceptives. *Journal of Obstetrics and Gynaecology of the British Commonwealth*, **77,** 1007 (1970)

98. WALTERS, W. A. W. and CAIN, D. Haemodynamic effects of low doses of female sex steroids. *Australian and New Zealand Journal of Obstetrics and Gynaecology*, **13,** 213 (1973)
99. BOSTON COLLABORATIVE DRUG SURVEILLANCE PROJECT. Oral contraceptives and venous thromboembolic disease, surgically confirmed gallbladder disease and breast tumours. *Lancet*, **1,** 1399 (1973)
100. LAYDE, P. M., VESSEY, M. P. and YEATES, D. Risk factors for gall-bladder disease: a cohort study of young women attending family planning clinics. *Journal of Epidemiology and Community Health*, **36,** 274 (1982)
101. BENNION, L. J., MOTT, D. M. and HOWARD, B. V. Oral contraceptives raise the cholesterol saturation of bile by increasing biliary cholesterol secretion. *Metabolism*, **29,** 18 (1980)
102. THORNTON, J. R., HEATON, K. W. and MACFARLANE. D. G. A relationship between high-density-lipoprotein cholesterol and bile cholesterol saturation. *British Medical Journal*, **283,** 1352 (1981)
103. LARSSON-COHN, V. Oral contraceptives and vitamins: A review. *American Journal of Obstetrics and Gynecology*, **121,** 84 (1975)
104. WEBB, J. L. Nutritional effects of oral contraceptive use – a review. *Journal of Reproductive Medicine*, **25,** 150 (1980)
105. TYRER, L. B. Nutrition and the pill. *Journal of Reproductive Medicine*, **29,** 547 (1984)
106. GAL, I., PARKINSON, C. and CRAFT, I. Effect of oral contraceptives on human plasma vitamin A levels. *British Medical Journal*, **2,** 436 (1971)
107. ADAMS, P. W., WYNN, ROSE, D. P. *et al.* Effect of pyridoxine hydrochloride (vitamin B6) upon depression associated with oral contraception. *Lancet*, **1,** 897 (1973)
108. NEWMAN, L. J., LOPEZ, R., COLE, H. S. *et al.* Riboflavin deficiency in women taking oral contraceptive agents. *American Journal of Clinical Nutrition*, **31,** 247 (1978)
109. SHOJANIA, A. M. and HORNADY, G. J. Oral contraceptives and folate absorption. *Journal of Laboratory and Clinical Medicine*, **82,** 869 (1973)
110. STREIFF, R. R. Folate deficiency and oral contraception. *Journal of the American Medical Association*, **214,** 105 (1970)
111. BLANCHINE, J. R., BONNLANDER, B., MACARAEG, P. V. *et al.* Serum B12 binding capacity and oral contraceptive hormones. *Journal of Clinical Endocrinology*, **29,** 1425 (1969)
112. SHOJANIA, A. M., HORNADY, G. J. and BARNES, P. H. The effect of oral contraceptives on folate metabolism. *American Journal of Obstetrics and Gynecology*, **111,** 782 (1971)
113. SMITH, J. L., GOLDSMITH, G. A. and LAWRENCE, J. D. Effects of oral contraceptive steroids on vitamin and lipid levels in serum. *American Journal of Clinical Nutrition*, **28,** 371 (1975)
114. WERTALIK, L. F., METZ, E. N., LOBUGLIO, A. F. *et al.* Decreased serum B12 levels with oral contraceptive use. *Journal of the American Medical Association*, **22,** 1371 (1972)
115. WYNN, V. Vitamins and oral contraceptive use. *Lancet*, **1,** 561 (1975)
116. RIVERS, J. M. Oral contraceptives and ascorbic acid. *American Journal of Clinical Nutrition*, **28,** 550 (1975)
117. HARRIS, A. B., HARTLEY, J. and MOOR, A. Reduced ascorbic acid excretion and oral contraceptives. *Lancet*, **2,** 201 (1973)
118. SAROJA, N., VAIYACHERI, R., MALLIKARHUNESWARA, V. R. *et al.* The effect of estrogens on ascorbic acid in the plasma and blood vessels of guinea pigs. *Contraception*, **3,** 269 (1971)
119. MCLEROY, V. J. and SCHENDEL, H. E. Influence of oral contraceptives on ascorbic acid concentrations in healthy, sexually mature women. *American Journal of Clinical Nutrition*, **26,** 191 (1973)
120. HORWITT, M. K., HARVEY, C. C. and DAHM, C. H. Relationship between levels of blood lipids, vitamins C, A, and E, serum copper compounds, and urinary excretions tryptophan metabolites in women taking oral contraceptive therapy. *American Journal of Clinical Nutrition*, **28,** 403 (1975)
121. RENAUD, S., CLAVATTI, M., PERROT, L. *et al.* Influence of vitamin E administration on platelet functions in hormonal contraceptive users. *Contraception*, **36,** 347 (1987)
122. BURTON J. L. Effect of oral contraceptives on haemoglobin, packed-cell volume, serum iron and total iron-binding capacity in healthy women. *Lancet*, **1,** 978 (1967)
123. JACOBI, J. M., POWELL, L. W. and GAFFNEY, T. J. Immunochemical quantitations of human transferrin in pregnancy and during the administration of oral contraceptives. *British Journal of Haematology*, **17,** 503 (1969)
124. MARGEN, S. and KING, J. Effect of oral contraceptive agents on the metabolism of some trace minerals. *American Journal of Clinical Nutrition*, **28,** 392 (1975)

125. O'LEARY, J. A. and SPELLACY, W. N. Zinc and copper levels in pregnant women and those taking oral contraceptives. *American Journal of Obstetrics and Gynecology*, **103,** 131 (1969)
126. HALSTED, J. A., HACKLEY, B. M. and SMITH, J. C. Plasma zinc and copper in pregnancy and after oral contraceptives. *Lancet*, **2,** 278 (1968)
127. SHENKER, J. G., HELLERSTEIN, S., JUNGREIS, E. *et al.* Serum copper and zinc levels in patients taking oral contraceptives. *Fertility and Sterility*, **22,** 229 (1971)
128. PRASAD, A. S., LEI, K. Y., OBERLEAS, D. *et al.* Effect of oral contraceptive agents on nutrients, I. Minerals. *American Journal of Clinical Nutrition*, **28,** 377 (1975)
129. REIMERS, D. and JEZEK, A. The simultaneous use of rifampicin and other antitubercular agents with oral contraceptives. *Praxis Pneumologie*, **25,** 255 (1971)
130. BACK, D. J. and BRECKENRIDGE, A. M. Drug interaction with oral contraceptives. *IPPF Medical Bulletin*, **12,** 1 (1978)
131. BOLT, H. M., KAPPUS, H. and BOLT, M. Effect of rifampicin treatment on the metabolism of oestradiol and 17-alpha-ethinyloestradiol by human liver microsomes. *European Journal of Clinical Pharmacology*, **8,** 301 (1975)
132. BACK, D. J., BRECKENRIDGE, A. M., CRAWFORD, F. E. *et al.* The effect of rifampicin on norethisterone pharmacokinetics. *European Journal of Clinical Pharmacology*, **15,** 193 (1979)
133. VAN DIJKE, C. P. H. and WEBER, J. C. P. Interaction between oral contraceptives and griseofulvin. *British Medical Journal*, **288,** 1125 (1984)
134. ORME, M. L'E., BACK, D. J. and BRECKENRIDGE, A. M. Drug interactions with oral contraceptive steroids. *British Journal of Family Planning*, **10,** 19 (1984)
135. BACK, D. J., BRECKENRIDGE, A. M., CHALLINER, M. *et al.* The effect of antibiotics on the enterohepatic circulation of ethinyloestradiol and norethisterone in the rat. *Journal of Steroid Biochemistry*, **9,** 527 (1978)
136. FRIEDMAN, C. I., HUNEKE, A. L., MOON, H. K. and POWELL, J. The effect of ampicillin on oral contraceptive effectiveness. *Obstetrics and Gynecology*, **55,** 33 (1980)
137. BACK, D. J., BRECKENRIDGE, A. M., MACIVER *et al.* The effects of ampicillin on oral contraceptive steroids in women. *British Journal of Clinical Pharmacology*, **14,** 43 (1982)
138. LAROSA, J. C. Effect of estrogen replacement therapy on lipids: Implications for cardiovascular disease risk. *Journal of Reproductive Medicine*, **30** [Suppl. 10], 811 (1985)

Chapter 3

Complications of combined oral contraception

J. Drife

Epidemiological methods

Side-effects of combined oral contraceptives (COCs) can be studied in various ways. The first and simplest is through case reports: unusual conditions occurring in COC-users may be reported to the manufacturers, to official bodies concerned with drug surveillance, or to medical journals. However, this gives little indication of the true incidence of complications, and because similar conditions may be under-reported in women who do not take COCs, may suggest a relationship which does not in fact exist.

Another method is to examine trends in national statistics such as mortality rates. Since the mid-1970s the number of COC users in Britain has been around three million [1], and if COCs carried a serious risk of life-threatening disease this should be reflected by a change in national mortality statistics. However, these statistics are affected by many factors – alterations in smoking habits, for example – and examination of mortality trends is a relatively crude method of assessing risk [2]. More refined epidemiological studies are therefore needed.

Two methods are used to quantify the risks of COCs: cohort studies and case-control studies. In cohort studies a large number of COC users are followed up over a long period of time, and the pattern of disease in this group of women is compared with a cohort of similar women using other methods of contraception. Two such studies have been in progress in Britain for almost 20 years. The Oxford Family Planning Association Study, which began in 1968, recruited 17 032 women of whom 57% were users of oral contraceptives, and is currently funded until mid-1989 [3, 4]. This study involves 17 family-planning clinics in different parts of England and Scotland. The other project is the Royal College of General Practitioners study, which also began in 1968, involved 1400 general practitioners and recruited about 46 000 women [5–7]. A third major cohort study in the United States of America, the Kaiser-Permanente Contraceptive Drug Study in Walnut Creek, California, began in 1969 and recruited about 18 000 women. It ended in 1977 [8].

One advantage of cohort studies is that the investigators do not need to have a clear idea of which complications they are looking for. The disadvantages include expense, organizational problems, and the fact that for rare complications large numbers of subjects are required to show any difference in incidence between the study group and controls. Another disadvantage of the COC studies currently in progress is that COCs have changed during the last 20 years, and the pills to which subjects were exposed at the beginning of the studies are different in formulation and dosage from those in current use. Nevertheless, these three cohort studies are of paramount importance in assessing the risks of COCs.

The other epidemiological method is the case-control study, which requires much smaller numbers of subjects, but can examine only one condition at a time and cannot detect previously unsuspected associations. Women with a particular disease ('cases') are matched with women who do not have the condition ('controls'), with a view to finding out differences between them – for example in duration of pill use, age at first exposure, type of formulation used, etc. In such studies cases and controls should be as similar as possible with respect to factors such as social class, parity or geographical location: if important differences exist, the study's conclusions may be weakened because of these so-called 'confounding variables'. For example, if COC-users tend to smoke more cigarettes than controls, smoking may confound the study's conclusions regarding respiratory or cardiovascular disease. Another possible problem with such retrospective studies is the accuracy of the women's memories. Recall of duration of COC use tends to be better than recall of the brands used [9]. Nevertheless, carefully carried out case-control studies are an essential way of checking suspicions generated by cohort studies.

As well as detecting complications, epidemiological studies attempt to answer more subtle questions about the nature of the association. For example, how soon after starting the pill does the side-effect become demonstrable? Is it related to the dosage of one or other of the steroids? Is there any interaction with other risk factors, and are any particular women susceptible? For how long does the effect persist after stopping the COC?

Carcinogenesis – See Chapter 4

Cardiovascular system

Cardiovascular complications were among the first side-effects of the COC to be reported in the 1960s, and the link between thromboembolism and the pill is well known to the public as well as to doctors. However, the epidemiological picture regarding cardiovascular disease is far from straightforward, particularly nowadays with the introduction of low-dose COC formulations, which appear to be safer than the pills prescribed in the 1960s. Confounding factors such as smoking are especially important with cardiovascular diseases, and information is still emerging about the interaction of COCs with smoking and other factors such as the woman's age.

Mortality rates from cardiovascular disease in England and Wales either remained stable or declined in women of reproductive age between 1968 and 1980, and Wiseman [10] has argued that this contradicts the conclusions of cohort and case-control studies discussed below. However, Mann and Vessey [2] concluded that although examination of vital statistics is not a particularly appropriate method for determining the vascular risks of oral contraceptives, the trends in mortality in England and Wales are not incompatible with a risk associated with the pill. In the USA, examination of mortality figures in Massachusetts in 1981 suggested that the number of preventable deaths related to pregnancy was almost the same as the number related to use of oral contraception, but COCs carried higher risks than pregnancy for women over the age of 35. Many of these older COC users, however, were smokers [11].

Realini and Goldzieher [12], in a long and detailed analysis of the available epidemiological data, argued that most of the cohort and case-control studies of COCs and cardiovascular disease have been affected by bias of one kind or another, and that there is little evidence of a true association. The majority of investigators, however, believe that a connection does exist, while acknowledging that the steady reduction in dosage of COCs during the last 20 years makes the risks of current formulations difficult to assess [13–19]. In spite of the large number of epidemiological studies, there is little if any reliable information relating to the risks of currently used COC formulations containing 30–35 μg of oestrogen [14].

Venous thrombosis

The first case history suggesting a link between venous thrombosis and COCs appeared in 1961, and in 1967 a report to the British Medical Research Council described evidence of a link between COCs and thromboembolic disease [14, 20]. In 1970 Inman et al. [20], in a paper based on reports to the Committee on Safety of Drugs and on similar reports in Sweden and Denmark, concluded that the risk of thromboembolism was related to the dose of oestrogen in the COC. It was therefore recommended in 1970 that the use of high-oestrogen pills should be discontinued, and this has made it difficult to confirm a dose-response relationship between oestrogen and venous thromboembolism [18].

In early studies the relative risk of venous thromboembolism associated with the COC varied between 11:1 and 2:1 in case-control studies, with an absolute risk of about 3–6 per 10 000 women per annum [14, 15]. However, the progressive reduction in dosage, together with improved selection of patients and better supervision have probably reduced this risk. A follow-up study of 65 000 women in Seattle in the early 1980s suggested a relative risk of 2.8 [21]. Vessey and his colleagues [22] recently published an analysis of the latest findings in the Oxford/FPA study. Because of fears that deep venous thrombosis (a condition notoriously difficult to diagnose with certainty on clinical grounds) might be diagnosed more readily in COC users, cases were divided into groups in which the diagnosis was (i) certain or probable, or (ii) possible, or (iii) involved superficial venous thrombosis only. The association between COC use and venous thromboembolism was strongest in women with a certain or probable diagnosis (relative risk: 7), and less strong in those in whom there was doubt about the diagnosis (relative risk: 3). There was little or no association with superficial venous thrombosis. The findings were consistent with the view that the risk is lower with COCs containing less than 50 μg oestrogen, but the data were too few to confirm this [22]. Previous data have also suggested, but not conclusively, that 30-μg pills carry less risk of fatal thromboembolism than those with 50 μg [14, 16].

The possibility of a link between progestogen content and the risk of venous thromboembolism has been examined, and no link has been found, apart from a possible link with superficial venous thrombosis [16, 18, 23]. The risk of venous thromboembolism is unrelated to the duration of use of COCs, and persists for only a week or so after stopping the pill [14, 22, 24]. Venous thromboembolism is more common in people of blood group A, and it has been suggested that this difference may be particularly marked for thromboembolism related to COC use. Smoking does not appear to affect the risk of venous thromboembolism, in contrast to its effect on arterial disease [18].

A French case-control study has concluded that hepatic-vein thrombosis is also more common among COC users, with a relative risk of approximately 2, similar to that for other types of venous thrombosis [25].

Stroke

The term 'stroke' includes both cerebral embolism and cerebral haemorrhage.

Haemorrhagic stroke

Subarachnoid haemorrhage is the commonest type of haemorrhagic stroke in women of reproductive age [26]. A report from the Walnut Creek study suggested that COCs increased the risk of subarachnoid haemorrhage by a factor of 6 [27], but more than half of the cases in this report were over 50 years old. More recent data from the Oxford/FPA study indicate that the increase in risk of subarachnoid haemorrhage in COC users is modest, probably not more than 1.5–2-fold [28]. The RCGP study suggests a slightly higher risk of subarachnoid haemorrhage, with relative risks of 3 in current users, and 4.5 in former users [7], but by contrast the Seattle study showed no increase in risk of stroke [21].

Smoking significantly increases the risk of subarachnoid haemorrhage [14, 27, 29] and hypertension is also an important risk factor. The risk is more strongly related to smoking and hypertension than to COC use [28]. The mechanism by which COCs could affect the risk of haemorrhage is uncertain. Possible causes of subarachnoid haemorrhage include arterial aneurysms, coagulation defects and hypertension, but it has recently been suggested that unrecognized venous thrombosis accounts for some of the excess cases among women using COCs [30]. Cerebral venous sinus thrombosis may be commoner among COC users [31].

Thrombotic stroke

With thrombotic stroke there is evidence of a larger effect than with haemorrhagic stroke [18, 28]. In the late 1960s there were case reports of COC users affected by cerebral thrombosis, and reports from neurological centres of a sharp increase in the numbers of cases of cerebral arterial insufficiency, mainly among COC users [14]. The increased risk was confirmed by case-control studies, which showed relative risks varying between 1.4:1 and 26:1, suggesting that the overall risk was increased several-fold [14, 18]. The numbers of cases in cohort studies were very small, making the estimation of absolute risk unreliable, but it appears that the overall mortality rate from stroke in COC users is around 1 in 10 000 woman years [7, 14], while the one-year risk of non-fatal stroke has been estimated as between 2 and 4 per 10 000 woman years [15].

Early reports suggested a relationship between the risk of stroke and the oestrogen content of COCs, and no strokes have been observed in the Oxford/FPA study in women using pills containing less than 50 μg of oestrogen: these data are, however, too few to be conclusive [28]. More interest has centred upon the effect of the progestogen dosage [32]. The data from the RCGP cohort study were analysed to assess the risks of different formulations containing the same dose of oestrogen but different doses of progestogen [7]. It was possible to study the number of reports of vascular disease in women using five different COC formulations: three contained 50 μg of ethinyloestradiol combined with either 1, 3 or 4 mg of norethisterone acetate, and the other two contained 30 μg ethinyloestradiol combined with either 150 or 250 mg levonorgestrel. At each oestrogen dose there was a relationship between the progestogen dosage and the rate of arterial disease: this applied to both cerebrovascular and cardiovascular disease, but the relationship was strongest for the former [7].

There is no conclusive evidence of a relationship between duration of use of COCs and cerebrovascular disease, though in the RCGP study a trend was seen which was not statistically significant [7]. The question of persistence of increased risk after stopping COCs remains difficult to answer; the RCGP study has suggested that the risk of cerebrovascular disease may remain increased in former pill users, but this has not been confirmed by other studies [7, 33]. Unlike haemorrhagic stroke, the risk of thrombotic stroke does not appear to be affected by smoking or hypertension. It has been suggested that the risk of cerebrovascular disease may be related to a pre-existing hypercoagulable state in some women [34].

Myocardial infarction

Myocardial infarction was the third type of cardiovascular disease to be linked with COC use. Early reports from case-control studies indicated that the relative risk associated with COC use was between 1 and 14, with most ratios being between 3 and 5, and data from cohort studies suggested that the absolute risk of fatal myocardial infarction was around 1 in 10 000 woman years [14, 15, 18]. There does not appear to be a relationship with oestrogen dosage, though most studies reporting an association relate to the time when preparations containing 50 μg or more were being used [14]. As mentioned above, there is firmer evidence of a relationship with progestogen dosage [7]. Data concerning duration of use are scanty, and there is little evidence of persisting increase in risk among ex-users of COCs, though one study has suggested that among long-term past users over the age of 40 a twofold increase in risk persists for up to ten years after COCs have been discontinued [17]. Reanalysis (same data) showed the ongoing risk to be mainly in the continuing-heavy smokers [17a].

It was quickly suspected that with myocardial infarction an interaction between COCs and other risk factors was important. Other risk factors include age, smoking, type II hyperlipoproteinaemia, hypertension, and diabetes. It seems likely that individual risk factors potentiate one another, and it has been suggested that the relative risk increases from 4:1 in women with one factor to 20:1 with two factors and 128:1 with three or more risk factors [14, 17]. Age and smoking are important risk factors for myocardial infarction [35, 36], and the interaction between age, smoking and COC use has been analysed in the RCGP study [7, 33]. The results indicate that the risk of circulatory death in smokers remains around 1 in 10 000 until the age of 35 (with the risk being even lower in non-smokers). Between the ages of 35 and 44, the risk is significantly increased in smokers to 1 in 2000, while for non-smokers the risk remains less than 1 in 6000 [7, 37]. Thus the suggestion that COCs should be discontinued by any woman reaching the age of 35 [38] does not necessarily apply to non-smokers [37]. Above the age of 45 the risk of death from circulatory disease in smokers is 1 in 550, while in non-smokers the risk is 1 in 2500. Thus the woman who smokes has a similar risk to that of a non-smoker ten years her senior [39]. However, it should be remembered that these figures relate to all brands of oral contraceptive, and that women who use brands containing low oestrogen and low progestogen almost certainly have a lower risk than the above figures suggest. The exact figures for low-dose pills are not available, because none of the cohort studies includes large enough numbers of women using these formulations.

Hypertension

The COC causes a rise in blood pressure in most women [40]. The mean increase is said to be 9 mmHg in systolic pressure and 5 mmHg in diastolic pressure [41], though the Walnut Creek study suggested that the figures were 4.5 and 1.5 mmHg respectively [8]. Severe hypertension is rare, but in the Walnut Creek study about 4% of users developed a diastolic blood pressure of over 90 mmHg, compared with a prevalence of less than 2% in non-users: these results were similar to those of the RCGP study, in which 5% of COC users developed hypertension over a 5-year period [15]. Those at risk of hypertension are older women and those with a past history or family history of hypertension, but, surprisingly perhaps, previous pre-eclampsia or being overweight are not risk factors [8, 15]. The mechanism of the effect is unclear, but there is some evidence that both the oestrogen and the progestogen components of the combined pill are involved with the production of hypertension [15, 41]. In most women the blood pressure returns to normal quickly after the COC is discontinued [26].

Summary of cardiovascular risks

COCs cause a three- to sixfold increase in the risk of venous thromboembolism. This is probably an oestrogen effect, and is unrelated to smoking. The excess risk disappears quickly when COCs are stopped. The overall risk of haemorrhagic stroke is doubled in COC-users, and this increase is related to smoking and hypertension. The risk of thrombotic stroke is increased several-fold, but this risk is not affected by smoking or hypertension. The risk of myocardial infarction is related to age and smoking, and COCs are contraindicated over the age of 35 in smokers, but not necessarily in non-smokers. COCs cause a slight increase in blood pressure and about 4–5% of users become hypertensive: this usually settles quickly after the pill is stopped. Finally, it should be emphasized that much of this information is based on studies involving high-dose COCs, and although there are encouraging signs that risks are lower with modern low-dose formulations, firm data on low-dose pills are scanty.

Reproductive system

Fibroids

Cohort studies initially provided inconsistent results regarding the effects of COCs on uterine fibroids. The RCGP study showed that fibroids were less commonly diagnosed in pill users, but early results from the Oxford/FPA study showed no effect. It is commonly thought that fibroids sometimes grow during pregnancy, although this has been questioned [42], and it has been suggested that high-oestrogen pills might also stimulate growth [39]. A recent case-control study based on women recruited to the Oxford/FPA study concluded that the risk of uterine fibroids decreased consistently with increasing duration of oral contraceptive use: there was a roughly 17% reduction in risk with each five years of oral contraceptive use, and the risk was reduced by about 30% in women who had used COCs for ten years [42].

Menstrual disorders

COCs suppress ovarian activity, and the incidence of functional ovarian cysts is therefore reduced. It has been estimated that among non-users of COCs the incidence of functional cysts requiring hospitalization is 38 per 100 000 women annually, and that this figure is reduced to three per 100 000 among COC users [43]. It is also thought that COC therapy makes functional cysts regress more quickly, although this has not been confirmed. The incidence of non-functional cysts does not appear to be altered by COCs. A small number of women may remain anovulatory after stopping COCs: the incidence of 'post-pill' amenorrhoea lasting more than one year is 0.6–1%, and it is estimated that of these women about 90% would have developed amenorrhoea whether or not they had taken the pill [44, 45]. See page 72.

The issue of subsequent fertility after discontinuing COCs is considered further in Chapter 5, pages 88–89.

According to the RCGP study, the incidence of menorrhagia, intermenstrual bleeding, and irregular bleeding is approximately halved by COCs [43], though it is possible that breakthrough bleeding has become more common since the introduction of lower-dose pills [45]. The amount of menstrual loss is reduced by COCs, and the incidence of iron-deficiency anaemia was reduced by about 50% in the RCGP study. Moderate anaemia can be improved by COC therapy, particularly if the number of withdrawal bleeds is reduced by the so-called 'tricycle' regimen (continuous use of COCs for 63 or 84 days at a time [26]).

The incidence of dysmenorrhoea was reduced by 40% in the RCGP study, and a survey in the United States showed that 8% of users take COCs solely to control menstrual disorders [26]. There is also an improvement in the incidence of premenstrual tension, although the extent of the reduction is uncertain because this symptom is difficult to quantify [26]. Beneficial effects such as the improvements in menstrual symptoms are often overlooked when side-effects of COCs are being discussed, and in 1982 the United States Food and Drug Administration attempted to rectify this by recommending that pill packages should describe the benefits of COCs [46].

Pelvic inflammatory disease

COCs reduce the risk of pelvic inflammatory disease by about 50% [47, 48], partly because the cervical mucus becomes thicker and less penetrable by bacteria, and possibly because of a direct inhibitory effect on the growth of gonococci in the tubes [26]. The protective effect, therefore, disappears soon after the pill is discontinued. Although there has been a suggestion that the protective effect applies to chlamydial as well as to gonococcal infection [48], evidence has recently been presented by the Centers for Disease Control in Atlanta that COCs might in fact promote chlamydial infection [49]. A two- to threefold increase in the prevalence of *cervical* chlamydial infection has been demonstrated in 12 of the 14 studies of this topic [49]. In a study of university students, endocervical *Chlamydia trachomatis* infection was lower among women using intrauterine or barrier contraception than among those who used COCs or no contraception [50]. It is possible, however, that these findings are due to variations in patterns of sexual activity rather than to a direct effect of COCs [51]. A case-control study of women with chlamydial salpingitis suggested that COCs might offer some protection against the perihepatitis that can occur in this condition [52]. It may be that COCs protect the upper genital tract (and peritoneum) without influencing the risk of cervical infection, which is related to lifestyle.

The risk of *ectopic pregnancy* is also reduced, partly because of the decreased incidence of salpingitis, and partly because COCs inhibit ovulation. An American study has estimated that the risk of ectopic pregnancy in COC users is as low as one-tenth of the risk faced by women who use no contraception. In the Oxford/FPA study, no unplanned pregnancies in COC users were ectopic, compared with 6.9% of pregnancies among users of the intrauterine contraceptive device, and 0.6% among women using other methods or none [26].

Candida and other vaginal infections

The effects of COCs on the incidence of candidal infections is difficult to assess because most studies have found it difficult to control for the number of sexual partners. In a controlled study, COC users had a slightly increased risk of candidal infection but a reduced risk of trichomonal infection [26]. The RCGP study found slightly increased rates of vaginal infections among COC users, but other cohort studies have found no effect. A recent study of over 1000 women attending three departments of genitourinary medicine in England suggested that there was no association between genital candidosis and COC use [53].

Subsequent pregnancy

Many studies have concluded that after the pill is discontinued there is no increased risk of miscarriage, congenital malformations, or sudden infant death [26]. If COCs are accidentally taken during early pregnancy there does not appear to be an increased risk of miscarriage or an increase in perinatal mortality, and according to most studies there is no increased risk of congenital malformations [8]. Three studies have suggested a higher rate of major malformations or neural-tube defects in women who used the pill during early pregnancy or just before conceiving, but other studies have not confirmed this [26, 54]. (See also page 86.)

Urinary system

Higher rates of proven urinary tract infection were found in COC users in the RCGP study: the annual rate of kidney infection was 1%, and of bladder infection 5%; 2.5% had other urinary infections. However, other cohort studies did not find increased rates of urinary infection. Asymptomatic bacteriuria is also slightly commoner in COC users. Whether these findings reflect a direct effect of COCs or an increased pattern of sexual activity is uncertain [26, 55].

Gastrointestinal disturbances

Chronic inflammatory bowel disease

In the RCGP cohort study the incidence of ulcerative colitis was approximately doubled among COC users, and the incidence of Crohn's disease was increased by 40%. The Walnut Creek study also suggested that the combined incidence of ulcerative colitis and Crohn's disease was approximately doubled among COC users. A recent case-control study in North America has suggested an overall doubling of the incidence of Crohn's disease among COC users: the risk was related to duration of COC use and disappeared four years after discontinuation of COCs [56]. Another small study in America suggested that COCs may increase the risk of Crohn's disease but decrease the risk of ulcerative colitis [57]. Recent analysis of the results of the Oxford/FPA study has suggested an association between COC use and both ulcerative colitis and Crohn's disease: the association was stronger for ulcerative colitis, but fell short of statistical significance [58]. The same study confirmed the association between smoking and chronic inflammatory bowel disease: the effect is negative for ulcerative colitis and positive for Crohn's disease [58].

Gallstones

Studies during the 1970s, including the RCGP study, indicated that COC use is associated with a risk of gallstones and cholecystitis [26]. However, the Walnut Creek study and the Oxford/FPA study did not find a significant excess risk, and the most recent results of the RCGP study do not confirm its earlier findings [7]. When the duration of COC use was re-examined in the RCGP study, it was found that there was an initial increase in the rate of gallbladder disease with a peak in the third year of use. After seven years, however, the rate was lower than that among control subjects. The rate appeared to be associated with the oestrogen dosage, but not with the dosage of progestogen [7]. These findings were interpreted as suggesting that COCs accelerate the presentation of symptoms of gallbladder disease in women who already have presymptomatic disease, but in the long term no more cases are reported among COC users than among non-users.

Duodenal ulcer

The FPA study and the RCGP study both suggest that duodenal ulcer is less common among pill users, though it is possible that this effect is due to selection of patients rather than to a true protective effect of the pill itself [39].

Central nervous system

Psychological effects

Patients often complain that the pill makes them depressed, but there is little epidemiological evidence that COCs cause depression. In the RCGP study, depression was commonly given as a reason for stopping the pill, but the excess risk of depression among COC users was about 1%, with an excess risk of attempted suicide of about 1 in 1000 [7]. There was a relationship with oestrogen dosage in the RCGP study, and among users of COCs containing 30–35 μg of oestrogen there was no excess risk of depression [7]. In the Oxford/FPA study, COC users did not have an increased risk of psychotic or neurotic mental disorders [59]. Studies have shown either an increase or a decrease of libido in COC users [13]: loss of libido is not correlated with specific hormonal changes, and treatment with androgens is unsuccessful [60].

Epilepsy

In animal studies, progestogens appear to have antiepileptic effects, and no clinical study has shown any worsening of seizures in women who use COCs. Indeed, improvement in seizure control may occur in cases of 'menstrual' or 'catamenial' epilepsy. Antiepileptic drugs may, however, reduce the effectiveness of COCs by inducing enzymes which metabolize the pill, and increased COC doses may therefore be necessary [61]. (See pages 80–82.)

Migraine

There is little epidemiological evidence that COCs have any consistent effect on the incidence of migraine. COCs may either improve or worsen the frequency or severity of the headaches, and there are indications that worsening is rather more common than improvement [62]. (See pages 83–84.)

Skin

No clear relationship between COC use and acne has been demonstrated in cohort studies. It has been suggested that this is because of variations in formulation between different types of pill, the more strongly progestogenic tending to increase sebum production, while the more oestrogenic tend to alleviate acne [26]. The RCGP study showed increases in the incidence of photosensitivity, rosacea, eczema, chloasma, erythema multiforme and erythema nodosum [5, 13].

Musculoskeletal system

Rheumatoid arthritis

The Royal College of General Practitioners' study showed a 50% reduction in the incidence of rheumatoid arthritis among COC users, and a retrospective case-control study in the Netherlands showed a similar decrease [26, 63]. One study has shown a decrease in the incidence of rheumatoid arthritis since 1965 in women but not in men, and this has been attributed to the introduction of COCs [63]. However, more recent case-control studies in the United States and in Sweden have failed to show any protective effect [63]. It has been suggested that the protective effects shown in the earlier studies may have been the result of bias, but the controversy remains unresolved.

Endocrine system

No association with the occurrence of diabetes was found in the Oxford/FPA study, but prolonged follow-up will be required to rule out this possibility completely. It is improbable that there is a causal relationship between COCs and pituitary adenomas; case-control studies have given conflicting results, and cohort studies have shown no evidence of an increase in risk [26]. (See also page 64.)

Respiratory system

There does not appear to be any relationship between asthma and COC use. Cases of allergic rhinitis have been reported but there is little evidence of a definite connection with COCs [39].

Immune system

A possible effect of COCs on the immune system has been suggested by the finding in cohort studies of higher risks of viral disease and infection of the urinary and respiratory tracts, and a slightly reduced resistance to malaria. In cases of pulmonary embolism, circulating levels of immune complexes are higher among COC users than among non-users [64]. However, there seems little evidence that the pill has a significant effect on the immune system.

Summary

The most important adverse effects of COCs are those on the cardiovascular system: the several-fold increases in venous thromboembolism and thrombotic stroke, and the increased risk of myocardial infarction among older women who smoke, although these risks may now be lower with modern low-dose formulations. The effects on the reproductive system are mainly beneficial, with reduced risks of fibroids, functional ovarian cysts, menstrual disorders, ectopic pregnancy and pelvic inflammatory disease. There is no convincing evidence of an adverse effect on subsequent pregnancy. COCs slightly increase the risk of inflammatory bowel disease but appear to accelerate the development of gallstones only in women who are already susceptible. There is no evidence that modern low-dose pills cause depression. Reports of a protective effect against rheumatoid arthritis have not been confirmed. Research into the long-term effects of COCs is continuing.

References

1. WELLINGS, K. and MILLS, A. Contraceptive trends. *British Medical Journal*, **289**, 939–940 (1984)
2. MANN, J. I. and VESSEY, M. P. Trends in cardiovascular disease mortality and oral contraceptives. *British Journal of Family Planning*, **6**, 99–104 (1981)
3. VESSEY, M., DOLL, R., PETO, R. *et al.* A long-term follow-up study of women using different methods of contraception – an interim report. *Journal of Biosocial Science*, **8**, 373–427 (1976)
4. VESSEY, M. P. and LAWLESS, M. The Oxford–Family Planning Association contraceptive study. *Clinics in Obstetrics and Gynaecology*, **11**, 743–757 (1984)
5. ROYAL COLLEGE OF GENERAL PRACTITIONERS. *Oral Contraceptives and Health*. Pitman Medical, London (1974)
6. ROYAL COLLEGE OF GENERAL PRACTITIONERS' ORAL CONTRACEPTION STUDY. Mortality among oral-contraceptive users. *Lancet*, **2**, 727–733 (1977)
7. KAY, C. R. The Royal College of General Practitioners' Oral Contraception Study: some recent observations. *Clinics in Obstetrics and Gynaecology*, **11**, 759–786 (1984)
8. RINEHART, W. and PIOTROW, P. T. OCs – update on usage, safety, and side effects. *Population Reports* Series A, No. **5**, A133–A186 (1979)
9. ROSENBERG, M. J., LAYDE, P. M., ORY, H. W. *et al.* Agreement between women's histories of oral contraceptive use and physician records. *International Journal of Epidemiology*, **12**, 84–87 (1983)
10. WISEMAN, R. A. Absence of correlation between oral contraceptive usage and cardiovascular mortality. *International Journal of Fertility*, **29**, 198–208 (1984)

11. SACHS, B. P., MASTERSON, T., JEWETT, J. F. and GUYER, B. Reproductive mortality in Massachusetts in 1981. *New England Journal of Medicine*, **311,** 667–670 (1984)
12. REALINI, J. P. and GOLDZIEHER, J. W. Oral contraceptives and cardiovascular disease: a critique of the epidemiologic studies. *American Journal of Obstetrics and Gynecology*, **152,** 729–798 (1985)
13. HAWKINS, D. F. and ELDER, M. G. *Human Fertility Control – Theory and Practice*. Butterworths, London (1979)
14. VESSEY, M. P. Female hormones and vascular disease – an epidemiological overview. *British Journal of Family Planning*, **6** [Supp.], 1–12 (1980)
15. DALEN, J. E. and HICKLER, R. B. Oral contraceptives and cardiovascular disease. *American Heart Journal*, **101,** 626–639 (1981)
16. STADEL, B. V. Oral contraceptives and cardiovascular disease (first of two parts). *New England Journal of Medicine*, **305,** 612– 618 (1981)
17. STADEL, B. V. Oral contraceptives and cardiovascular disease (second of two parts). *New England Journal of Medicine*, **305,** 672–677 (1981)
17a. LAYDE, P. M., ORY, H. W. and SCHLESSELMAN, J. J. The risk of myocardial infarction in former users of oral contraceptives. *International Family Planning Perspectives*, **2,** 79–81 (1982)
18. SARTWELL, P. E. and STOLLEY, P. D. Oral contraceptives and vascular disease. *Epidemiologic Reviews*, **4,** 95–109 (1982)
19. SHAPIRO, S. Oral contraceptives – time to take stock. *New England Journal of Medicine*, **315,** 450–451 (1986)
20. INMAN, W. H. W., VESSEY, M. P., WESTERHOLM, B. and ENGELUND, A. Thromboembolic disease and the steroidal content of oral contraceptives: a report to the Committee on Safety of Drugs. *British Medical Journal*, **2,** 203–209 (1970)
21. PORTER, J. B., HUNTER, J. R., JICK, H. and STERGACHIS, A. Oral contraceptives and nonfatal vascular disease. *Obstetrics and Gynecology*, **66,** 1–4 (1985)
22. VESSEY, M., MANT, D., SMITH A. and YEATES, D. Oral contraceptives and venous thromboembolism: findings in a large prospective study. *British Medical Journal*, **292,** 526 (1986)
23. FOTHERBY, K. Oral contraceptives, lipids and cardiovascular disease. *Contraception*, **31,** 367–394 (1985)
24. EDITORIAL. Cardiovascular catastrophes. *British Journal of Family Planning*, **6,** 97 (1981)
25. VALLA, D., LE, M. G., POYNARD, T. *et al.* Risk of hepatic vein thrombosis in relation to recent use of oral contraceptives – a case-control study. *Gastroenterology*, **90,** 807–811 (1986)
26. KOLS, A., RINEHART, W., PIOTROW, P. T. *et al.* Oral contraceptives in the 1980s. *Population Reports*, **10,** A191– A222 (1982)
27. PETITTI, D. B. and WINGERD, J. Use of oral contraceptives, cigarette smoking, and risk of subarachnoid haemorrhage. *Lancet*, **2,** 234–236 (1978)
28. VESSEY, M. P., LAWLESS, M. and YEATES, D. Oral contraceptives and stroke: findings in a large prospective study. *British Medical Journal*, **289,** 530–531 (1984)
29. LONGSTRETH, W. T. and SWANSON, P. D. Oral contraceptives and stroke. *Stroke*, **15,** 747–750 (1984)
30. CHILVERS, E. and RUDGE, P. Cerebral venous thrombosis and subarachnoid haemorrhage in users of oral contraceptives. *British Medical Journal*, **292,** 524 (1986)
31. IMAI, W. K., EVERHART, F. R. and SANDERS, J. M. Cerebral venous sinus thrombosis: report of a case and review of the literature. *Pediatrics*, **70,** 965–970 (1982)
32. MANN, J. I. Progestogens in cardiovascular disease: an introduction to the epidemiologic data. *American Journal of Obstetrics and Gynecology*, **142,** 752–757 (1982)
33. ROYAL COLLEGE OF GENERAL PRACTITIONERS' ORAL CONTRACEPTION STUDY. Incidence of arterial disease among oral contraceptive users. *Journal of the Royal College of General Practitioners*, **33,** 75–82 (1983)
34. ELAM, M. B., VIAR, M. J., RATTS, T. E. and CHESNEY, C. M. Mitral valve prolapse in women with oral contraceptive-related cerebrovascular insufficiency: associated persistent hypercoagulable state. *Archives of Internal Medicine*, **146,** 73–77 (1986)
35. SALONEN, J. T. Oral contraceptives, smoking and risk of myocardial infarction in young women: a longitudinal population study in Eastern Finland. *Acta Medica Scandinavica*, **212,** 141–144 (1982)
36. JUGDUTT, B. I., STEVENS, G. F., ZACKS, D. J. *et al.* Myocardial infarction, oral contraception, cigarette smoking and coronary artery spasm in young women. *American Heart Journal*, **106,** 757–761 (1983)
37. KAY, C. R. Latest views on Pill prescribing. *Journal of the Royal College of General Practitioners*, **34,** 611–614 (1984)

38. KUENSSBERG, E. V. and DEWHURST, J. Mortality in women on oral contraceptives. *Lancet*, **2,** 757 (1977)
39. GUILLEBAUD, J. *The Pill* (3rd edn), Oxford University Press (1984)
40. CAIRNS, V., KEIL, V., DOERING, A. *et al.* Oral contraceptive use and blood pressure in a German metropolitan population. *International Journal of Epidemiology*, **14,** 389–395 (1985)
41. LEADING ARTICLE. Hypertension and oral contraceptives. *British Medical Journal*, **1,** 1570–1571 (1978)
42. ROSS, R. K., PIKE, M. C., VESSEY, M. P. *et al.* Risk factors for uterine fibroids: reduced risk associated with oral contraceptives. *British Medical Journal*, **293,** 359–362 (1986)
43. MISHELL, D. R. Noncontraceptive health benefits of oral steroidal contraceptives. *American Journal of Obstetrics and Gynecology*, **142,** 809–816 (1982)
44. PEPPERELL, R. J. Beneficial and adverse side-effects of hormonal contraception. *Medical Journal of Australia*, **144,** 169–170 (1986)
45. SHEARMAN, R. P. Oral contraceptive agents. *Medical Journal of Australia*, **144,** 201–205 (1986)
46. KUBBA, A. A. The benefits of oral contraceptives. *Journal of the Royal Society of Health*, **105,** 73–74 (1985)
47. HIGGINS, J. E., WILKENS, L. R., CHI, I. and HATCHER, R. A. Hospitalizations among black women using contraceptives. *American Journal of Obstetrics and Gynecology*, **153,** 280–287 (1985)
48. GRIMES, D. A. Reversible contraception for the 1980s. *Journal of the American Medical Association*, **255,** 69–75 (1986)
49. WASHINGTON, A. E., GOVE, S., SCHACHTER, J. and SWEET, R. L. Oral contraceptives, *Chlamydia trachomatis* infection, and pelvic inflammatory disease: a word of caution about protection. *Journal of the American Medical Association*, **253,** 2246–2250 (1985)
50. HARRISON, H. R., COSTIN, M., MEDER, J. B. *et al.* Cervical *Chlamydia trachomatis* infection in university women: relationship to history, contraception, ectopy, and cervicitis. *American Journal of Obstetrics and Gynecology*, **153,** 244–251 (1985)
51. GALL, S. A. Oral contraceptives and *Chlamydia* infections. *Journal of the American Medical Association*, **255,** 38 (1986)
52. WOLNER-HANSSEN, P. Oral contraceptive use modifies the manifestations of pelvic inflammatory disease. *British Journal of Obstetrics and Gynaecology*, **93,** 619–624 (1986)
53. DAVIDSON, F. and OATES, J. K. The pill does not cause 'thrush'. *British Journal of Obstetrics and Gynaecology*, **92,** 1265–1266 (1985)
54. KASAN, P. N. and ANDREWS, J. The effects of recent oral contraceptive use on the outcome of pregnancy. *European Journal of Gynecology, Obstetrics and Reproductive Biology*, **22,** 77–83 (1986)
55. GUILLEBAUD, J. Combined oral contraceptive pills. In: *Handbook of Family Planning* (ed. N. B. Loudon and J. R. Newton), Churchill Livingstone, Edinburgh, pp. 53–98 (1985)
56. LESKO, S. M., KAUFMAN, D. W., ROSENBERG, L. *et al.* Evidence for an increased risk of Crohn's disease in oral contraceptive users. *Gastroenterology*, **89,** 1046–1049 (1985)
57. CALKINS, B. M., MENDELOFF, A. I. and GARLAND, C. Inflammatory bowel disease in oral contraceptive users. *Gastroenterology*, **91,** 523–524 (1986)
58. VESSEY, M., JEWELL, D., SMITH, A. *et al.* Chronic inflammatory bowel disease, cigarette smoking, and use of oral contraceptives: findings in a large cohort study of women of childbearing age. *British Medical Journal*, **292,** 1101–1103 (1986)
59. VESSEY, M. P., MCPHERSON, K., LAWLESS, M. and YEATES, D. Oral contraception and serious psychiatric illness: absence of an association. *British Journal of Psychiatry*, **146,** 45–49 (1985)
60. BANCROFT, J., DAVIDSON, D. W., WARNER, P. and TYRER, G. Androgens and sexual behaviour in women using oral contraceptives. *Clinical Endocrinology*, **12,** 327–340 (1980)
61. MATTSON, R. H., CRAMER, J. A., DARNEY, P. D. and NAFTOLIN, F. Use of oral contraceptives by women with epilepsy. *Journal of the American Medical Association*, **256,** 238–240 (1986)
62. BENSON, M. D. and REBAR, R. W. Relationship of migraine headache and stroke to oral contraceptive use. *Journal of Reproductive Medicine*, **31,** 1082–1088 (1986)
63. DEL JUNCO, D. J., ANNEGERS, J. F., LUTHRA, H. S. *et al.* Do oral contraceptives prevent rheumatoid arthritis? *Journal of the American Medical Association*, **254,** 1938–1941 (1985)
64. PLOWRIGHT, C., ADAM, S. A., THOROGOOD, M. *et al.* Immunogenicity and the vascular risk of oral contraceptives. *British Heart Journal*, **53,** 556–561 (1985)

Chapter 4

Oral contraception and cancer*

M. P. Vessey

Oral contraceptives first became available in the United States in 1959 and since that time they have been widely adopted by women in many different countries. Well over 50 million women worldwide are currently 'on the pill' while many millions more have used oral contraceptives in the past. Accordingly, a proper assessment of the possible relationship between oral contraceptive use and cancer is of great public health importance.

In this chapter, attention is concentrated on combined oral contraceptives, although there are also a few references to sequential preparations. Reliable human data on progestogen-only pills and on injectable progestogen contraceptives (medroxyprogesterone acetate and norethisterone oenanthate) are sparse, and these preparations are not discussed here.

A number of important general considerations need to be borne in mind when studying the literature on the relationship between oral contraceptives and cancer.

Latent period

There is usually an appreciable 'latent period' between first exposure to a carcinogen and the development of overt malignant disease. In addition, the cumulative effects of prolonged exposure or repeated exposure are likely to be of importance. Steroid contraceptives have been in widespread use for little more than 20 years; relatively few women have had both the prolonged exposure and the extended period of follow-up required to evaluate carcinogenic effects with confidence.

Changes in preparation

The types and doses of steroid in common use have changed markedly since the introduction of the pill. For example (a) the dosages of both oestrogens and progestogens have been progressively reduced, (b) some new progestogens (e.g. levonorgestrel, desogestrel) have been introduced, (c) other progestogens (e.g. chlormadinone acetate, megestrol acetate) have been withdrawn, and (d) sequential preparations have largely disappeared while triphasic and biphasic preparations have been developed. From this it follows that even recent studies of the possible carcinogenic effects of oral contraceptives largely relate to discontinued products.

*Some sections of this chapter are based on material included in an article entitled 'Exogenous hormones' which appeared in a book entitled *Cancer Risks and Prevention* edited by M. P. Vessey and J. A. Muir Gray and published by Oxford University Press in 1985.

Time of exposure

Exposure to contraceptive steroids at particular times of life, such as during adolescence, before the first term pregnancy, or during the perimenopausal years might be of special importance. In this context it must be remembered that over the years women have tended to adopt the pill at younger and younger ages, and to use hormonal contraception to delay the first birth as well as to space or limit later births. Again, during the last few years there has been a sharp fall in the numbers of women over 35 years of age who use the pill. It is important not to extrapolate the results of epidemiological studies to groups of women to whom they do not relate.

High-risk groups

It is possible that oral contraceptives might have no relationship with a particular cancer in the generality of women, but nonetheless might have an effect on risk in those with predisposing factors: for example, in the case of breast cancer, in those with a history of benign disease or a positive family history. To draw a well-known analogy from another field, it seems that the pill has an important effect on the risk of acute myocardial infarction only in the presence of other risk factors such as cigarette smoking.

Breast cancer

The use of oral contraceptives seems to be associated with a protective effect against clinically detectable benign breast disease. This topic has been reviewed in detail by Vessey [1]. The protective effect increases with duration of use, is largely confined to current or very recent users, and is probably attributable to the progestogen component of the pill. Some studies have suggested that the protective effect may be restricted to the less serious forms of disease in which epithelial atypia are minimal or absent [2]. This observation provides a possible explanation for the apparent paradox that oral contraceptives protect against benign breast disease, but not (as we shall see) against breast cancer.

As oral contraceptives are used by more and more women, any major effect on the risk of breast cancer might be reflected in temporal trends in age-specific rates or mortality rates. No changes in trend have yet been reported in the United Kindom which might be attributed to the influence of the pill. Mortality data for England and Wales are given in Table 4.1. As can be seen, there has been a substantial increase in

Table 4.1 Breast cancer mortality, England and Wales 1955–1984

	Rate per 100 000 population				
Year	*15–24 years*	*25–44 years*	*45–64 years*	*65–74 years*	*75+ years*
1955	0.04	12	64	106	164
1960	0.20	12	66	105	161
1965	0.12	13	70	104	161
1970	0.23	14	78	109	158
1975	0.21	14	80	120	174
1980	0.05	13	83	122	183
1984	0.15	13	84	134	209

mortality during the last 30 years in women over the age of 44 years, but little change below that age.

Vital statistical data, however, have obvious limitations, and to make further progress we need to examine the results of analytical epidemiological studies which are of two main kinds: case-control studies and cohort studies.

Case-control studies

Some features of the ten largest case-control studies conducted to date are given in Table 4.2, while Table 4.3 summarizes the overall findings in these studies about breast cancer risk in relation to total duration of oral contraceptive use. Apart from the results reported by Meirik et al. [11], the data are clearly reassuring, and the same is true for analyses relating risk to interval since first oral contraceptive use (not shown). In fact there is now strong evidence from case-control studies that the use of oral contraceptives in the middle of the fertile years (say between the ages of 25 and 39) has no effect whatsoever on breast cancer risk. Such use, of course, dominates the exposure accumulated by the women included in the studies considered in Tables 4.2 and 4.3. Data are sparse (and not consistently negative) with regard to oral contraceptive use by women in their forties and beyond [13], but the main concern at present centres round the use of the preparations at a young age.

Anxiety about a possible harmful effect of prolonged oral contraceptive use *before first term pregnancy* followed publication of the data shown in Table 4.4 by Pike et al. in 1981 [14]. The study involved 163 women in Los Angeles County, USA, in whom breast cancer had been diagnosed at age 32 years or less. In 1983 Pike et al. published a further report from Los Angeles [15]. Their series of cases now included 314 women with breast cancer aged 36 years or less, and their primary analyses concerned oral contraceptive use *before age 25 years* rather than before a first term pregnancy. Their main findings are summarized in Table 4.5. Pike et al. [15] also related breast cancer risk in their study to the 'progestogen potency' of the oral contraceptives used as measured by the delay in menses test, claiming that the adverse effect was largely

Table 4.2 Some features of large-scale case-control studies of oral contraceptives and breast cancer

Authors	*Place*	*Age range (years)*	*Time cases diagnosed*	*No. of cases*	*No. of controls*
Paffenbarger *et al.* [3]	San Francisco, USA	All ages	1973–77	1432	2560
Brinton *et al.* [4]	Multicentre USA	All ages 35 up	1973–77	963	858
Vessey *et al.* [5]	London and Oxford, UK	16–50	1968–80	1176	1176
Rosenberg *et al.* [6]	Multicentre USA and Canada	20–59	1976–81	1191	5026
Hennekens *et al.* [7]	Eleven states in USA	30–55	1960–76	989	9890
La Vecchia *et al.* [8]	Milan, Italy	Up to 59	1982–85	776	1282
Cancer and Steroid Hormones Study [9]	Multicentre USA	20–54	1980–82	4711	4676
Paul *et al.* [10]	New Zealand (national study)	25–54	1983–85	433	897
Meirik *et al.* [11]	Sweden and Norway (national study)	Up to 45	1984–85	422	722
McPherson *et al.* [12]	London, Oxford, Edinburgh, UK	16–64	1980–84	1125	1125

Table 4.3 Breast cancer risk in case-control studies in relation to total duration of oral contraceptive use

<table>
<tr><th rowspan="2">Study</th><th rowspan="2">0</th><th colspan="20">Total duration of oral contraceptive use (years)</th></tr>
<tr><th>1</th><th>2</th><th>3</th><th>4</th><th>5</th><th>6</th><th>7</th><th>8</th><th>9</th><th>10</th><th>11</th><th>12</th><th>13</th><th>14</th><th>15</th><th>16</th><th>17</th><th>18</th><th>19</th><th>20</th></tr>
<tr><td>Paffenbarger et al. [3]</td><td>1.0</td><td>1.1</td><td>1.2</td><td colspan="2">1.4</td><td colspan="2">1.3</td><td colspan="14">1.4</td></tr>
<tr><td>Brinton et al. [4]</td><td>1.0</td><td colspan="4">0.9</td><td>1.2</td><td></td><td colspan="6">1.5</td><td colspan="8">1.0</td></tr>
<tr><td>Vessey et al. [5]</td><td>1.0</td><td>0.9</td><td colspan="3">1.0</td><td colspan="4">1.2</td><td colspan="12">1.0</td></tr>
<tr><td>Rosenberg et al. [6]</td><td>1.0</td><td>0.9</td><td colspan="3">1.0</td><td colspan="5">1.3</td><td colspan="11">0.8</td></tr>
<tr><td>Hennekens et al. [7]</td><td>1.0</td><td>1.1</td><td colspan="2">1.1</td><td colspan="2">0.7</td><td colspan="6">1.1</td><td colspan="9">0.7</td></tr>
<tr><td>La Vecchia et al. [8]</td><td>1.0</td><td colspan="2">1.0</td><td colspan="18">1.1</td></tr>
<tr><td>Cancer & Steroid Hormones Study [9]</td><td>1.0</td><td>0.9</td><td>0.9</td><td colspan="3">1.0</td><td colspan="4">1.0</td><td colspan="5">1.1</td><td colspan="6">0.6</td></tr>
<tr><td>Paul et al. [10]</td><td>1.0</td><td colspan="2">1.1</td><td colspan="3">0.8</td><td colspan="4">0.8</td><td colspan="11">1.0</td></tr>
<tr><td>Meirik et al. [11]</td><td>1.0</td><td colspan="3">1.1</td><td colspan="4">1.2</td><td colspan="4">1.4</td><td colspan="9">2.2</td></tr>
<tr><td>McPherson et al. [12]</td><td>1.0</td><td colspan="4">0.9</td><td colspan="9">1.1</td><td colspan="7">0.8</td></tr>
</table>

The figures given are relative risks taking non-users of oral contraceptives as the reference group. The listing of 20 years as the upper limit of use is arbitrary

Table 4.4 Risk of breast cancer in relation to use of oral contraceptives before first full term of pregnancy. (Modified from Pike *et al.* [14])

Duration of oral contraceptive use (months)	*Cases*		*Controls*		*Relative risk*
	No.	*%*	*No.*	*%*	
0	79	48.5	141	52.2	1.0
1–48	53	32.5	103	38.2	1.0
49–96	24	14.7	22	8.1	2.2
97+	7	4.3	4	1.5	3.5
Total	163	100.0	270	100.0	

Test for linear trend, $P = 0.009$

Table 4.5 Risk of breast cancer in relation to use of oral contraceptives before age 25. (Modified from Pike *et al.* [15]

Duration of oral contraceptive use (months)	*Cases*		*Controls*		*Relative risk*
	No.	*%*	*No.*	*%*	
0	65	20.7	93	29.6	1.0
1–24	106	33.8	118	37.7	1.3
25–48	79	25.2	67	21.3	1.7
49–72	40	12.7	29	9.2	2.0
73+	24	7.6	7	2.2	4.9
Total	314	100.0	314	100.0	

Test for linear trend, $P = 0.001$

attributable to pills with a 'potency score' of 5 or more. Subsequent publications (see, for example, Swyer [16]) have made it clear that the classification of progestogen potency used by the Los Angeles group is invalid, but this, of course, does nothing to alter the basic findings shown in Table 4.5.

A number of other groups have been able to collect sufficient data to address the questions raised by Pike and his colleagues. Table 4.6 summarizes the most important results concerning oral contraceptive use before first term pregnancy. It can be seen that the studies by Meirik et al. [11] and by McPherson et al. [12] support the results from Los Angeles while, in general, the other studies do not. Table 4.7 considers use of oral contraceptives before the age of 25 years. Only the study by Meirik et al. [11] shows a clear positive association between risk and duration of use.

Clearly the findings in different studies, at least with regard to use before first term pregnancy, are markedly heterogeneous. What are the possible explanations for this state of affairs? First, chance could be responsible, but this seems highly unlikely in view of the strength and statistical significance of the associations reported by Pike et al. [14], Meirik et al. [11], and McPherson et al. [12]. Secondly, it has been suggested that the negative studies are well designed, conducted, and analysed, and therefore correct and that the positive studies are less satisfactory in these respects and therefore wrong. Criticisms can, however, be levelled at all of these studies and this does not seem to be a very fruitful line of argument. Finally, there might be important differences between the studies with regard to oral contraceptive preparations used,

Table 4.6 Case-control studies of breast cancer risk and oral contraceptive use before first term pregnancy. (See also Table 4.4)

<table>
<tr><th rowspan="2">Study</th><th rowspan="2">No. of cases</th><th colspan="9">Duration of oral contraceptive use before first term pregnancy (years)</th></tr>
<tr><th>0</th><th>1</th><th>2</th><th>3</th><th>4</th><th>5</th><th>6</th><th>7</th><th>8 +</th></tr>
<tr><td>Vessey et al. [17]</td><td>1176</td><td>1.0</td><td>0.7</td><td colspan="3">0.8</td><td colspan="4">0.8</td></tr>
<tr><td>Cancer and Steroid Hormones Study [18]</td><td>1874</td><td>1.0</td><td>1.3</td><td colspan="3">1.1</td><td colspan="4">1.2</td></tr>
<tr><td>Paul et al. [10]</td><td>433</td><td>1.0</td><td>0.8</td><td colspan="2">0.8</td><td colspan="2">0·7</td><td colspan="3">0.6</td></tr>
<tr><td>Meirik et al. [11]</td><td>411
194*</td><td>1.0
1.0</td><td colspan="3">1.2
0.9</td><td colspan="4">1.0
1.5</td><td>2.0
4.4</td></tr>
<tr><td>Miller et al. [19]</td><td>521</td><td>1.0</td><td>0.7</td><td>1.4</td><td colspan="2">0.8</td><td colspan="2">1.5</td><td colspan="2">1.4</td></tr>
<tr><td>McPherson et al. [12]</td><td>351</td><td>1.0</td><td>1.0</td><td colspan="3">2.0</td><td colspan="4">2.6</td></tr>
</table>

* Swedish cases <40 years of age with controls matched for year of birth and age at first term pregnancy

Table 4.7 Case-control studies of breast cancer risk and oral contraceptive use before age 25 years. (See also Table 4.5

<table>
<tr><th rowspan="2">Study</th><th rowspan="2">No. of cases</th><th colspan="9">Duration of oral contraceptive use before age 25 years (years)</th></tr>
<tr><th>0</th><th>1</th><th>2</th><th>3</th><th>4</th><th>5</th><th>6</th><th>7</th><th>8+</th></tr>
<tr><td>Cancer and Steroid Hormones Study [18]</td><td>726</td><td>1.0</td><td colspan="2">1.2</td><td colspan="2">1.3</td><td colspan="2">1.1</td><td colspan="2">1.3</td></tr>
<tr><td>Paul et al. [10]</td><td>433</td><td>1.0</td><td>1.2</td><td colspan="2">1.0</td><td colspan="2">0.7</td><td colspan="3">0.6</td></tr>
<tr><td>Meirik et al. [11]</td><td>422</td><td>1.0</td><td colspan="3">1.1</td><td colspan="4">1.1</td><td>2.7</td></tr>
<tr><td>Miller et al. [14]</td><td>521</td><td>1.0</td><td>0.8</td><td>1.0</td><td colspan="2">1.3</td><td colspan="4">1.1</td></tr>
<tr><td>McPherson et al. [12]</td><td>351</td><td>1.0</td><td>0.8</td><td colspan="3">0.9</td><td colspan="4">1.3</td></tr>
</table>

precise patterns of use, the distribution of known (or unknown) risk factors for breast cancer and so on. It can only be said that the investigators involved in the major studies have conducted many supplementary analyses of their data and have met twice in the USA under the auspices of the National Institutes of Health to try to resolve the discrepancies between the studies along these lines, but without success.

One idea put forward by McPherson et al. [20] deserves special mention. These workers have suggested that the variation in the results might be accounted for by a latency effect, i.e. that after completion of a critical amount of exposure before the first term pregnancy (say 4 years or more), a latent period (perhaps 15 years or more) has to elapse before any adverse effect on the breast is apparent. An obvious implication of this hypothesis is that studies concerning women with *recent* early exposure, even if long-term, would yield negative results. The idea is clearly of importance, but it has to be admitted that little evidence has been unearthed from the different studies so far to support it. Accordingly, the question of the possible relationship between early oral contraceptive use and breast cancer remains unresolved at the time of writing.

Before leaving the case-control studies, it is worth mentioning that several authors have studied breast cancer risk in pill users in relation to the type of oral contraceptive formulation taken and in relation to the presence or absence of breast cancer risk factors such as a positive family history or previous benign disease. Space precludes a detailed review of the findings here and it must suffice to say that no consistent associations have emerged.

Cohort studies

Data on oral contraceptive use and breast cancer have been reported from five large cohort studies: (a) the Royal College of General Practitioners Study which includes 46 000 British women recruited by 1400 family doctors [21], (b) the Oxford/Family Planning Association Contraceptive Study which includes 17 000 British women recruited at 17 family planning centres [22], (c) the Walnut Creek Contraceptive Drug Study which includes 16 500 North American women who joined the study by having a general health check in an automated multitest laboratory [23], (d) a study conducted in Eastern Massachusetts which includes 96 000 women who were identified from residence lists and mailed a questionnaire [24], and (e) a study conducted in the USA involving 122 000 nurses aged 30 to 55 years [25]. The findings have, in general, been reassuring but, save for the American nurses study [25], the numbers of cases involved are rather small. In the Royal College of General Practitioners Study [21], however, there was some evidence that breast cancer risk might be increased in oral contraceptive users under 35 years of age (relative risk; ever users to never users 2.8 to 1, $P = 0.05$). There was no indication of any such effect in the other four studies. Trapido [24] found the relative risk associated with oral contraceptive use in nulliparous women to be 2.1, but statistically the figure was not significantly different from unity.

The Royal College of General Practitioners Study, the Oxford/Family Planning Association Contraceptive Study and the American nurses study, all of which are still continuing, will eventually yield a very large amount of information about the risk of breast cancer in oral contraceptive users. None of these studies, however, will be able to provide a significant quantity of data about early use of the pill. Accordingly, it is to case-control studies that we must look for a resolution of the problems discussed in the previous section.

Oral contraceptive use and prognosis of breast cancer

Spencer et al. [26] compared 44 newly diagnosed breast-cancer patients with recent oral contraceptive use with 44 other newly diagnosed breast-cancer patients who were non-users of the pill, and found prognosis to be better in the former group. Similar findings were later reported by the same workers in an investigation involving an additional 93 breast-cancer patients who had been taking the pill, and 93 'controls', studied in an identical way [27]. Vessey et al. [5] reported on the clinical stage of breast cancer at diagnosis in 572 breast-cancer patients included in their case-control study. As is shown in Table 4.8, women who had never used oral contraceptives presented with more advanced tumours than those who had used them during the year before detection of cancer, while past users were in an intermediate position. These

Table 4.8 Stage classification of 572 patients with breast cancer. (Modified from Vessey *et al.* [5])

	Use of oral contraceptives					
	Never used		*Used only in past**		*Used recently**	
Clinical stage	*No.*	%	*No.*	%	*No.*	%
I	196	55.4	83	64.4	66	74.2
II	74	20.9	23	17.8	11	12.4
III–IV	84	23.7	23	17.8	12	13.4
Total	354	100.0	129	100.0	89	100.0

*'Used recently' indicates use during year before detection of lump. 'Used only in past' indicates use only before that time

differences in staging were reflected in the pattern of survival. Possible explanations put forward by the authors for these observations included 'surveillance bias' among oral contraceptive users leading to earlier diagnosis or a beneficial effect of oral contraceptives on tumour growth and spread.

Two more recent papers from the United States have reported little difference between pill users and non-users with regard to breast cancer stage at presentation or prognosis, suggesting perhaps that the earlier results were attributable to surveillance bias [28, 29].

Ovarian cancer

The first data to suggest that oral contraceptives might protect against epithelial ovarian cancer appeared in a paper from the United Kingdom by Newhouse et al. [30]. Among 300 women with the disease (the great majority with epithelial tumours), only 19 (6.3%) had ever used the pill, while in each of two control groups of 300 women, 31 (10.3%) had done so. Since then at least eight additional case-control studies have been published and, as can be seen from Table 4.9, all have yielded results pointing in the same direction. As epithelial ovarian tumours tend to be more common in less fertile women, it was at first thought that the apparent protective effect of the pill might be attributable to confounding, but the more recent studies make it clear that this explanation is extremely unlikely.

Ovarian cancer is rare below the age of 40 years, while present teaching about oral contraceptive use recommends discontinuation of medication in the majority of women at about the age of 40 years because of the risk of cardiovascular adverse effects. For the protective effect of the pill against ovarian cancer to be of major practical value, it follows that it must persist in ex-users, and persist for many years. Table 4.10 summarizes the available findings on this point and also provides information about the effect of duration of contraceptive use. The results so far look encouraging, but clearly more extensive data are required.

The major cohort studies concerned with the long-term effects of oral contraceptive use still include too few cases of ovarian cancer for firm conclusions to be drawn. Such data as are available, however, are in support of the findings in the case-control studies [38].

Table 4.9 Case-control studies of oral contraceptive use and ovarian cancer

Authors	*Country*	*Ovarian cancer cases*		*Relative risk: ever use to never use of pill*
		Age range	*Number*	
Newhouse *et al.* [30]	UK	All ages	300	0.6
Casagrande *et al.* [31]	USA	25–49	150	0.7*
Weiss *et al.* [32]	USA	35–54	112	0.6
Willett *et al.* [33]	USA	30–55	47	0.8 (0.4–1.5)
Hildreth *et al.* [34]	USA	45–74	62	0.5 (0.2–1.5)
Rosenberg *et al.* [35]	USA	–59	136	0.6 (0.4–0.9)
Cramer *et al.* [36]	USA	–59	144	0.4 (0.2–1.0)
La Vecchia *et al.* [8]	Italy	–60	209	0.6 (0.3–1.0)
Cancer and Steroid Hormones Study [37]	USA	20–54	546	0.6 (0.5–0.7)

*Use for more than 6 months

Figures in brackets indicate 95% confidence limits (not always given by author)

Table 4.10 Case-control studies of oral contraceptive use and ovarian cancer. Data on duration of use and recency of use

Authors	*Increasing protection with duration of use?*	*Persistent protection after stopping use?*
Newhouse *et al.* [30]	Not stated	Not stated
Casagrande *et al.* [31]	Yes	Not stated
Weiss *et al.* [32]	Not after 3 years use	Not stated
Willett *et al.* [33]	No	Not stated
Hildreth *et al.* [34]	No data	No data
Rosenberg *et al.* [35]	Yes	For at least 10 years
Cramer *et al.* [36]	Not after 3 years use	For at least 10 years
La Vecchia *et al.* [8]	Yes	For at least 6 years
Cancer and Steroid Hormones Study [37]	Yes	For at least 15 years

Endometrial cancer

In view of the fact that unopposed oestrogen replacement therapy is a well-established cause of endometrial cancer, it is not surprising that the highly oestrogenic sequential oral contraceptives also have this effect [39, 40]. The earliest data to indicate that combined preparations might protect against this disease were reported by Weiss and Sayvetz in 1980 [40]. These workers, in a case-control study including 117 women aged 35–54 years with endometrial cancer and 395 healthy controls, found combined oral contraceptives to reduce the risk of cancer by 50%. As Table 4.11 shows, six other case-control studies published since then have produced equally encouraging results. As with ovarian cancer, it seems clear that the apparent protective effect is not merely a reflection of the fact that women at risk of endometrial cancer are less fertile than other women.

Endometrial cancer is rare below the age of 45 years, so the comments made previously about the public health importance of a persistent protective effect against ovarian cancer in ex-users of the pill apply even more strongly for this tumour. The data summarized in Table 4.12 offer a certain amount of encouragement in this respect.

Table 4.11 Case-control studies of combined oral contraceptive use and endometrial cancer

Authors	*Country*	*Endometrial cancer cases*		*Relative risk: ever use to never use combined pills*
		Age range	*Number*	
Weiss and Sayvetz [40]	USA	35–54	117	0.5 (0.1–1.0)
Kaufman *et al.* [41]	USA	–59	154	0.5 (0.3–0.8)
Kelsey *et al.* [42]	USA	45–74	167	0.6
Hulka *et al.* [43]	USA	–59	79	0.4
Henderson *et al.* [44]	USA	–45	127	0.5
La Vecchia *et al.* [8]	Italy	–60	170	0.6 (0.2–1.3)
Cancer and Steroid Hormones Study [45]	USA	20–54	433	0.6 (0.3–0.9)

Figures in brackets indicate 95% confidence limits (not always given by author)

Table 4.12 Case-control studies of combined oral contraceptive use and endometrial cancer. Data on duration of use and recency of use

Authors	*Increasing protection with duration of use?*	*Persistent protection after stopping use?*
Weiss and Sayvetz [40]	Not after 1 year's use	For a year or two
Kaufman *et al.* [41]	Yes	For at least 5 years
Kelsey *et al.* [42]	Yes	Not stated
Hulka *et al.* [43]	Yes	Effect wanes
Henderson *et al.* [44]	Yes	Not stated
La Vecchia *et al.* [8]	No data	No data
Cancer and Steroid Hormones Study [45]	Yes	For at least 15 years

Some authors have found that the protective effect against endometrial cancer is more prominent with the strongly progestogenic pills and that use of oestrogen replacement therapy can eliminate the benefit. Henderson et al. [44] found clear evidence of reduced risk only in women who had had less than three live births and who weighed less than 170 lb.

As with ovarian cancer, the preliminary results from the large cohort studies are generally encouraging. Recent data from the Oxford/Family Planning Association Contraceptive Study also indicate that prolonged use of combined pills offers considerable protection against fibromyomata of the uterus, tumours which have a similar epidemiology to endometrial cancer [46].

Choriocarcinoma

In a small study in the Philippines of women with choriocarcinoma, a higher proportion of cases than controls had previously used oral contraceptives [47]. In a larger study in England of 611 women who had had a hydatidiform mole, the need for subsequent chemotherapy was increased two- to threefold among women who took oral contraceptives [48]. Oral contraceptives also delayed the fall in human chorionic gonadotrophin excretion in women who did not need chemotherapy. This oral contraceptive related delay was not shown in a study of 194 patients from Vancouver [49]; it was nevertheless found that the proportion of women who ingested oral contraceptive preparations containing more than 50 μg oestrogen was higher among 17 patients with invasive complications in the post-molar phase than among women without invasive complications. The most recent study of 149 cases of molar pregnancy managed at the Women's Hospital in Los Angeles provides no evidence that the use of oral contraceptives prior to human chorionic gonadotrophin remission increases the risk of either invasive mole or choriocarcinoma [50].

Bagshawe's unit continues to recommend that neither oestrogen nor progestogen preparations (including under this heading depo-medroxyprogesterone acetate and hormone-replacement therapy) should be taken between the evacuation of a hydatidiform mole and the return to normality of gonadotrophin values [48]. This is a prudent policy, although it is not established that the modern low-dose OCs would pose a significant risk; and the data do not suggest that oral contraceptives increase the initial risk of trophoblastic disease itself.

Cancer of the cervix uteri

There is evidence that all three tissue components of the normal cervix (stroma, columnar epithelium, and squamous epithelium) respond to the influence of endogenous sex hormones, and oestrogen receptors have been described in a high proportion of squamous carcinomas [51]. Despite this, the epidemiology of cervical cancer gives little hint that endogenous hormones are of much aetiological importance.

Studies attempting to relate the risk of neoplasia of the cervix uteri to the use of oral contraceptives are beset by many difficulties [52]. First, it is extremely difficult to make adequate allowance for the effect of confounding variables, especially age at first sexual intercourse and number of sexual partners, which are powerful predictors of cervical neoplasia risk. Secondly, it is reasonably well established that occlusive methods of contraception offer some protection against cervical neoplasia. Thirdly, since almost all preinvasive lesions and many invasive ones are detected by cervical cytology, any substantial difference in the pattern of smear examinations between groups being compared may easily lead to incorrect conclusions. Fourthly, histopathologists vary greatly in their interpretation and classification of preinvasive lesions of the cervix, and this can lead to serious bias if any one pathologist receives a disproportionate amount of material from women using a particular contraceptive method.

Early case-control studies of cervical cancer (or cervical intraepithelial neoplasia – CIN) in relation to oral contraceptive use were mostly negative but, of necessity, they included few women with long-term exposure [53–55]. Studies published since 1980 are summarized in Table 4.13. It can be seen that the great majority have suggested a modest increase in risk, especially in women with long-term use of oral contraceptives. Cohort studies have also tended to give positive results. Thus in the Walnut Creek Study, a statistically significant association between the incidence of carcinoma-in-situ and duration of pill use was reported [63], although it was subsequently suggested that this result was, to some extent, attributable to confounding by differences in sexual activity, both between users and non-users of oral contraceptives and among women with different durations of oral contraceptive use [64]. More recent data have come from the Oxford/Family Planning Association Contraceptive Study [65, 66]. In this analysis, the incidence of biopsy-proven cervical neoplasia during a ten-year follow-up period was determined in 6838 parous women who entered the study while using oral contraceptives, and 3154 parous women who

Table 4.13 Case-control studies of cervical cancer and oral contraceptives published since 1980

Study	*Country*	*No. of cases*	*Control for no. sexual partners*	*Relative risk for longest duration of use group*
Harris *et al.* [56]	UK	190 (CIN)	Yes	10 + years, 2.1
World Health Organization [57]	Many	698 (Inv)	Yes	>5 years, 1.5
Hellberg *et al.* [58]	Sweden	140 (CIN)	Yes	>5 years, 1.0
Clarke *et al.* [59]	Canada	250 (CIN)	Yes	Ever, 1.7
Reeves *et al.* [60]	Panama	156 (mostly Inv)	Yes	Ever, 1.8
Brinton *et al.* [61]	USA	481 (Inv)	Yes	5 + years, 1.9
La Vecchia *et al.* [8]	Italy	225 (Inv)	Yes	>2 years, 2.9
		202 (CIN)	Yes	>2 years, 0.9
Ebeling *et al.* [62]	GDR	129 (Inv)	Yes	7 + years, 1.8

CIN, Cervical intraepithelial neoplasia; Inv, Invasive cancer

entered the study while using an intrauterine device. Risk factors for cervical neoplasia and frequency of examination by cervical cytology were similar in the two groups. All 13 cases of invasive cancer occurred in women in the oral contraceptive group; nine had more than six years use of the pill. CIN also occurred more frequently in the oral contraceptive group than in the intrauterine device group and there was a trend in incidence with duration of oral contraceptive use. The incidence of all forms of neoplasia combined rose from 0.9 per 1000 woman-years in those with up to two years pill use to 2.2 per 1000 woman-years in those with more than eight years pill use. Amongst the IUD users there was no such trend in incidence with duration of use; the rate fluctuated around 1.0 per 1000 woman-years.

Some interesting papers have been published concerning the rate of progression of CIN in users of different contraceptive methods. Stern et al. [67] working in Los Angeles, found rates of progression from dysplasia to carcinoma-in-situ to be much higher in women using Ovulen than in women using intrauterine devices. Bamford et al. [68] on the other hand examined the records concerning 105 women in whom cervical cytology exhibited progression from mild or moderate dyskaryosis to severe dyskaryosis together with the records concerning 152 control women, and could find no effect of contraceptive method on the speed of progression.

Dallenbach-Hellweg [69] has described a series of 21 adenocarcinomas of the endocervix, the majority of which occurred in women with prolonged oral contraceptive use. Some authors have also suggested that the rising incidence of adenocarcinoma of the cervix in young women in the United States is related to oral contraceptive use [70, 71].

Although the balance of evidence suggests quite strongly that prolonged oral contraceptive use slightly increases the risk of cervical cancer, in the author's view it is impossible to be sure that the effect is not due to incompletely controlled confounding by sexual factors. Nonetheless, it seems a wise precaution to suggest that, where possible, long-term oral contraceptive users should be screened at regular intervals by cervical cytology.

Other tumours

There is little doubt that *hepatocellular adenomas* occur much more frequently in oral contraceptive users than in other women, although their incidence among the former is still extremely low (at most, 1–2 per 100 000 users per annum). Evidence in support of this association has been derived from numerous case-reports and (more importantly) from two case-control studies [72, 73]. The risk seems to be greatest in older women using oral contraceptives of high biological activity over a long period of time [73].

It has long been suspected that long-term oral contraceptive use might, on very rare occasions, also lead to the occurrence of *hepatocellular carcinoma*. Three case-control studies, one conducted in Los Angeles and two in Britain, lend support to this idea [74–76]. It may be noted that the association seems strongest in women developing hepatocellular carcinoma in a non-cirrhotic liver in the absence of evidence of hepatitis B infection, so the results obtained may well not be applicable in developing countries. Neuberger et al. [75] have estimated that the maximum number of cases of hepatocellular carcinoma attributable to long-term oral contraceptive use in England and Wales is 12 per year.

The possibility that oral contraceptive use might increase the risk of *malignant melanoma* of the skin was first raised by Beral et al. in 1977 on the basis of data collected in the Walnut Creek area in California [77]. Subsequent studies have given conflicting results [78–80]. However, no investigation has yet been reported which includes a sufficiently large number of cases with long-term oral contraceptive use for any firm conclusions to be drawn.

For many years it has been widely held that oral contraceptive use increases the risk of certain *benign tumours of the pituitary gland*, particularly prolactinoma. Two recently reported case-control studies have provided strong evidence against this association [81, 82]. Shy et al. [81] have suggested that previous reports of an association between pill use and prolactinoma may have resulted from oral contraceptive treatment of menstrual irregularity in women with an undiagnosed tumour.

Comment

As anticipated, oral contraceptives are proving to have effects on a wide variety of tumours. The risks of benign breast lumps, endometrial cancer, uterine fibroids and epithelial cancer of the ovary are almost certainly reduced by the use of combined preparations. Protection against cancer of the ovary in particular is of great potential importance, since this terrible disease commonly presents at an advanced stage and the results of treatment are depressing. On the other hand, the evidence that early use of oral contraceptives may increase breast cancer risk and that prolonged use generally may increase cervical cancer risk, while certainly not conclusive, is nonetheless disturbing. In comparison, the risk of occasionally inducing hepatocellular adenoma and extremely rarely, hepatocellular carcinoma, is of much lesser consequence.

Further research into the effects of oral contraceptive use on cancer is obviously of great importance. It should focus on defining the risks and benefits according to patterns of use and types of preparation. Clearly the long-term aim must be to develop a pill or pills which will retain the known benefits of existing preparations, but not be associated with serious hazards. A major handicap at present for epidemiologists working in this field is the absence of useful information from the laboratory and from clinical research about the ways in which different oral contraceptives might be grouped together when attempting to assess their effects on certain end organs, particularly the breast. In this respect, the painstaking histological approach to the study of cell turnover in the human breast, developed by Anderson and his colleagues in Edinburgh, seems promising [83].

References

1. VESSEY, M. P. Contraception and benign breast disease – epidemiological studies. In *Contraception et Sein* (eds. R. Renaud and B. Gairard), Masson, Paris p. 63 (1983)
2. LI VOLSI, V. A., STADEL, B. V., KELSEY, J. L. *et al.* Fibrocystic disease in oral contraceptive users. A histopathological evaluation of epithelial atypia. *New England Journal of Medicine*, **299,** 381 (1978)
3. PAFFENBARGER, R. S., KAMPERT, J. B. and CHANG, H.-G. Oral contraceptives and breast cancer risk. *Les Editions de l'INSERM*, **83,** 93 (1979)
4. BRINTON, L. A., HOOVER, R., SZKLO, M. and FRAUMENI, J. F. Oral contraceptives and breast cancer. *International Journal of Epidemiology*, **11,** 316 (1982)
5. VESSEY, M., BARON, J., DOLL, R. *et al.* Oral contraceptives and breast cancer: final report of an epidemiological study. *British Journal of Cancer*, **47,** 455 (1983)
6. ROSENBERG, L., MILLER, D. R., KAUFMAN, D. W. *et al.* Breast cancer and oral contraceptive use. *American Journal of Epidemiology*, **119,** 167 (1984)
7. HENNEKENS, C. H., SPEIZER, F. E., LIPNICK, R. J. *et al.* A case-control study of oral contraceptive use and breast cancer. *Journal of the National Cancer Institute*, **72,** 39 (1984)
8. LA VECCHIA, C., DECARLI, A., FASOLI, M. *et al.* Oral contraceptives and cancers of the breast and of the female genital tract. Interim results from a case-control study. *British Journal of Cancer*, **54,** 311 (1986)
9. CANCER AND STEROID HORMONES STUDY. Oral contraceptive use and the risk of breast cancer. *New England Journal of Medicine*, **315,** 405 (1986)
10. PAUL, C. SKEGG, D. C. G., SPEARS, G. F. S. and KALDON, J. M. Oral contraceptives and breast cancer: a national study. *British Medical Journal*, **293,** 723 (1986)
11. MEIRIK, O., LUND E., ADAMI, H.-O. *et al.* Oral contraceptive use and breast cancer in young women. A joint national case-control study in Sweden and Norway. *Lancet*, **2,** 650 (1986)
12. MCPHERSON, K., VESSEY, M., NEIL, A. *et al.* Early oral contraceptive use and breast cancer: results of another case-control study. *British Journal of Cancer*, **56,** 653 (1987)
13. JICK, H., WALKER, A. M., WATKINS, R. N. *et al.* Oral contraceptives and breast cancer. *American Journal of Epidemiology*, **112,** 577 (1980)
14. PIKE, M. C., HENDERSON, B. E., CASAGRANDE, J. T. *et al.* Oral contraceptive use and early abortion as risk factors for breast cancer in young women. *British Journal of Cancer*, **43,** 72 (1981)
15. PIKE, M. C., HENDERSON, B. E., KRAILO, M. D. *et al.* Breast cancer in young women and use of oral contraceptives: possible modifying effect of formulation and age at use. *Lancet*, **2,** 926 (1983)
16. SWYER, G. I. M. Oral contraceptives and cancer. *Lancet*, **2,** 1019 (1983)
17. VESSEY, M. P., MCPHERSON, K., YEATES, D. and DOLL, R. Oral contraceptive use and abortion before first term pregnancy in relation to breast cancer risk. *British Journal of Cancer*, **45,** 327 (1982)
18. STADEL, B. V., RUBIN, G. L., WEBSTER, L. A. *et al.* Oral contraceptives and breast cancer in young women. *Lancet*, **2,** 970 (1985)
19. MILLER, D. R., ROSENBERG, L., KAUFMAN, D. W. *et al.* Breast cancer in relation to early oral contraceptive use. *Obstetrics and Gynecology*, **68,** 863 (1986)
20. MCPHERSON, K., COOPE, P. A. and VESSEY, M. P. Early oral contraceptive use and breast cancer: theoretical effects of latency. *Journal of Epidemiology and Community Health*, **40,** 289 (1986)
21. ROYAL COLLEGE OF GENERAL PRACTITIONERS. Breast cancer and oral contraceptives: findings in Royal College of General Practitioners Study. *British Medical Journal*, **282,** 2089 (1981)
22. VESSEY, M. P., MCPHERSON, K. and DOLL, R. Breast cancer and oral contraceptives: findings in the Oxford/Family Planning Association Contraceptive Study. *British Medical Journal*, **282,** 2093 (1981)
23. RAMCHARAN, S., PELLEGRIN, F. A., RAY R. and HSU, J. P. *The Walnut Creek contraceptive drug study: a prospective study of the side effects of oral contraceptives*, Vol. III. U.S. Government Printing Office, Washington DC (1981)
24. TRAPIDO, E. J. A prospective cohort study of oral contraceptives and breast cancer. *Journal of the National Cancer Institute*, **67,** 1011 (1981)

25. LIPNICK, R. J., BURING, J. E., HENNEKENS, C. H. *et al.* Oral contraceptives and breast cancer: a prospective cohort study, *Journal of the American Medical Association*, **255,** 58 (1986)
26. SPENCER, J. D., MILLIS, R. R. and HAYWARD, J. L. Contraceptive steroids and breast cancer. *British Medical Journal*, **1,** 1024 (1978)
27. MATHEWS, P. N., MILLIS, R. R. and HAYWARD, J. L. Breast cancer in women who have taken contraceptive steroids. *British Medical Journal*, **282,** 774 (1981)
28. ROSNER, D., LANE, W. W. and BRETT, R. P. Influence of oral contraceptives on prognosis of breast cancer in young women. *Cancer*, **55,** 1556 (1985)
29. ROSNER, D. and LANE, W. W. Oral contraceptive use has no adverse effect on the prognosis of breast cancer. *Cancer*, **57,** 591 (1986)
30. NEWHOUSE, M. L., PEARSON, R. M., FULLERTON, J. M. *et al.* A case control study of carcinoma of the ovary. *British Journal of Preventive and Social Medicine*, **31,** 148 (1977)
31. CASAGRANDE, J. T., LOUIE, E. W., PIKE, M. C. *et al.* "Incessant ovulation" and ovarian cancer. *Lancet*, **2,** 170 (1979)
32. WEISS, N. S., LYON, J. L., LIFF, J. M. *et al.* Incidence of ovarian cancer in relation to the use of oral contraceptives. *International Journal of Cancer*, **28,** 669 (1981)
33. WILLETT, W. C., BAIN, C., HENNEKENS, C. H. *et al.* Oral contraceptives and risk of ovarian cancer. *Cancer*, **48,** 1684 (1981)
34. HILDRETH, N. G., KELSEY, J. L., LI VOLSI, V. A. *et al.* An epidemiological study of epithelial carcinoma of the ovary. *American Journal of Epidemiology*, **114,** 398 (1981)
35. ROSENBERG, L., SHAPIRO, S., SLONE, D. *et al.* Epithelial ovarian cancer and combination oral contraceptives. *Journal of the American Medical Association*, **247,** 3210 (1982)
36. CRAMER, D. W., HUTCHINSON, G. B., WELCH, W. R. *et al.* Factors affecting the association of oral contraceptives and ovarian cancer. *New England Journal of Medicine*, **307,** 1047 (1982)
37. CANCER AND STEROID HORMONES STUDY. The reduction in risk of ovarian cancer associated with oral contraceptive use. *New England Journal of Medicine*, **316,** 650 (1987)
38. VESSEY, M., METCALFE, A., WELLS, C. *et al.* Ovarian neoplasms, functional ovarian cysts and oral contraceptives. *British Medical Journal*, **294,** 1518 (1987)
39. SILVERBERG, S. G. and MAKOWSKI, E. L. Endometrial carcinoma in young women taking oral contraceptive agents. *Obstetrics and Gynecology*, **46,** 503 (1975)
40. WEISS, N. S. and SAYVETZ, T. A. Incidence of endometrial cancer in relation to the use of oral contraceptives. *New England Journal of Medicine*, **302,** 551 (1980)
41. KAUFMAN, D. W., SHAPIRO, S., SLONE, D. *et al.* Decreased risk of endometrial cancer among oral contraceptive users. *New England Journal of Medicine*, **303,** 1045 (1980)
42. KELSEY, J. L., LI VOLSI, V. A., HOLFORD, T. R. *et al.* A case-control study of cancer of the endometrium. *American Journal of Epidemiology*, **116,** 333 (1982)
43. HULKA, B. S., CHAMBLESS, L. E., KAUFMAN, D. G. *et al.* Protection against endometrial carcinoma by combination-product oral contraceptives. *Journal of the American Medical Association*, **247,** 475 (1982)
44. HENDERSON, B. E., CASAGRANDE, J. T., PIKE, M. C. *et al.* The epidemiology of endometrial cancer in young women. *British Journal of Cancer*, **47** 749 (1983)
45. CANCER AND STEROID HORMONES STUDY. Combination oral contraceptive use and the risk of endometrial cancer. *Journal of the American Medical Association*, **257,** 796 (1987)
46. ROSS, R. K., PIKE, M. C., VESSEY, M. P. *et al.* Risk factors for uterine fibroids: reduced risk associated with oral contraceptives. *British Medical Journal*, **293,** 359 (1986)
47. BALTAZAR, J. C. Epidemiological features of choriocarcinoma. *Bulletin of the World Health Organisation*, **54,** 523 (1976)
48. STONE, M., DENT, J., KARDANA, A. and BAGSHAWE, K. D. Relationship of oral contraception to development of trophoblastic tumour after evacuation of a hydatidiform mole. *British Journal of Obstetrics and Gynaecology*, **83,** 913 (1976)
49. YUEN, B. H. and BIRCH, P. Relationship of oral contraceptives and the intrauterine contraceptive devices to the regression of concentrations of the beta sub-unit of human chorionic gonadotrophin and invasive complications after molar pregnancy. *American Journal of Obstetrics and Gynecology*, **145,** 214 (1983)
50. MORROW, P., NAKAMURA, R., SCHLAERTH, J. *et al.* The influence of oral contraceptives on the post molar

human chorionic gonadotrophin regression curve. *American Journal of Obstetrics and Gynecology*, **151**, 906 (1985)

51. SOUTTER, W. P., PEGORARO, R. J., GREEN THOMPSON, R. W. *et al.* Nuclear and cytoplasmic oestrogen receptors in squamous carcinoma of the cervix. *British Journal of Cancer*, **44**, 154 (1981)
52. SWAN, S. H. and PETTITI, D. B. A review of problems of bias and confounding in epidemiologic studies of cervical neoplasia and oral contraceptive use. *American Journal of Epidemiology*, **115**, 10 (1982)
53. WORTH, A. J. and BOYES, D. A. A case-control study into the possible effects of birth control pills on pre-clinical carcinoma of the cervix. *Journal of Obstetrics and Gynaecology of the British Commonwealth*, **79**, 673 (1972)
54. THOMAS, D. B. Relationship of oral contraceptives to cervical carcinogenesis. *Obstetrics and Gynecology*, **40**, 508 (1972)
55. BOYCE, J. G., LU, T., NELSON, J. H. and FRUCHTER, R. G. Oral contraceptives and cervical carcinoma. *American Journal of Obstetrics and Gynecology*, **128**, 761 (1977)
56. HARRIS, R. W. C., BRINTON, L. A., COWDELL, R. H. *et al.* Characteristics of women with dysplasia or carcinoma-in-situ of the cervix uteri. *British Journal of Cancer*, **42**, 359 (1980)
57. WORLD HEALTH ORGANIZATION COLLABORATIVE STUDY OF NEOPLASIA AND STEROID CONTRACEPTIVES. Invasive cervical cancer and combined oral contraceptives. *British Medical Journal*, **290**, 961 (1985)
58. HELLBERG, D., VALENTIN, J. and NILSSON, S. Long term use of oral contraceptives and cervical neoplasia: an association confounded by other risk factors? *Contraception*, **32**, 337 (1985)
59. CLARKE, A. E., HATCHER, J., MCKEOWN-EYSSEN, G. E. and LICKRISH, G. M. Cervical dysplasia: association with sexual behavior, smoking and oral contraceptive use? *American Journal of Obstetrics and Gynecology*, **151**, 612 (1985)
60. REEVES, W. C., BRINTON, L. A., BRENES, M. M. *et al.* Case-control study of cervical cancer in Herrera Province, Republic of Panama. *International Journal of Cancer*, **36**, 55 (1985)
61. BRINTON, L. A., HUGGINS, G. R., LEHMAN, H. F. *et al.* Long term use of oral contraceptives and risk of invasive cervical cancer. *International Journal of Cancer*, **38**, 339 (1986)
62. EBELING, K., NISCHAN, P. and SCHINDLER, C. Use of oral contraceptives and risk of invasive cervical cancer in previously screened women. *International Journal of Cancer*, **39**, 427 (1987)
63. PERITZ, E., RAMCHARAN, S., FRANK, J. *et al.* The incidence of cervical cancer and duration of oral contraceptive use. *American Journal of Epidemiology*, **106**, 462 (1977)
64. SWAN, S. H. and BROWN, W. L. Oral contraceptive use, sexual activity and cervical carcinoma. *American Journal of Obstetrics and Gynecology*, **139**, 52 (1981)
65. VESSEY, M. P., LAWLESS, M., MCPHERSON, K., and YEATES, D. Neoplasia of the cervix uteri and contraception: a possible adverse effect of the pill. *Lancet*, **2**, 930 (1983)
66. VESSEY, M. P., LAWLESS, M., MCPHERSON, K. and YEATES, D. Oral contraception and cervical cancer. *Lancet*, **2**, 1358 (1983)
67. STERN, E., FORSYTHE, A. B., YOUKELES, L. and COFFELT, C. F. Steroid contraceptive use and cervical dysplasia: increased risk of progression. *Science*, **196**, 1460 (1977)
68. BAMFORD, P. N., FORBES-SMITH, P. A., ROSE, G. L. *et al.* An analysis of factors responsible for progression or regression of mild and moderate cervical dyskaryosis. *British Journal of Family Planning*, **11**, 5 (1985)
69. DALLENBACH-HELLWEG, C. Incidence and histologic structure of adenocarcinoma of the cervical mucosa after prolonged use of ovulation inhibitors. *Geburtshilfe und Frauenheilkunde*, **42**, 249 (1982)
70. PETERS, R. K., CHAO, A., MACK, T. M. *et al.* Increased frequency of adenocarcinoma of the uterine cervix in young women in Los Angeles County. *Journal of the National Cancer Institute*, **76**, 423 (1986)
71. SCHWARTZ, S. M. and WEISS, N. S. Increased incidence of adenocarcinoma of the cervix in young women in the United States. *American Journal of Epidemiology*, **124**, 1045 (1986)
72. EDMONDSON, H. A., HENDERSON, B. and BENTON, B. Liver cell adenomas associated with use of oral contraceptives. *New England Journal of Medicine*, **294**, 470 (1976)
73. ROOKS, J. B., ORY, H. W., ISHAK, K. G. *et al.* Epidemiology of hepatocellular adenoma. The role of oral contraceptive use. *Journal of the American Medical Association*, **242**, 644 (1979)
74. HENDERSON, B. E., PRESTON-MARTIN, S., EDMONDSON, H. A. *et al.* Hepatocellular carcinoma and oral contraceptives. *British Journal of Cancer*, **48**, 437 (1983)
75. NEUBERGER, J., FORMAN, D., DOLL, R. and WILLIAMS, R. Oral contraceptives and hepatocellular carcinoma. *British Medical Journal*, **292**, 1355 (1986)

76. FORMAN, D., VINCENT, T. J. and DOLL, R. Cancer of the liver and the use of oral contraceptives. *British Medical Journal*, **292,** 1357 (1986)
77. BERAL, V., RAMCHARAN, S. and FARIS, R. Malignant melanoma and oral contraceptive use among women in California. *British Journal of Cancer*, **36,** 804 (1977)
78. ADAM, S. A., SHEAVES, J. K., WRIGHT, N. H. *et al.* A case-control study of the possible association between oral contraceptives and malignant melanoma. *British Journal of Cancer*, **44,** 45 (1981)
79. BAIN, C., HENNEKENS, C. H., SPEIZER, F. E. *et al.* Oral contraceptive use and malignant melanoma. *Journal of the National Cancer Institute*, **68,** 537 (1982)
80. HOLLY, E. A., WEISS, N. S. and LIFF, J. M. Cutaneous melanoma in relation to exogenous hormones and reproductive factors. *Journal of the National Cancer Institute*, **70,** 827 (1983)
81. SHY, K. K., MCTIERNAN, A. M., DALING, J. R. and WEISS, N. S. Oral contraceptive use and the occurrence of pituitary prolactinoma. *Journal of the American Medical Association*, **249,** 2204 (1983)
82. PITUITARY ADENOMA STUDY GROUP. Pituitary adenomas and oral contraceptives: a multicenter case-control study. *Fertility and Sterility*, **39,** 753 (1983)
83. ANDERSON, T. J., FERGUSON, D. J. P. and RAAB, G. M. Cell turnover in the "resting" human breast: influence of parity, contraceptive pill, age and laterality. *British Journal of Cancer*, **46,** 376 (1982)

Chapter 5

Practical prescribing of the combined oral contraceptive pill

J. Guillebaud

The purpose of this chapter is to provide practical guidelines to clinicians who wish to utilize the 'science' of this contraceptive method, as described in the preceding three chapters, in their 'practice': thus minimizing the systemic risks while maximizing the benefits. Much of the metabolic and epidemiological data available are contradictory or mainly of academic interest, with as yet little practical application. There remains room for some disagreement and considerable need for personal judgement regarding the relative weight to be placed on different data. Hence the frequent use in this practical chapter of the personal pronoun. The views expressed are my own though backed with references when available.

In selecting a combined oral contraceptive (COC) for an individual woman, few would disagree with the recommendations of the British National Association of Family Planning Doctors (NAFPD) which are as follows:

'The pill of choice should be the one containing the lowest suitable dose of oestrogen and progestogen which:

1. provides effective contraception,
2. produces acceptable cycle control (a concept expanded below),
3. is associated with fewest side-effects and
4. has the least known effect on carbohydrate and lipid metabolism and haemostatic parameters' [1].

Furthermore, few would disagree with the extension of number 4 by Victor Wynn (Personal communication) to read: 'If we can measure any substance in a pill-user, we would like it to be normal, or as near normal as possible.'

To achieve these desiderata requires careful consideration of absolute and relative contraindications, to select what I have elsewhere called the 'safer women'. [2] The aim then is to prescribe 'safer pills'. But since there is no certainty which are the safest among the currently available products, one should take into consideration the fact of biological variation in the pharmacokinetics for each woman. A possible way this can be done is discussed below (using bleeding from the uterus as a 'threshold bioassay'). Practical prescribing also requires decisions about the 'best second choice' of COC, based either on bleeding side-effects or on the others, most of which are pregnancy-mimicking. Thereafter, monitoring requires alertness for the development of new risk factors, regular blood pressure checks and, as will be stressed below, specific attention to the important side-effect of headache.

Selection of users

Women (and their partners) must be allowed to retain the right to choose either this method or an alternative. The absolute and relative contraindications are listed in Tables 5.1–5.3 but will not be discussed further here, since they follow so logically from data discussed in other chapters as well as in my books [2, 3]. Note that the pill might be *absolutely* contraindicated by the possession of more than one *relative* contraindication, e.g. a diabetic who smokes cigarettes or with hypertension or any diabetic tissue damage; or a cigarette smoker above the age of 35. Young otherwise healthy diabetics may use the combined pill, with careful monitoring: even then short-term use is advised, and the progestogen-only pill (POP) is usually preferable [4].

There is another important message, far from sufficiently accepted by either women or doctors, from all the post-1980 pill research. This is that women free of other risk factors may routinely continue to use the COC until the mid-forties—or even longer in selected cases, especially for therapeutic indications such as gynaecological disorders including menorrhagia and endometriosis . It is proving enormously difficult to dispel the myth that the upper age limit of 35 applies to all women. This limit certainly

Table 5.1 Absolute contraindications to combined oral contraception

A. Past or present circulatory disease

1. Arterial or venous thrombosis*
2. Ischaemic heart disease or angina
3. Hyperlipidaemia
4. *Severe* or *combined* risk factors for arterial disease. See Table 5.2.
5. Known prothrombotic abnormality of coagulation/fibrinolysis, including post-splenectomy if the platelet count is above 500×10^9/l (Dr Sam Machin, 1987, personal communication)
6. Other conditions predisposing to thrombosis, including elective major or leg surgery; during recumbent immobilization or varicose-vein treatments; and residence above 4000 metres which is associated with raised blood viscosity due to haemoconcentration in the short term and polycythaemia later (Dr Michael Ward, alpinist, 1986, personal communication to NAFPD)
7. Focal migraine, migraine requiring ergotamine treatment
8. Transient ischaemic attacks even without headache
9. Past cerebral haemorrhage, which can be secondary to cerebral venous thrombosis, also to avoid hypertension
10. Most types of valvular heart disease (discuss with cardiologist); pulmonary hypertension

B. Disease of the liver

1. Active liver disease, recurrent cholestatic jaundice or a history of cholestatic jaundice in pregnancy. Dubin–Johnson and Rotor syndromes. (NB after infectious hepatitis, COC may be used 3 months after liver function tests have returned to normal)
2. Liver adenoma
3. Gallstones (but COC may be used after cholecystectomy)
4. The porphyrias

C. History of serious condition affected by sex steroids or related to previous COC use, e.g.
herpes gestationis
haemolytic uraemic syndrome
trophoblastic disease (until βHCG levels are undetectable)

D. Pregnancy

E. Undiagnosed genital-tract bleeding

F. Oestrogen-dependent neoplasms
e.g. breast cancer (but discuss with oncologist)

G. Woman's anxiety unrelieved by counselling

Several of the above are not necessarily permanent contraindications
*Includes past definite thrombosis in varicose vein(s)

Table 5.2 Risk factors for cardiovascular system (CVS) disease

Risk factor	*Absolute contraindication*	*Relative contraindication*	*Remarks*
Family history (FH) of CVS disease (arterial or venous) in a first-degree relative $\leqslant 45$	Known atherogenic lipid profile or prothrombotic haemostatic profile, or tests not available	Normal blood profiles or first attack in relative >45	NB If FH of *arterial* disease, must test *both* for lipids & haemostasis Blood group also relevant (see text)
Diabetes mellitus (DM)	Severe, or diabetic complications present (e.g. retinopathy, renal damage)	Not severe/labile, & no complications, young patient with short duration of DM	POP usually a better hormonal method
Hypertension	Diastolic BP $\geqslant 95$ mmHg on repeated testing	Diastolic BP 85–95 mmHg see text	POP better choice
Cigarette smoking	$\geqslant 40$ cigarettes per day	5–40 cigarettes per day	
Increasing age	See Table 5.10	35–45 non-smokers	Smokers should avoid or discontinue COCs *10 years earlier*
Excess weight	$>50\%$ above ideal for height	20–50% above ideal	

Some of the numbers selected are necessarily a little arbitrary and relate to use solely for contraception. COCs for medical indications entail a different risk-benefit analysis (see text)

Table 5.3 Relative contraindications to COC use

1. First see Table 5.2, i.e. risk factors for arterial disease are relative contraindications, provided normally that only one is present, and not to so marked a degree that it would become an absolute contraindication. For interaction between age, smoking and duration of COC use see Table 5.10
2. Migraine, of any kind other than as Table 5.1
3. Homozygous sickle-cell disease (see text)
4. Long-term partial immobilization (e.g. in a wheelchair)
5. Sex-steroid-dependent cancer. Seek the specialist's advice: most will permit COC use after treatment for melanoma. A history of breast cancer is almost invariably considered an absolute contraindication. Past breast biopsy showing the premalignant epithelial atypia is considered by some a relative, and by others an absolute, contraindication
6. Oligo-/amenorrhoea should be investigated but the pill may subsequently be prescribed [6]
7. Hyperprolactinaemia: this is now considered only a relative contraindication for patients under specialist supervision
8. Very severe depression, if likely to be exacerbated by COCs. But unwanted pregnancies can be very depressing!
9. Chronic systemic diseases. Crohn's disease is now considered a relative contraindication, as are diabetes and chronic renal disease. In both the latter HDL-cholesterol is lowered. For other conditions with no apparent COC association, see text
10. Diseases requiring long-term treatment with drugs which might interact with the pill (see text for special management)
11. Conditions which impair absorption of COCs, such as some operations for obesity. Moreover, HDL-C is reduced in chronic malabsorption states, with a well-recognized increased risk of arterial thrombosis
12. New relative contraindications now under consideration include:
    (a) if a first-degree relative has had breast cancer;
    (b) during the monitoring of mildly abnormal cervical smears;
    (c) following definitive treatment for cervical intraepithelial neoplasia, CIN.
    After counselling the decision may well be taken to prescribe the COC, but women in categories (b) and (c) will need special monitoring, at least by annual smears

applies to smokers. But even using the data of the RCGP study which relates to 50 μg or stronger COCs, there should be no more anxiety about a non-smoker of 44 years using the method than about a smoker of 34 [5]. NB See the US FDA committee statement on page 236, which extends the upper age limit for non-smokers, free of all other risk factors.

Note also that secondary amenorrhoea which has resolved is no contraindication, and if it is current the COC may, after full investigation, even be recommended. Reasons for this include the need for oestrogenic protection of the bones, or to suppress the symptoms of polycystic ovarian disease in a woman not yet wanting to conceive [6].

Blood group O is associated with a reduced risk of both venous thromboembolism and myocardial infarction [6a]. Hence a woman with this blood group might sometimes be allowed to continue using the COC despite other less favourable factors. Blood grouping is also useful in all cases with a relevant family history (Table 5.2)

Medical conditions in which the COC may be used

According to current information, the following diseases come into the category of medical conditions in which the COC may be used with caution, since there is no evidence that deterioration may be caused (the order is alphabetical): asthma, Gilbert's disease, Hodgkin's disease, multiple sclerosis, myasthenia gravis, pre-existing Raynaud's disease, renal dialysis, rheumatoid arthritis, sarcoidosis, spherocytosis and thalassaemia major. In most cases the prescriber should, nevertheless, consult with the hospital specialist(s) supervising treatment for the main disorder, to obtain their support and to guard against unforeseen drug interactions. Reliable protection from pregnancy is often particularly important when other diseases are present [7].

If the COC is used in the disorders listed in Table 5.3 (*Relative contraindications*), this, unlike the above, does entail some known risk due to the method. But the added risk obtaining in pregnancy may justify this, primarily because the COC is so very effective. This thinking does not apply however to the *absolute contraindications*.

Sickle-cell disorders

Sickle-cell trait has no bearing on the COC. The situation regarding the homozygous conditions (SS and SC genes) is more uncertain. Both sickle-cell disease and the COC individually lead to an increased risk of thrombosis, possibly superimposed during the arterial stasis of a crisis [8]. Hence many authorities and most of the pill manufacturers have for many years included the frank sickling diseases among the absolute contraindications to the COC. However, Serjeant [9], reviewing studies in West Africa and the West Indies suggests that sickle-cell disease should only be considered a relative contraindication, especially when balanced against the particularly serious risks of pregnancy. Pending further information, injectables or the POP may be even better choices [8].

For a more complete discussion of contraception and disease, the reader is referred to the excellent chapter with that title and Table 35 in the book by Sapire [10].

The pill of first choice

There is effectively only one oestrogen, ethinyloestradiol (EE) (see Chapter 2). Until more controlled epidemiological data are available, it remains impossible to decide the '*best buy*' among the available progestogens. Hence for practical purposes, the first pill brand tried can be according to the prescriber's choice, so long as the dose of oestrogen is normally ≤35 μg combined with the lowest acceptable dose of whichever progestogen is chosen. This policy excludes brands with more than 150 μg levonorgestrel or 1.5 mg of norethisterone (or its pro-drugs) for routine contraception, since they adversely affect plasma lipids (see Chapter 2; also page 90 for the choice of pill in older women or when a risk factor is present).

But what is the lowest acceptable dose?

Individual variation – the uterus as a threshold bioassay for blood levels

Until recently an important point with regard to acceptability has been overlooked, namely biological variation. There is an up to tenfold interindividual variation in the achieved blood levels of both oestrogen and progestogen (see page 16, and Figure 5.1, which is a schema based on a large body of work on the levels of both hormones). It is a false expectation that any single pill will be found to suit all women.

On the one hand (Figure 5.1) it follows that some women will have suboptimal blood levels. It is likely that they are at increased risk of breakthrough pregnancy, especially if they omit pills. (But the fact that they also tend to manifest the problem by breakthrough bleeding (BTB) and absence of withdrawal bleeding (WTB) [11] can be utilized, see below.)

On the other hand it is a very tenable hypothesis that those with exceptionally high blood levels of the exogenous hormones may be at higher risk of both annoying and dangerous side-effects (Figure 5.1). One confirmatory study is that of Ahluwalia et al. [12], discussed in Chapter 2. A major project is in progress at the Margaret Pyke Centre to confirm their finding of higher blood artificial steroid levels in pill-takers with hypertension, and to test the hypothesis for a range of metabolic variables and subjective symptoms.

Absence of BTB, therefore, may not be innocuous; it could mean a woman is receiving a stronger COC than she requires for the desired (contraceptive) effect.

How then can we avoid giving the woman who tends to the highest levels a stronger

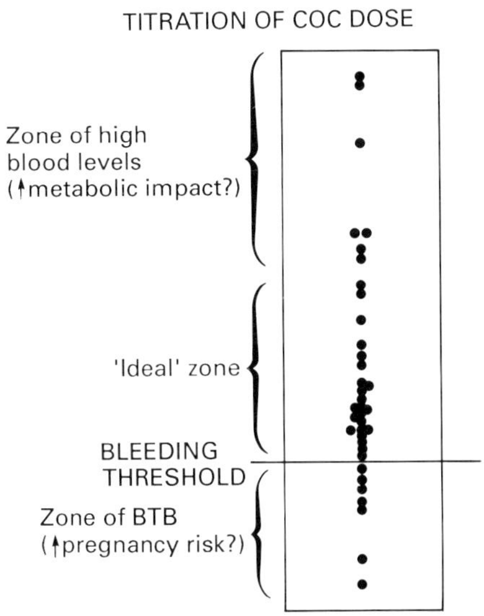

Figure 5.1. Schematic representation of approx tenfold variability in blood levels of both contraceptive steroids, and rationale of suggested 'titration'.

formulation than she requires? In the absence of any easy clinical test for blood levels, I have been suggesting for some years that during early follow-up after initial pill-prescribing, one should titrate the dose downwards against BTB as a threshold bioassay [13]. In other words, one attempts to 'give each woman the lowest dose combination pill that her uterus will allow'. This may be, but need not necessarily be, a phasic pill. The latter are only widely available for levonorgestrel and norethisterone-containing COCs, and these do tend to give a better bleeding pattern for lowered mean doses with reduced metabolic effects. Desogestrel- and gestodene-containing pills are at present usually monophasic, and yet cycle control is adequate and metabolic changes are acceptable.

The fundamental point being made here is that one should not necessarily represcribe the same brand for years if a lower dose in the same progestogen 'ladder' has never been tried.

One's ability to follow this principle – arranging that, for a given progestogen, one's patients are all given the lowest dose which is just (but only just) above their bleeding threshold – is obviously prejudiced by the fact that for the newer progestogens there may be only one or at the most two dosage levels available. Hopefully this will be corrected by the manufacturers in due course.

Other causes of BTB

To sound a note of caution, if BTB occurs one should first eliminate other possible causes. The following check-list is modified from Sapire [14]:

Default – poor compliance
Diarrhoea and/or vomiting
Disturbance of absorption (e.g. after gut resection in the treatment of obesity)
Diet – vegetarianism alters the gut flora in such a way as to lead to diminished recycling of oestrogen[6]
Drugs – interacting (see below)
Disease – examine the cervix (the bleeding symptoms of invasive cancer have been known to be attributed to BTB)
Disorder of pregnancy causing bleeding (e.g. abortion, trophoblastic tumour)
Duration – too short, since minimal BTB which is tolerable may resolve in 2–3 months
and finally
Dose – after the above have been excluded change to a phasic or higher-dose pill

Once other explanations have been eliminated, prescribers should not be disturbed if satisfactory cycle control can only be obtained for a particular woman by a 'stronger' regimen than would usually be prescribed. If all $\leqslant$35-μg ethinyloestradiol pills produce BTB, one could try a 50-μg brand. On the working hypothesis here, such women have unusually low blood levels of the hormone, and hence a strong pill is equivalent, for them, to an ordinary low-dose pill. Indeed, it may well be appropriate to give two COCs per day in selected cases, bearing in mind the tenfold variation in blood levels of the ingested hormones referred to above.

End-organ effects

It may be objected that BTB is not a totally accurate marker of blood levels, and indeed variability in BTB or WTB with the same blood level could be caused by variation at the end-organ [15]. This is indubitably true. But it would not significantly alter the suggested policy in practice. BTB is annoying in any event, and women will always wish to have the symptom removed. The dose administered for that purpose should be only just above (and not enormously above) the bleeding threshold, whether mediated by low blood level or an unusually susceptible end-organ. Hence, titration downwards in those *without* BTB is still logical.

Risk of pregnancy during BTB
It has been argued that attempting to find the best initial choice of pill by titrating downwards at follow-up will lead to breakthrough conceptions. That these rarely occur is, I believe, for the following reasons. First, even the current low-dose pills are so highly effective, with back-up contraceptive mechanisms (notably the progestogen 'block' to cervical mucus penetration by sperm) operating even if ovulation should occur. Second, it appears that BTB is a symptom which appears when there is more circulating artificial steroid than the minimum to permit conception – in compliant women. (It may well be true that BTB does imply a reduced margin for error; as discussed below, the pill-taking errors that matter are those that lead to lengthening of the pill-free interval.) Thirdly, it is likely that bleeding from the uterus itself temporarily enhances the anti-implantation contraceptive mechanism.

To conclude, I would stress that this prescribing system is based on a hypothesis, which is only now being rigorously tested. I would ask the reader to judge its plausibility and my view that it should be followed, pending the discovery of any better scheme.

What notice should by taken of the pre-existing symptomatology of a woman, during initial pill selection?
Dickey [16] and others [17] have made much of this approach, producing elaborate rules, based on symptoms in the woman's pre-existing menstrual cycle which are presumed to be caused by too much or too little progestogen or oestrogen. I have always considered that since the combined pill will remove a woman's normal menstrual cycle anyway and replace it with an artificial one, the important thing is to produce as good an artificial cycle as possible. With modern low-dose 'balanced' pills this can usually be achieved – for all hormone-related symptoms, not solely bleeding – by arranging the lowest biological impact on the system that the uterus will allow, in the manner described above.

However, there are differences at the end-organs, and clearly at the margins of choice one would tend to select an oestrogen-dominant pill for a woman with severe pre-existing acne, and a progestogen-dominant pill for someone with pre-existing fibroids or benign breast disease. In the majority, however, I recommend that that type of adjustment is reserved until (non-bleeding) symptoms appear during use of the first or subsequent pill (Tables 5.8, 5.9) – the latter having been selected according to the bleeding threshold, in the way described above.

Starting routines for the combined pill

Several workers [18–20] have shown that the combined pill appears to develop its contraceptive efficacy within less than seven days of the first tablet being taken. In view of the unlikelihood of a fertile ovulation before day 7 of any cycle, starting routines can be as shown in Table 5.4. The day 1 start is preferred. But starting on any day of the cycle later than day 5 is permissible, provided the woman is not actually or

Table 5.4 Starting routines

	Start when?	*Extra precautions?*
1. Menstruating	On or after 5th day of cycle	Yes (see text)
	First day	No*
2. Post-partum		
(a) No lactation	21–28th day postpartum	No
(b) Lactation	Not normally recommended at all (POP preferred)	
3. Postinduced abortion/miscarriage	Same day	No
4. Post-trophoblastic tumour	One month after no human chorionic gonadotrophin detected	As 1
5. Post-higher dose COC	Instant switch	No (see text)
6. Post-lower or same dose COC	After usual 7-day break	No
7. Post-POP	First day of period	No
8. Post-POP with secondary amenorrhoea/during lactation	After last packet of POP	No

*Except in the case of Logynon ED (triphasic levonorgestrel 50/75/125 μg with ethinyloestradiol (EE) 30/40/30 μg), since the starting routine entails the taking of a variable number of placebos. With other COCs, starting active treatment as late as day 3 of the cycle without extra precautions has proved effective in clinical practice (p. 140)

potentially pregnant and additional contraception (for just seven days) is advised. In that event she should be warned of cycle irregularity and followed up after no more than one month.

The recommendation in Table 5.4 to switch directly from a higher- to a lower-dose COC is based solely on anecdotal reports of 'rebound' conceptions at that time. An alternative is to recommend additional contraception for the first seven days of the new lowered-dose packet. Both recommendations are probably over-cautious, in the light of modern experience with those phasic pills whose first phase regularly has a lower dose than the preceding third phase.

Postpartum contraception

In the absence of lactation. the earliest potentially fertile ovulations have been reported at the end of the fourth week of the puerperium [21]. It is preferable not to commence oestrogen treatment much earlier for fear of thromboembolism. If the COC is started during the fourth week no extra contraceptive precautions are required. A certain degree of individualization can be practised. Thus, for an obese woman one might wait until the end of the fourth week (or later with additional contraception). On the other hand in a woman thought to be at above average risk of conceiving, commencement about day 21 would be preferred.

The combined pill should not of course be chosen at all in lactating women, as the progestogen-only pill is sufficient for near 100% contraception [21]. The earliest ovulation reported in a fully lactating woman is about day 43 [22].

The paramount importance of the pill-free interval

It is now well-established that in many women on current low-dose COCs there is a variable degree of restoration of endogenous ovarian function during the pill-free interval [23]. See Figure 5.2 for a summary of the findings. Not only do the levels of gonadotrophins plus oestradiol rise [15, 19, 20, 24], but also in many women serial ultrasound scanning of the ovaries shows regular return of follicular activity [18]. Killick et al. [20] conclude that:

> 'the seven day gap between pill packets is analogous to starting the very first pack of pills on Day 7 of a normal cycle, in the sense that the hypothalamo–pituitary axis and ovary are allowed seven days to initiate follicle development. The withdrawal bleed in the middle of this seven day gap is inconsequential and in no way inhibits follicular development.'

Given this information, it follows that breakthrough ovulation is most likely to occur at the end of any pill-free interval which is lengthened, the lengthening being caused by omitted pills either just prior to the 7-day break or immediately following it. Seven days is almost always insufficient to permit ovulation, but in some women (unknown to the prescriber) anything more will do so. Moreover the progestogenic effect of her pill on the cervical mucus will also be at its lowest at the end of any lengthened pill-free interval (PFI).

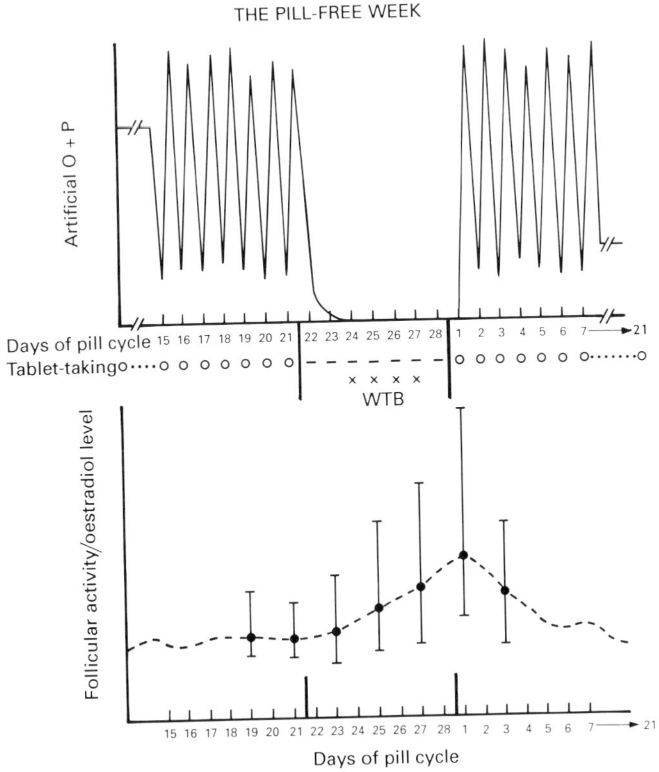

Figure 5.2. Changes through the pill-taking cycle in the blood levels of both the ingested artificial hormones (oestrogen (O) and progestogen (P)), and in follicular activity as demonstrated by growth of the dominant follicle by ultrasound, with special reference to the pill-free week.

The practical implications relate in the first place to the advice given to women who miss their contraceptive pills. In the United Kingdom the Family Planning Association (FPA) and the NAFPD have agreed new advice which is now routinely given and printed on Patient Instruction Leaflets. The content of the new advice is as follows although a more 'user-friendly' presentation is planned:

If you forget a pill

'Take it as soon as you remember, and the next one at your normal time. If you are 12 or more hours late with any pill, especially the first or last in the pack, the pill may not work. As soon as you remember, continue normal pill taking. However, you will not be protected for the *next seven days* and must either not have sex, or use another method such as the condom.

'*If, and only if*, these seven days run beyond the end of your packet, start the next packet as soon as you have finished the present one, i.e. do not have a gap between packs, or – if you are using everyday (ED) pills – miss out the seven inactive pills. This will mean you may not have a period until the end of two packs but this does you no harm. Nor does it matter if you see some bleeding on tablet-taking days.' [25]

Seven days of pill-taking appears to give sufficient time for restoration of contraception in the vast majority of cases [23]. When pills are omitted at the end of a packet, the new advice also avoids the illogicality of permitting the woman to take a further seven day break – from the contraceptive effects of her method – on top of the break she has already inadvertently taken by missing pills.

The bleeding referred to at the end of the advice is of course even more likely if the woman has missed triphasic pills at the end of a pack and switches directly (as instructed) to the first, lower-dose, phase. But contraceptive efficacy is maintained, which is the object of the exercise. If the prescriber prefers to recommend one of the alternative 'instant switch' procedures depicted in Figure 5.3, this will only reduce the risk of bleeding. It will not make an important contribution to contraception.

Vomiting, diarrhoea, drug interactions

The same advice is recommended in other situations where the bioavailability of contraceptive steroids is temporarily reduced: such as vomiting and severe diarrhoea, and – with modifications to be described below – in the short-term use of interacting drugs. 'Stomach upsets' have been shown to be particularly important in this context, accounting for one in three breakthrough conceptions in ostensibly compliant women [26].

Advantages of the pill-free interval

Elsewhere [23] I have assessed all the available scientific data supporting the importance of the pill-free interval (PFI) – something that was overlooked for many years. It is clear that having regular PFIs, as devised originally by Pincus, is of greater importance than is implied by the simple imitation of the normal menstrual cycle and the regular reassurance of withdrawal bleeds. It leads to a smaller total quantity of artificial steroids being ingested per year than if no breaks were taken. But possibly more significant, some of the metabolic variables altered by the COC show a tendency to return to normal by the end of the pill-free week. This was shown for HDL-cholesterol by Demacker and colleagues [27]. The latter work requires confirmation, and is indeed being extended to other metabolic variables in studies at the Margaret

Pyke Centre. But it implies a possible important benefit to health, and possibly to COC reversibility, as a consequence of the monthly 'rest' from systemic actions of the method.

Disadvantages of the pill-free interval
There are also disadvantages of the PFI, chiefly, as already shown, that it potentially impairs the efficacy of the method. It can also be associated with certain side-effects such as withdrawal headaches. In the short term it can certainly be eliminated with impunity for women who wish to postpone bleeding, e.g. because of an impending holiday. This is simple with monophasic brands, but specific procedures are necessary for most phasic pills, as explained in Figure 5.3.

Tri-cycle regimens
Because of the likely benefits of the PFI as just discussed, and the fact that the epidemiological studies which show the method is acceptably safe have all been based upon pill-taking with a PFI, it is felt that the generality of women should continue to take the COC in that way. There are strong arguments for making it shorter: a 6-day pill-free gap would be contraceptively safer than the present norm of 7 days – if the manufacturers would oblige [23].

However, there are indications for eliminating the PFI, as shown in Table 5.5. Even then most authorities – and, indeed, most pill-takers – prefer that there should be periodic breaks from pill taking. In the medium-to-long term, it is therefore usual to recommend that the woman takes three or alternatively four packets continuously (63 or 84 tablets), followed by a four- to seven-day break. This is known as 'tri-cycling' [28]. It means that if symptoms such as severe headaches occur regularly during the PFI, they will occur just four times a year instead of every month.

Phasic pills cannot of course be used in this way. Indeed for some conditions, such as non-focal migraine and epilepsy, such pills are inappropriate because part of the

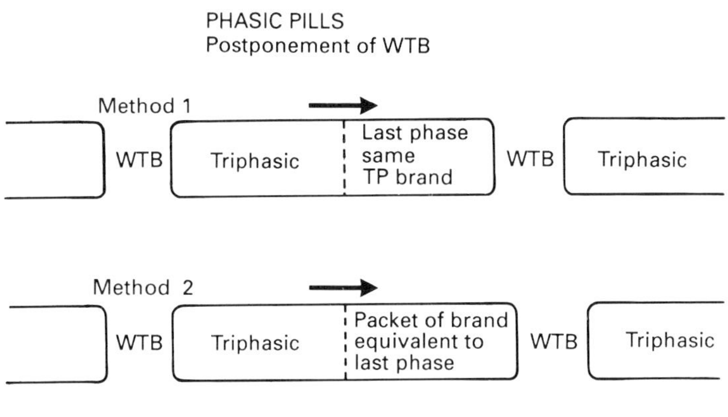

Figure 5.3. Two possible methods for short-term postponement of withdrawal bleeding (WTB) by women using phasic pills. The brand 'equivalent to the last phase' will be a monophasic pill with a (near-) identical formulation, e.g. Microgynon/Nordette in the case of triphasic levonorgestrel pills.

Table 5.5 COCs: Indications for eliminating the pill-free interval (PFI)

Short-term Holidays, etc
Long-term Tricycle regimens
1. Severe headache occurring during hormone withdrawal in the PFI
2. The occurrence of heavy withdrawal bleeding, especially in women given the COC to help menorrhagia
3. Non-focal migraine (see text)
4. Epilepsy (see text)
5. Endometriosis, especially when using a progestogen-dominant pill for maintenance treatment
6. Any cause for the suspicion of reduced efficacy of the COC, e.g. past 'breakthrough' pregnancy, or during long-term use of an enzyme-inducing drug
   Alternative: shorten the pill-free interval
7. At the woman's choice

object of the exercise is to keep hormone levels as steady as possible (as fluctuations tend to precipitate symptoms).

Drug interactions

As described in Chapter 2, enzyme-inducing drugs are capable of reducing the contraceptive efficacy of combined pills, with lowered blood levels and a concomitant increase in the incidence of breakthrough bleeding and absent withdrawal bleeding. Enzyme-inducing drugs can affect both the oestrogen and the progestogen, whereas broad-spectrum antibiotics have a lesser effect since they only influence the recycling of ethinyloestradiol. This also means that they can have no significant interaction with the progestogen-only pill.

Vitamin C (ascorbic acid) is a drug that competitively raises blood levels of the oestrogen (see Chapter 2), and since co-trimoxazole is an enzyme inhibitor it also somewhat raises levels. See Table 5.6 for the clinically more important drug interactions with COCs.

Note that very few interactions in the reverse direction, in which COCs influence the actions of other drugs, are believed to have clinical significance. COCs are weak inhibitors of hepatic microsomal enzymes, causing some inhibition of the metabolism of, for example, caffeine [29], some benzodiazepines [29], and cyclosporin [30]. The reported case of severe hepatotoxicity due to the last-mentioned suggests an important interaction. For most other examples the degree of change is very small compared with the interindividual differences in drug metabolism [29].

Enzyme inducers – practical implications

Short-term use

If treatment is commenced with a drug such as rifampicin or griseofulvin, then either abstinence or extra contraceptive precautions should follow for the duration of the treatment and for at least seven days thereafter: omitting the PFI if the seven days extend beyond the end of the packet.

In fact, enzyme induction shows marked individual variation. It may take numerous days to reach its peak when the inducer drug is introduced and from four to 12 weeks to disappear when it is withdrawn [31]. Hence, on the one hand the advice just given may be somewhat overcautious for very short-term treatments; on the other hand, if the enzyme inducer is used for a month or more loss of contraceptive activity must be assumed to continue for several further weeks, and appropriate advice given (i.e. as for long-term use, see below).

Table 5.6 Drug interactions with COCs

Clinically relevant enzyme-inducing drugs	
Anticonvulsants	Barbiturates
	Phenytoin
	Primidone
	Carbamazepine
	NB. NOT *sodium valproate or clonazepam*
Antibiotics	Rifampicin
Antifungals	Griseofulvin
Anti-inflammatory drugs	Phenylbutazone
Diuretics	Spironolactone
Hypnotics	Chloral hydrate
	Dichloralphenazone
Tranquillizers	Chlorpromazine
Broad-spectrum antibiotics	
	Ampicillin and relatives
	Tetracyclines
	Neomycin
	NB NOT *Co-trimoxazole*

Long-term use of enzyme inducers

This chiefly applies to epileptics and women being treated for tuberculosis. All common antiepileptic treatments are enzyme inducers apart from sodium valproate and clonazepam. An alternative method of contraception such as an intrautcrinc device may be offered.

But if the combined pill is preferred it is appropriate to prescribe initially a 50 µg oestrogen-containing preparation, recommending that the pill-free interval is shortened. This can be most easily arranged by issuing a menstrual diary card on which the woman marks each day of tablet taking and crosses off the (suggested) four pill-free days. She needs to understand that the WTB may extend somewhat into the start of each new packet, and that her starting day will vary from month to month, though neither of these are important. If sufficient time is taken to explain this system, compliance and efficacy can be ensured in most cases. Appropriate placebo-packaging, with four placebos and 24 active tablets, would help – if the drug companies were to oblige.

A very satisfactory alternative is the *tri-cycle regimen* described above. This is particularly appropriate for epileptics, since the frequency of attacks is often reduced by the maintenance of steady hormone levels [32]. At the end of each tri-cycle I would still recommend that the PFI be shortened to four or five days, in view of the work previously reviewed. The rate of restoration of ovarian activity appears to bear little relation to the duration of previous suppression by COC taking [19, 23].

With or without a monthly or three-monthly (shortened) PFI, if the woman develops BTB the next step is to give two tablets a day of 30 µg or 35 µg oestrogen pills. The combined oestrogen content of the two pills per day can be increased if necessary to 80 or 100 µg (maximum), titrated against the BTB. In this way the usual policy, giving the minimum dose of both hormones to finish just above the threshold for bleeding, can be followed. I reassure the woman that she is metaphorically 'climbing a down escalator'. In other words her increased liver metabolism means that her system is still basically receiving a low-dose regimen. She is exposed to more metabolites, but this is not known to be harmful (and for some women the available alternatives to the COC are just not acceptable).

Caution is necessary when enzyme inducers are withdrawn, since it takes some weeks for the liver's level of excretory function to revert to normal. After long-term use it is therefore recommended (M. Orme, 1986, personal communication to NAFPD) that there is a delay of about four weeks before the woman returns to a standard low-dose pill regimen. This might reasonably be increased to eight weeks after very prolonged use of barbiturates [31]. And as usual there should be no PFI between the higher- and the low-dose packets (Table 5.4).

Broad-spectrum antibiotic treatment

Short-term use

Use of broad-spectrum antibiotics such as those listed should lead to extra contraceptive precautions during treatment and for seven days thereafter, with no gap between packets as and if indicated by the advice suggested earlier. The likelihood of contraceptive failure with antibiotics is small (see Chapter 2), but from the practical point of view one never knows which woman is in the most susceptible group.

Long-term use of antibiotics

Here there is the useful fact that the large-bowel flora responsible for recycling oestrogens is reconstituted with resistant organisms in about three to four weeks (Orme, 1986, personal communication). In practice therefore, if the COC is commenced in a woman who has been taking a tetracycline long term for acne, for example, there is no need to advise extra contraceptive precautions. There is a problem only in the reverse situation, when the tetracycline is first introduced to treat an established pill-taker. Even then extra precautions need to be sustained only for say one month (or a higher oestrogen dose given for that time).

Follow-up arrangements and monitoring

In routine cases, the first follow-up visit should be scheduled for 3 months, and subsequent prescriptions made out for 6 months – or up to a year in selected low-risk cases. But women with cardiovasular system (CVS) risk factors (Table 5.2), and those with any medical condition not known to be completely unaffected by sex steroids, need to be seen more frequently, say after one month and then regularly every 3–6 months.

In all cases, having selected the 'safest' pill brand in the manner described above (which may require a trial of several varieties) the main aspects of monitoring are as follows:

1. Be alert for the onset of any new risk factors, especially if one is already present.
2. Look for the warning signs of circulatory disease risk, particularly a rise in *blood pressure* or the onset of or change in the character of *migraine headaches*.
3. Try alternative formulations should there be non-bleeding side-effects.
4. Arrange regular cervical cytology.
5. Teach breast self-examination, with annual medical examination and mammography as indicated.
6. Give advice concerning special situations such as immobilization, proposed minor surgery to the legs, etc.

7. Advise about continuation of the method according to age achieved and total duration of use.

The importance of blood pressure

Blood pressure (BP) should be measured pretreatment and thereafter at every routine visit. Studies have shown that mean systolic and diastolic blood pressures both increase among pill-taking populations [33]. Such elevations by no more than about 5 mmHg in women without other risk factors are of no concern. However *clinical* hypertension should be detected, since (rarely) irreversible, malignant hypertension can occur [34], whereas it is fully reversible if the pill is discontinued in time. Repeated readings at or above 160/95 would be too high both for commencing and for continuing the COC method. A progestogen-only method may however be used (see Chapter 2).

At all elevated levels of BP there is an increased risk of haemorrhagic strokes, including subarachnoid haemorrhage. Thus, mild degrees of hypertension should be taken seriously, especially if there are circulatory risk factors, and regarded as a *marker* for an increased risk of arterial disease. Studies by the life-insurance companies of large populations [35] have shown that raised BP is associated with a small but measurable reduction in life expectancy – even in women. While it is not certain that pill-induced mild hypertension has the same significance as the idiopathic variety, it would be prudent to assume that it does. Faced with a 33-year-old heavy-smoking woman with a BP repeatedly around 135/85 – especially if prior to pill-taking the BP is known to have been say 100/65 – one would therefore recommend the use of an alternative method of birth control sooner rather than later, and specifically without waiting for the absolute upper age limit, for smokers, of 35 years.

I have maintained for some years now that the blood pressure can thus be used as an ongoing test of liability to arterial disease. A normal or low reading can be considered as a 'green test' and provide some reassurance that there is no extra risk in continuing with the method, although 'trouble can still strike out of a clear blue sky'.

Young non-smokers (who reject other methods) with established non-pill-induced hypertension, well controlled by treatment, may be given the COC. This should only be done after full consultation with the physician supervising control of the hypertension. The progestogen-only pill would normally be a better choice.

Past severe pre-eclampsia

Previous pregnancy-related hypertension does not correlate with the appearance of COC-induced hypertension [36]. If the BP rises or stays elevated in pill-takers with this history, it is most probably due to underlying chronic vascular disease or essential hypertension which initially became apparent late in the earlier pregnancy [36]. Pre-eclampsia does not therefore contraindicate a supervised trial of the COC. There are disturbances of coagulation in severe cases, including a rebound elevation of the platelet count as much as six weeks postnatally (C. Redman, 1987, personal communication). For these women it may therefore be safest to recommend alternative contraception until eight weeks: and during the first three months of COC use to check the BP monthly, then three-monthly.

The importance of migraine

In my opinion vascular headaches of the migraine type should always be considered a relative contraindication to the combined pill. Migraine sufferers as a group have an increased incidence of thrombotic strokes, even without the added effects on haemostatic variables caused by oestrogen. However, the COC may be offered, under supervision, to women with non-migraine headaches or migraines which are free of features to be described shortly, if they are found tolerable by the woman herself. Should such headaches occur during the PFI, tri-cycling may be advised (see above). Also, all sufferers should have their attention specifically drawn to the warning symptoms mentioned below, which might presage a preventable stroke.

Migraine types which contraindicate oestrogen

In my opinion the types of migraine which indicate that (oestrogen in) the combined pill should be avoided or discontinued are:

1. Focal migraine, that is, with transient cerebral ischaemia (see below).
2. Crescendo migraine, meaning a migrainous headache which is unduly severe and sustained for several days.
3. The woman's first-ever attack while taking the COC; this is not always a permanent contraindication.
4. The concurrent use of ergotamine (since the drug is a cerebral vasoconstrictor and prothrombotic changes caused by oestrogen might lead to thrombosis of a constricted artery).

In 1975 Bickerstaff wrote an important monograph [37] which drew attention to preventable aspects of cerebral arterial insufficiency. As well as a history of a past thrombotic event, CVS risk factors such as diabetes and heavy smoking, blood dyscrasias and pre-existing hypertension, he also drew attention to the important factor of transient vasoconstriction. This can occur during a crescendo migraine attack, but is also the cause of focal migraine. During the latter there are symptoms of transient cerebral ischaemia with lateralization (but unilateral *headache* is a feature of most migraines and not relevant). Important symptoms are: transient hemiparesis, hemianaesthesia or marked paraesthesiae, perhaps mainly in one limb; transient loss of a field of vision (but not blurring, fortification spectra or flashing lights, which are common in non-focal migraine); transient difficulty in speaking (nominal dysphasia or slurred speech); acute vertigo; or focal epilepsy.

Should any of these symptoms occur and have no other valid explanation, the message is in practical terms 'stop the COC today, and probably forever'. This vigorous response is necessary because of the reports by many neurologists, including Bickerstaff, that a number of those (very few) young pill-takers admitted with strokes give such a history, during the weeks or days leading up to their admission. It is a very reasonable hypothesis that these women would not have suffered irreversible cerebral arterial insufficiency had the oestrogen in the combined pill been stopped sooner [37]. This has not been proved by controlled trial, but prudence surely dictates the action suggested here.

What method should the patient use in future? The main medical concern is that prothrombotic blood changes caused by oestrogen might, superimposed on transitory cerebral ischaemia, cause an irreversible thrombotic stroke. Hence there need be no contraindication to use of the progestogen-only modalities, including the POP and injectables. One cannot promise the woman that she will not continue to have the migraine headaches themselves, perhaps even occasionally with focal symptoms. On those grounds she may well decide to discontinue all varieties of hormonal contraception. But if she can live with her headaches, with the POP for example, there should be no added risk of cerebral thrombosis.

Table 5.7 Reasons to stop oestrogen, pending advice

Reason	*Worst diagnosis* or risk*
Pain	
Pain in calf	Deep venous thrombosis
in chest	Pulmonary embolus
	Myocardial infarction
in abdomen	Thrombosis of major vessel
Dyspnoea/haemoptysis	Pulmonary embolus
Migraine	
± Loss of visual field	Retinal thrombosis/Impending stroke
± Unilateral numbness	Impending stroke
± Unilateral weakness	Impending stroke
± Dysphasia	Impending stroke
Blood pressure	
BP ≥ 160/95	Haemorrhagic stroke
Other	
Immobilization after accident or emergency surgery	Deep venous thrombosis/Pulmonary embolus
Jaundice	Cholestasis or hepatitis

*But usually not the most probable diagnosis

Table 5.7 lists the symptoms about which a pill-taker should request urgent advice, so a clinician may decide whether (or not) the oestrogen in the combined pill should be discontinued. This information should be made available to all users.

Major elective surgery

Here there is already an increased risk of deep venous thrombosis (DVT) and pulmonary embolism. In view of the independent and likely synergistic association with oestrogen therapy, it remains my firm opinion [38] that the combined pill should be discontinued, although that view has recently been questioned [39]. One should follow the principle of 'primum non nocere'. Moreover, the cautious policy will protect those women in any community who have an extra predisposition to thrombosis because of an as yet undiagnosed coagulopathy, such as congenital protein C deficiency [40].

Anxiety that the morbidity due to unwanted pregnancy would outweigh that prevented by this policy is misplaced; there are alternative methods of contraception. It is not a 'pill or nothing' choice. One very good option which we offer at the Margaret Pyke Centre is (after counselling) to use an injectable such as depot medroxyprogesterone acetate [40]. One or more injections will cover the time on any waiting-list and the COC can be restarted at any convenient time more than two weeks following mobilization, even if this antedates the expiry of contraception from the last injection. This is particularly useful if the injection causes irregular bleeding (about which women should always be forewarned). Indeed, the COC is often used as a convenient source of oestrogen for treating bleeding problems in longer-term injectable users.

The advisability of avoiding oestrogen exposure also applies to any elective minor procedures with an above-average risk of DVT, notably to the legs, such as surgery or injection sclerotherapy for varicose veins, and operative arthroscopy.

However, the case should not be overstated. The risk is vanishingly small in young women having non-leg-associated minor surgery with a short anaesthetic and early mobilization, such as most dentistry and sterilization whether by laparoscopy or minilaparotomy. It also does not apply to the progestogen-only pill (POP) – another contraceptive option, indeed, to cover elective major procedures.

Emergency major surgery or recumbent immobilization following an accident
In these situations the woman should be positively instructed to discontinue pill-taking (which she will otherwise continue out of habit) from the day of admission, and some consideration should be given to the use of prophylactic subcutaneous low-dose heparin (5000 units six-hourly). The morbidity of the latter is small but needs to be balanced against the total background risk of DVT in each individual.

Summary

Major elective surgery, or minor operative procedures to the legs
Discontinue all oestrogen-containing preparations four weeks preoperatively. Recommence the COC at the first menstrual period which is at least two weeks after mobilization. The rule does not apply to other minor surgery. The POP and injectables are satisfactory alternative contraceptives.

Emergency surgery, immobilization after an accident
Discontinue the COC and consider subcutaneous heparin.

Outcome of pregnancy following or associated with COC use

After discontinuing the COC, there is no increased risk of miscarriage, ectopic gestation, stillbirth, or alteration in the sex ratio or birthweight [41]. In 1981 an expert scientific group of the WHO declared categorically that there was no evidence of any adverse effect on the fetus of pill-use prior to conception [42]. No subsequent publications have seriously challenged this view.

COC exposure during pregnancy
Here it is believed that the attributable risk of teratogenesis is extremely small, though not proven to be non-existent. The evidence has been well reviewed by Sapire [43]. The rate of birth defects in the Oxford/FPA and RCGP studies following COC exposure and delivery was no higher than expected among any group of women having a planned baby. There is some persistent anxiety regarding limb reduction deformities [44], but otherwise no single abnormality has been identified in association with hormone usage during pregnancy.

Practical implications
The rule that a pregnant woman should avoid all drugs, especially in the first trimester, remains the ideal. If a woman becomes pregnant and continues taking the COC during organogenesis she cannot be promised a normal baby. Although it is so well agreed that the commoner fetal abnormalities are not more frequent in pill-takers, there has to remain some uncertainty about rare anomalies. Moreover, two percent of all babies show an important abnormality. But what can be clearly stated is that the risk is small enough to be considered negligible by most people. The concept of COC-related teratogenesis should not be used as the sole grounds for recommending therapeutic abortion.

Note that the fetal risk after failure of postcoital hormone treatment, which is given before implantation, would be expected to be even less than the low risk estimated for COC-users (see Chapter 8).

Some authorities advise that women should discontinue the pill and use a mechanical method of contraception for two to three cycles before a wanted conception. This may be reasonable for the most pessimistic. It should certainly do no harm, but there is no objective evidence that it is worth the effort. The advent of diagnostic ultrasound has minimized the dating advantage; and certainly any woman who does find herself pregnant less than three months after pill discontinuation should be strongly reassured. For the generality of women there are also no grounds for specific vitamin supplementation, though all pregnant women should be advised to take a fully balanced diet, including green vegetables and citrus fruits.

Management of so-called minor side-effects [45]

First and foremost, these often do not seem minor to the woman affected. But many of them are common in the general population, so it is difficult to be sure that the COC is to blame in any individual case. The frequency of complaint depends on many factors including anxiety about possible harm due to the therapy. Most of the problems can be classified under two main headings: those related to cycle control (which were dealt with earlier) and those which are also commoner in pregnancy.

The relatively common, pregnancy-mimicking, minor side-effects include (in alphabet order):

> breast enlargement, bloating, cramps and pains in the legs, cystitis and other urinary infections, depression with or without loss of libido, gingivitis, headaches, nausea, vaginal discharge (non-specific) with or without cervical 'erosion' and weight gain. Less common problems include pain in the breasts, chloasma, galactorrhoea and superficial thrombophlebitis.

Note that the last-mentioned, though minor in itself, implies a tendency to DVT, and the COC would be absolutely contraindicated for the future.

A general point about management is that it is preferable not to use another drug to get rid of reversible side-effects which are believed to be caused by the first drug (the COC in this case). It is usually bad medicine to prescribe diuretics, anti-migraine treatments, anti-hypertensives or anti-depressants for pill-induced weight gain, migraine, hypertension or depression, respectively. However, for the last of these, pyridoxine is worth a try (see Chapter 2). Chloasma can be masked with cosmetics, and 'erosions' if symptomatic can be treated (after cytology) by outpatient techniques.

Otherwise there are two general and two more specific approaches to the selection of an alternative formulation for women who wish to continue using the method.

Empirical (general) courses of action

1. *Decrease the dose*, if the manufacturer has in fact provided a range of doses for the particular progestogen, and if it is still possible after earlier titrating downwards. If appropriate, *oestrogen* can be eliminated altogether by a trial of the progestogen-only pill.

2. *Change to a different progestogen*, and again move down the new progestogen 'ladder' as symptoms dictate and if a range of doses exists.

More specific approaches (Tables 5.8 and 5.9)
Certain side-effects and conditions have become associated, mainly anecdotally, with relative excess of either steroid [16, 45]. The remedy is to prescribe either a more progestogen- or a more oestrogen-dominant formulation, as exemplified in the Tables.

Duration of use and taking breaks

Should the COC be discontinued for, say, six months every two or every five years?
No: from the point of view of preservation of fertility, and in particular the subsequent occurrence of secondary amenorrhoea, duration of use seems irrelevant

Table 5.8 Which second choice of pill? (Relative oestrogen excess)

Symptoms	*Conditions*
Nausea	Benign breast disease
Dizziness	Fibroids
'Premenstrual tension' and irritability	Endometriosis
Cyclical weight gain (fluid)	
'Bloating'	
Vaginal discharge (no infection)	
Some cases of breast tenderness	

Treat with progestogen-dominant COC such as
Loestrin 30 (EE 30 μg + NEA 1.5 mg
Eugynon 30 (EE 30 μg + LNG 250 μg (Second choice because of effects on HDL-cholesterol, but may be first choice for endometriosis)

Key: See Table 5.9

Table 5.9 Which second choice of pill? (Relative progestogen excess)

Symptoms	*Conditions*
Dryness of vagina	Acne/seborrhoea
Some cases of:	Hirsutism
sustained weight gain	
depression	
loss of libido	
lassitude	

Treat with oestrogen-dominant COC, such as

Ovysmen/Brevinor	(EE 35 μg + NET 1 mg)
Marvelon	(EE 30 μg + DSG 150 μg)
Dianette	(EE 35 μg + CPA 2 mg)

(Dianette is an acne treatment which is also contraceptive, and now preferred to Diane)

Key to Tables 5.8 and 5.9. EE, Ethinyloestradiol; NEA, Norethisterone acetate; LNG, Levonorgestrel; NET, Norethisterone; DSG, Desogestrel; CPA, Cyproterone acetate and breaks of no benefit [6, 46]. In general, when women stop the COC they regain after a short (one to three months) delay the fertility that they would have had if they had never taken the medication [47].

Vessey's 1986 report [48] implies an exception to that statement relating to the group of nulliparous women discontinuing the COC above age 30. But note that firstly the report itself provides no evidence (even in that category of pill-takers) for any permanent loss of fertility, as compared with the controls. Secondly, there was a clinically important delay in conception – above that due to being over the age of 30 – only in half the population; compare the top with the bottom half of Figure 4 in that study [48]. Hence I disagree with the view that nulliparous pill-takers reaching the age of 30 should necessarily be encouraged to switch to barrier methods on fertility grounds. Of course they may wish to do so after discussion, and all should be warned of the possibility of some pill-associated delay, which could amount to an extra year in some cases.

There is no evidence in Vessey's studies that duration of pill-use prior to discontinuation was relevant, nor in any study that women conceive sooner if they have taken breaks.

Of great potential relevance is the fact that any woman who has been on the pill for 10 years has in fact taken 130 breaks each of a week in duration. They may well be beneficial to metabolism and perhaps to overall health (see above). At present there are no reasons for believing that longer breaks need to be taken. The main problem with breaks of any duration is the number of unwanted pregnancies that result.

Duration of use and cardiovascular system (CVS) disease risk

There remains some uncertainty about duration of use and CVS disease risk (see Chapter 3), whether for current takers or for ex-takers. However, even if the limited evidence on that issue is believed, there is no value to be expected from simply taking breaks, unless the breaks are long enough to make a real difference to the total accumulated duration of use [49].

Duration of use and cancer risk

There exist studies showing a beneficial effect on cancer of the ovary and endometrium, and others showing a possible harmful effect on cancer of the cervix and breast. But in each of these opposite categories the effect described is greater with increasing duration of use. Since at present it is impossible to say whether, overall, the beneficial effects of pill-use on cancer outweigh the adverse effects (see Chapter 4), it is equally impossible to assess the changes on both sides of the equation caused by increased duration of use. But relatively short breaks of six months are again unlikely to signify. The evidence suggests that, as for the CVS, the accumulated total duration of COC use is likely to be more relevant.

Summary

We are forced to base our decisions about duration of use primarily on the better (though still incomplete) evidence concerning CVS disease. Table 5.10 suggests a scheme, erring on the side of caution, for pill prescribing according both to the age reached by the woman and the total accumulated duration of use. It is important that the two matters are not considered in isolation. Age is the more important factor. Fifteen years' use by a woman under 30 would be considered of less importance than if she were over 40. Even in that older age group, it may be considered acceptable by

Table 5.10 Management by age, smoking, and duration of COC use

	Age and COC use (years)			
	30	35	40	45
Smoker	Review	Change method	—	—
Non-smoker		Review	2nd review	Change method

Above 45 (35 in smokers): COCs contraindicated solely for contraception. **May be usable if also indicated as therapy (e.g. for gynaecological disorders in selected cases, Table 12.3, p. 228)**. Consider also POP.

	Accumulated duration of COC use (years)			
	5	*10*	*15*	*20*
Smoker	Review	2nd Review	Change method	—
Non-smoker	—	Review	2nd review	Change method (? – see text)

some prescribers to continue beyond the suggested 20 years at the woman's expressed request, and provided there are no risk factors. See also p. 70–72.

For the older woman, or at any age if a CVS risk factor is present, most recent metabolic studies support the use of low dose oestrogen plus a 'selective, third generation' progestogen (pages 12–26). Though others may follow, currently only a desogestrel combination also provides the minimum available oestrogen dose (20 μg). On metabolic grounds, and pending more data, this is in my view a suitable COC for selected older women, especially above age 45.

In the 'contraceptive gap' of the years leading to the menopause, potentially fertile women would like to continue to be allowed some kind of oestrogen-plus-progestogen hormonal contraception for the prevention of gynaecological pathology, as well as for the reassurance of regular bleeds (see pages 227–230). Current teaching is largely based on the epidemiological data of the RCGP study. I argue that that study, of rather high-dose pill brands by modern standards, does not apply to a modern contraceptive/hormone replacement regimen. That modern ideal would probably provide natural oestrogen, combined with the most appropriate progestogen given in the lowest dose necessary for contraception and to prevent carcinoma of the uterus – and provide both by a portal of entry by-passing the liver. Various options are under investigation (see page 230).

It will take time and further research to prove that the benefits of these proposed regimens do outweigh the risks. But they would improve the present bizarre situation in which older women are prescribed hormone replacement pills which may not be fully contraceptive and may be no *safer* than their previous contraceptive pills. Yet years earlier they stopped the latter because careful doctors told them they were too old!

Pill myths

This chapter on practical prescribing may appropriately be concluded by summarizing (Tables 5.11 and 5.12) some of the myths which still have widespread credence [50]. They may need to be dispelled when counselling prospective or current pill-takers.

Table 5.11 Some myths about modern low-dose COCs

Myth *Do not prescribe if:*	*Fact* *The low-dose COC is:*
1. Desire to optimize future fertility	Beneficial, by protecting against pelvic infection, fibroids etc. (p. 44, 45)
2. Desire to reduce risk of birth defects	No excess risk of birth defects (p. 86)
3. Fibroids	Beneficial* (p. 44)
4. Benign breast disease	Beneficial* (p. 53)
5. Past amenorrhoea	Neutral, *may* be beneficial (p. 72)
6. Recent menarche	Neutral, if periods established [3]
7. Varicose veins	Neutral (unless with obesity = RC, past thrombophlebitis = AC) (p. 70)
8. Thrush	Neutral (p. 46)
9. Sickle-cell trait	Neutral (p. 72)
10. Sickle-cell disease	RC (fairly strong) (p. 72)
11. Abnormal cervical cytology, during and after any treatment	RC* (Table 5.3 and pp. 62–63)
12. Epilepsy	RC (But special handling of drug interactions) (pp. 48, 81–82)
13. Migraine, tolerable and non-focal	RC (If focal = AC) (p. 84)
14. Past hypertension in pregnancy	RC

RC, Relative contraindication; may use COC with careful monitoring
AC, Absolute contraindication
See this chapter for discussion and references, or Chapters 3 and 4

Table 5.12 Some myths about follow-up management of the COC

Myth *Women should discontinue the COC:*	*Fact*
1. If they have not had a break in last 5 years	Breaks convey no known benefit
2. If they are past age 35	Non-smokers without risk factors may continue to 45 or longer if a therapeutic indication
3. If they have used it altogether for more than 10 years	20 years' use is acceptable for non-smokers upon request (maybe more)
4. If they are about to have *any* surgery	Need only stop before elective major surgery and surgery to legs
5. If they do not see withdrawal bleeds (WTB), to preserve future fertility	This is a pointless action as WTB is related only to the response of the end-organ (the endometrium)
And, finally, perhaps the most interesting myth:	
6. That if pills are forgotten the most 'risky' is one in the middle of a packet	This is hardly a problem: what matters is what women often refer to as 'starting my pack a bit late'

See text of this chapter for full discussion of all these myths

References

1. NATIONAL ASSOCIATION OF FAMILY PLANNING DOCTORS. Interim guidelines for doctors following the pill scare. *British Journal of Family Planning*, **9**, 120–122 (1984)
2. GUILLEBAUD, J. *Contraception – Your Questions Answered*. Churchill Livingstone, Edinburgh, p. 119 (1985)
3. GUILLEBAUD, J. *The Pill*. Oxford University Press, Oxford (1987)
4. STEEL, J. M. and DUNCAN, L. J. The progestogen-only contraceptive pill in insulin dependent diabetics. *British Journal of Family Planning*, **6**, 108–110 (1981)

5. KAY, C. Present perspectives and clinical implications. *Journal of Obstetrics and Gynaecology*, **4** [Suppl.], S98–S102 (1984)
6. JACOBS, H. S. The care of patients with past and present amenorrhoea. *British Journal of Family Planning*, **4** [Suppl.], S2–S5 (1987)
6a. JICK, H., DINAH, B, HERMAN, R. and ROTHMAN, K. J. Myocardial infarction and other vascular diseases in young women. *Journal of the American Medical Association*, **240,** 2548–2552 (1978)
7. GUILLEBAUD, J. *Contraception – Your Questions Answered.* Churchill Livingstone, Edinburgh, pp. 111–115 (1985)
8. EVANS, D. I. Sickle cells and hormonal contraception. *British Journal of Family Planning*, **3,** 80–81 (1984)
9. SERJEANT, G. R. Pregnancy and contraception. In *Sickle Cell Disease*. Oxford University Press, Oxford, pp. 287–288 (1985)
10. SAPIRE, K. E. *Contraception and Sexuality in Health and Disease.* McGraw-Hill, Johannesburg, pp. 255–262 (1986)
11. ORME, M. L'E., BACK D. J., BRECKENRIDGE, A. M. Drug interactions with oral contraceptive steroids. *British Journal of Family Planning*, **10** [Suppl.], 19–26 (1984)
12. AHLUWALIA, D. V., CURRY, C. L., CROCKER, C. L. and VERMA, P. S. Evidence of higher ethynylestradiol blood levels in human hypertensive oral contraceptive users. *Fertility and Sterility*, **28,** 627–630 (1977)
13. GUILLEBAUD, J. *Contraception – Your Questions Answered.* Churchill Livingstone, Edinburgh, pp. 126–131 (1985)
14. SAPIRE, K. E., *Contraception and Sexuality in Health and Disease.* McGraw-Hill, Johannesburg, p. 70 (1986)
15. GILLMER, M. D., BOUNDS, W., GUILLEBAUD, J. *et al.* Failure of withdrawal bleeding on oral contraception. Workshop on Fertility Control. *Royal Society of Medicine International Congress and Symposium Series*, **31,** 32–37 (1980)
16. DICKEY, R. P. Initial pill selection and managing the contraceptive pill patient. *International Journal of Gynaecology and Obstetrics*, **16,** 547–555 (1979)
17. SAPIRE, K. E. *Contraception and Sexuality in Health and Disease*, McGraw-Hill, Johannesburg, pp. 62–63 (1986)
18. MOLLOY, B. G., COULSON, K. A., LEE, J. M., WATTERS, J. K. "Missed pill" conception: fact or fiction? *British Medical Journal*, **290,** 1474–1475 (1985)
19. SMITH, S. K., KIRKMAN, R. J., ARCE, B. B. *et al.* The effect of deliberate omission of Trinordiol or Microgynon on the hypothalamo–pituitary–ovarian axis. *Contraception*, **34,** 513–522 (1986)
20. KILLICK, S., EYONG, E. and ELSTEIN, M. Ovarian follicular development in oral contraceptive cycles. *Fertility and Sterility*, **48,** 409–413 (1987)
21. GUILLEBAUD, J. Contraception and Sterilisation in the Puerperium. In *Textbook of Obstetrics:* (ed Turnbull A. C. and Chamberlain G. V.), Churchill Livingstone, Edinburgh (in press)
22. HATHERLEY, L. I. Lactation and post partum infertility: the use-effectiveness of natural family planning (NFP) after term pregnancy. *Clinical Reproduction and Fertility*, **3,** 319–334 (1985)
23. GUILLEBAUD, J. The forgotten pill – and the paramount importance of the pill-free week. *British Journal of Family Planning*, **12** [Suppl.], S35–S43 (1987)
24. WANG, E., SHI, S., CEKAN, S. Z. *et al.* Hormone consequences of 'missing the pill'. *Contraception*, **26,** 545–566 (1982)
25. FAMILY PLANNING INFORMATION SERVICE. *How to Take the Combined Oral Contraceptive Pill (Method Instruction Sheet)*. Family Planning Association and Health Education Authority, London (1987)
26. SPARROW, M. J. Pill method failures. *New Zealand Medical Journal*, **100,** 102–105 (1987)
27. DEMACKER, P. N., SCHADE, R. W., STALENHOEF, A. F. *et al.* Influence of contraceptive pill and menstrual cycle on serum lipids and high-density lipoprotein cholesterol concentrations. *British Medical Journal*, **284,** 1213–1215 (1982)
28. LOUDON, N. B., FOXWELL, M., POTTS, D. M. *et al.* Acceptability of an oral contraceptive that reduces the frequency of menstruation: the tricycle pill regimen. *British Medical Journal*, **2,** 487–490 (1977)
29. GRIMMER, S. F. and ORME, M. L'E. The basic pharmacology, pharmacokinetics and drug interactions of hormonal contraceptives. *British Journal of Family Planning*, **12,** 38–42 (1986)
30. DERAY, G., LE HOANG, P., CACOUB, P. *et al.* Oral contraceptive interaction with cyclosporin. *Lancet* **1,** 158–159 (1987)

31. BRECKENRIDGE, A. and ORME, M. L'E. Measurement of plasma warfarin concentrations. In *Biological Effects of Drugs in Relation to Their Plasma Concentrations*. (ed. Davis, D. S. and Pritchard, B. N.) Macmillan, London, pp. 145–154 (1973)
32. MATTSON, R. H., CRAMER, J. A., DARNEY, P. D. and NAFTOLIN, F. Use of oral contraceptives by women with epilepsy. *Journal of the American Medical Association*, **256,** 238–248 (1986)
33. KHAW, K. T. and PEART, W.S. Blood pressure and contraceptive use. *British Medical Journal*, **285,** 403–406 (1982)
34. LIM, K. G., ISLES, C. G., HODSMAN, G. P. *et al.* Malignant hypertension in women of childbearing age and its relation to the contraceptive pill. *British Medical Journal*, **294,** 1057–1059 (1987)
35. STATISTICAL BUREAU. Metropolitan Life Insurance Company – based on the experience of 26 companies, 1935–1954 (1956).
36. PRITCHARD, J. A. and PRITCHARD, S. A. Blood pressure response to estrogen–progestin oral contraceptive after pregnancy-induced hypertension. *American Journal of Obstetrics and Gynecology*, **129,** 733–739 (1977)
37. BICKERSTAFF, E. R. *Neurological Complications of Oral Contraceptives*. Oxford University Press, Oxford, pp. 16–39, 81–86 (1975)
38. GUILLEBAUD, J. Surgery and the pill. *British Medical Journal*, **291,** 498–499 (1985)
39. SUE-LING, H. and HUGHES, L. E. Should the pill be stopped preoperatively? *British Medical Journal*, **296,** 447–448 (1988)
40. GUILLEBAUD, J. Should the pill be stopped preoperatively? *British Medical Journal*, **296,** 786–787 (1988)
41. VESSEY, M. P., MEISLER, Z. and FLAVEL, R. Outcome of pregnancy in women using different methods of contraception. *British Journal of Obstetrics and Gynaecology*, **86,** 548 (1979)
42. WORLD HEALTH ORGANISATION (WHO). *The Effect of Female Sex Hormones on Fetal Development and Infant Health.* Report of a WHO scientific group. WHO Technical Report Series, **657.** WHO, Geneva (1981)
43. SAPIRE, K. E. *Contraception and Sexuality in Health and Disease*. McGraw-Hill, Johannesburg, pp. 110–111 (1986)
44. KRICKER, A., ELLIOTT, J. W., FORREST, J. M. and MCCREDIE, J. Congenital limb reduction deformities and use of oral contraceptives. *American Journal of Obstetrics and Gynecology*, **155,** 1072–1078 (1986)
45. GUILLEBAUD, J. *Contraception – Your Questions Answered.* Churchill Livingstone, Edinburgh, pp. 152–153 (1985)
46. JACOBS, H. S., KNUTH, D. A., HULL, M. G. and FRANKS, S. Post-pill amenorrhoea – cause or coincidence? *British Medical Journal*, **2,** 940–942 (1977)
47. VESSEY, M. P., WRIGHT, M. H., MCPHERSON, K. and WIGGINS, P. Fertility after stopping different methods of contraception. *British Medical Journal*, **1,** 265–267 (1978)
48. VESSEY, M. P., SMITH, M. A. and YEATES, D. Return of fertility after discontinuation of oral contraceptives. *British Journal of Family Planning*, **11,** 120–124 (1986)
49. GUILLEBAUD, J. *Contraception – Your Questions Answered.* Churchill Livingstone, Edinburgh, pp. 135–137 (1985)
50. GRUBB, G. S. Women's perceptions of the safety of the pill: a survey in eight developing countries. *Journal of Biosocial Science*, **19,** 313–321 (1987)

Chapter 6

The progestogen-only pill

K. Fotherby

'The Minipill – a limited alternative for certain women' was the title of a review of the progestogen-only pill (POP) in 1975 [1]. Unfortunately, the subsequent decade has seen little change in this viewpoint, although the POP with its many advantages deserves to be more widely used. Currently, its share of the oral contraceptive market is less than 7% in the UK, about 4% in Australia and less than 0.5% in the USA. In 1983, about 300 000 women in the UK were using a POP. This low usage largely reflects a reluctance on the part of the pharmaceutical companies to actively promote the POP. However, the advantages of the POP become more relevant as the limitations on the use of combined oestrogen–progestogen contraceptives increase, and the POP should be offered an equal place with other contraceptive methods.

Two comprehensive reviews of the POP have been published [1, 2] and these are supplemented by two further articles [3, 4].

Four progestogens (Figure 6.1) are formulated as POPs. All are 19-nor-steroids and two, lynoestrenol and ethynodiol diacetate, are rapidly converted *in vivo* in humans to norethisterone.

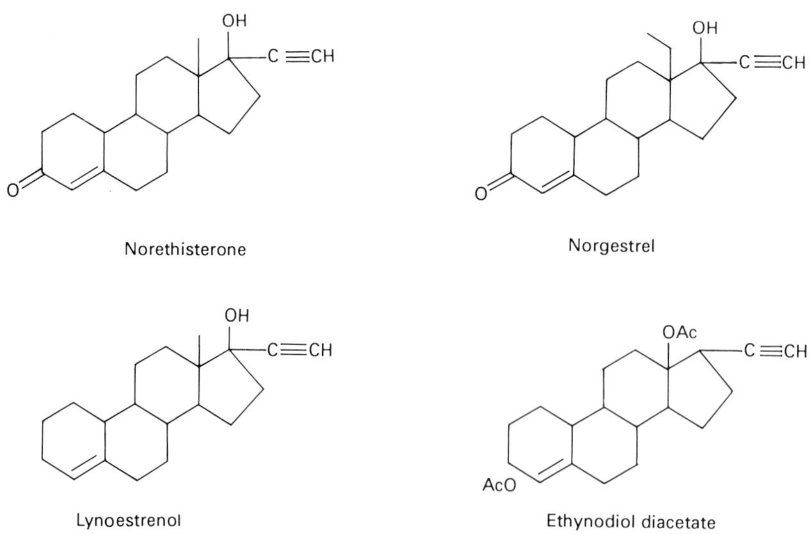

Figure 6.1 Progestogens formulated as progestogen-only pills.

Efficacy

Cumulative results from a number of multicentre trials of the POP are shown in Table 6.1. Since 1976 when these values were tabulated, only three large-scale clinical trials have been reported. The values in Table 6.1 are still the most relevant ones because they involve large numbers of woman-years of treatment and give a realistic idea of failure rates. A failure rate of less than 3 per 100 woman-years of use would appear to be acceptable for a contraceptive method (Table 6.1), particularly if it has advantages over a method with a higher efficacy. Reduction of the daily dose below that shown in Table 6.1 usually leads to an increased pregnancy rate although, suprisingly, Ruis-Velasco *et al.* [5] found that doses of ethynodiol diacetate of 250 to 500 μg/day were equally effective. Increasing the daily dose usually leads to an increased incidence of irregular bleeding.

The results of a few further clinical trials of the POP have been reported since the values in Table 6.1 were published in 1977. Postlethwaite [6] studied 309 women using ethynodiol diacetate for a total of 9566 cycles; six pregnancies occurred, two in women who missed tablets for 1 and 2 weeks. Based on the four tablet failures, the pregnancy rate (Pearl index) was 0.52 (confidence limits 0.14–1.33) per 100 woman-years. Lawson [7] reported the results of a multicentre trial involving 11 921 cycles of norethisterone 350 μg daily in 913 women. Of the 22 pregnancies which occurred, eight were in women who omitted to take the formulation and the remaining 14 in women who reported that they took the tablets regularly. The overall and method failure rates (Pearl index) were 2.2 and 1.4 per 100 woman-years respectively.

In a randomized double-blind trial carried out in two centres in Yugoslavia and India [8], two POPs (norethisterone 350 μg and levonorgestrel 30 μg) were compared with two combined oral contraceptives (COC) containing the same progestogens (150 μg levonorgestrel + 30 μg ethinyloestradiol and 1 mg norethisterone + 50 μg mestranol) in 518 women over 6092 cycles. Of the 34 pregnancies, 28 occurred in the Indian centre and 22 of these resulted from poor compliance with the instructions, whereas only one of the six pregnancies in Yugoslavia resulted from poor compliance. Twenty-two pregnancies occurred in women taking the POP, and the cumulative net life-table pregnancy rates after two years of use of the POP (9.5 for levonorgestrel and 19.6 for norethisterone) were not significantly different from those of the corresponding combined oral contraceptive. From the data supplied it is not possible to compute the Pearl index without making certain assumptions, but approximate values would be less than 2 per 100 woman-years for levonorgestrel and less than 4 for norethisterone.

Table 6.1 Cumulative results of multicentre trials of progestogens administered daily (from [2])

Progestogen	*Dose (μg daily)*	*Trade name*	*No. of woman-months of treatment*	*No. of women*	*Pregnancy rate (Pearl index)*
Ethynodiol diacetate	500	Femulen	24 534	2 420	2.1
Lynoestrenol	500	Exluton	37 405	4 731	0.9
Norethisterone	350	Micronor, Noriday	26 173	2 925	2.3
dl-Norgestrel	75	Neogest	20 006	2 202	2.4
Levonorgestrel	30	Microval, Norgeston	36 118	3 318	3.0

Vessey *et al.* [9] obtained an overall failure rate of 0.9 pregnancies per 100 woman-years during a total period of use of 3303 woman-years; about one-half of the 30 pregnancies which occurred might have been due to incorrect pill taking. Most of the women were using norethisterone 350 μg daily. In a recent trial of Femulen [10] involving 425 women, the overall pregnancy rate was 1.6 per 100 woman-years (0.6 method failure, 1.0 patient failure); the total number of woman-years of use was not stated.

Although for most of the trials the efficacy appears to be satisfactory, in some trials unacceptably high pregnancy rates have been reported. The cause of this variation is not apparent, but may reflect inadequate counselling of the subjects and non-compliance with the strict regime of tablet taking. As discussed below, it may be necessary with the POP to ingest it regularly at the same time each day, to relate administration to the pattern of sexual behaviour of the subjects, and to ensure that no tablets are missed. Also, the large variations between subjects in their metabolism of the POP and in their sensitivity at the target-organ level may imply that the dose, which is critical, whilst suitable for most women, may be inadequate for a few.

The pregnancy rate with the POP appears to decrease with age [11]. In women aged 25–29 years the pregnancy rate was reported to be 3.8 per 100 woman-years falling to 2.9 in women aged 30–34 years and to only 0.8 in women over 35 years of age. This finding has been confirmed in a more recent analysis of the Oxford/FPA study [9]. Failure rates decreased from 3.1 pregnancies per 100 woman-years in women aged 25–29 to only 0.3 in those over 40 years of age.

There is still controversy regarding the incidence of ectopic pregnancies in women using POPs. Bonnar [12] and Hawkins [13], and more recently WHO [8], found an incidence of 1–2 ectopic pregnancies per 100 woman-years of use, whereas Lawson [7] reported an incidence of only 0.3 per 100 woman-years. In the Oxford/FPA study [9], only one of 23 pregnancies which were not terminated was ectopic in 3303 woman-years of use. Bergsjo et al. [14] encountered nine tubal pregnancies in Norwegian women using 300 μg norethisterone daily, and although they could not relate these to the total use of this steroid, they considered that this figure represented an increased incidence, a conclusion also arrived at by Liukko et al. [15] for Finnish women. The latter authors further suggested that whereas the risk was about one ectopic pregnancy per 250–300 woman-years of use with 300 μg norethisterone or 30 μg levonorgestrel, it was very much lower (1 per 1170 woman-years) for 500 μg lynoestrenol; this finding is surprising in view of the known conversion of lynoestrenol to norethisterone *in vivo* and, if true, must result from the higher dose of lynoestrenol compared to norethisterone.

These findings have been interpreted to suggest that the POP might be less effective in preventing ectopic pregnancies than intrauterine ones or, by inhibiting the mobility of the Fallopian tubes, might delay ovum transport and provide an increased opportunity for extrauterine implantation. However, the overall incidence of ectopic pregnancies appears to have increased in most countries during the past two decades [16, 17] and this has to be taken into account in assessing the incidence of ectopic pregnancies in POP users. From the clinical point of view women using POPs who present with symptoms of abdominal pain occurring after a light, delayed or missed period should be adequately investigated to exclude an ectopic pregnancy, and the possibility of pregnancy should not be dismissed just because she is using a steroidal contraceptive. A previous ectopic pregnancy is not an absolute contraindication to the POP, but clearly a combined oral contraceptive is preferred to protect the remaining Fallopian tube.

Clinical side-effects

Non-menstrual side-effects

Non-menstrual side-effects appear to be minor and are usually considered to be less than those observed with combined oral contraceptives. Many women who have discontinued combined oral contraceptives because of side-effects appear not to have experienced them on using the POP. However, comparative trials of the POP and combined oral contraceptives show little difference in the incidence of non-menstrual side-effects [8, 18, 19]. In the WHO study there was little difference between the four preparations tested (norethisterone 1 mg + mestranol 50 μg, levonorgestrel 150 μg + ethinyloestradiol 30 μg, norethisterone 350 μg, and levonorgestrel 30 μg), except that discontinuations were highest for gastrointestinal symptoms (nausea, vomiting) with the levonorgestrel–oestrogen formulation and lowest with this formulation for central nervous system symptoms (headache, dizziness). In assessing the significance of the incidence of side-effects in contraceptive trials, the findings of trials such as those performed by Aznar-Ramos et al. [20] and Goldzieher et al. [21, 22], which showed no significant difference between women taking an oral contraceptive and those taking a placebo, are important.

The POP does not appear to affect either the systolic or diastolic blood pressure. This was apparent from the early short-term (6 months) longitudinal study of Spellacy and Birk [23], using either norgestrel or ethynodiol diacetate. No changes were found in prospective studies over 2 years in women using norethisterone (350 μg) or norgestrel (75 μg) daily [7, 24]. An increased frequency of functional ovarian cysts often associated with pain has been demonstrated by ultrasound in women using a POP [25]. These cysts seem to disappear on discontinuation of the POP.

Menstrual side-effects

Disturbance of the menstrual pattern is regarded as the major disadvantage of the POP, and irregular bleeding, usually with an increase in the frequency, is the main cause of women discontinuing use. These changes in menstrual bleeding have been examined in detail [1, 2]. In women using the POP, the proportion of cycles of 25–35 days in length is about 55–65% compared to more than 80% in untreated women, whereas the proportion of cycles of less than 24 days is increased up to 30% compared to less than 5% in untreated women. Comparative trials also show the difference between POPs and combined oral contraceptives; Vessey et al. [18] found the proportion of cycles of length 25–31 days in women using POPs to be about 30% lower than in women using combined oral contraceptives. However, the high-dose oral contraceptives in use at that time would have magnified the difference between the two types of contraceptives. In the WHO Study [8], discontinuation for bleeding disturbances amongst women using POPs was similar to that of women using norethisterone 1 mg + mestranol 50 μg, but significantly higher than that of women using levonorgestrel 150 μg + ethinyloestradiol 30 μg. There was no significant difference, however, between the two POPs in the incidence of irregular bleeding or discontinuations for menstrual disturbances.

Another important aspect of the menstrual disturbances noted in trials is that as use of the POP continues, the percentage of short cycles shows a decrease. This partly reflects that women who experience a marked effect or find it inconvenient discontinue use of the POP, and is partly an actual decrease in the menstrual irregularity. In the trial of Postlethwaite [6], about 100 women completed 36 cycles of treatment and 22 completed 84 cycles, but only 15% of the women discontinued because of irregular bleeding. This suggests that, for the majority of the women, disturbance of the menstrual pattern was not marked enough to be considered important. An increased proportion of cycles of normal length and a decrease in short cycles with duration of treatment is evident from the data of Lawson [7]. Ferrari et al. [26] also suggested that the increasing proportion of cycles of normal length with continued treatment was *not* an artefact due to women with irregular cycles withdrawing, and in a group of women who had used norgestrel for 28–88 months [27] the frequency distribution of cycle lengths was similar to that of normal women. In respect of the duration and quality of the menstrual flow a summary of the findings [1] suggests that there are no major changes compared to pretreatment values.

From the clinical point of view what is important is the group of women who show very prolonged cycles (greater than 45 days, up to 12% of women) or amenorrhoea (varying from 3% to 15% depending upon definition), since the possibility of pregnancy would arise. Now that simple, quick methods of pregnancy testing are available, this possibility is easily checked. Although there is no evidence to suggest that administration of low doses of progestogens as in the POP is associated with a teratogenic effect [28], it would of course be good practice not to continue the POP if the woman were pregnant.

Oestrogen administration should not be used to attempt the control of irregular bleeding since this would negate one of the advantages of the POP and, more importantly, may counteract the chief contraceptive effect of the progestogen on the cervical mucus. Changes in the vasculature of the endometrium in women using a POP have recently been described [29], and may be related to the high incidence of irregular bleeding in these women.

Return of fertility after discontinuation

The POP does not produce a delay in the return of fertility after discontinuation, and prolonged post-pill amenorrhoea, occasionally reported after discontinuation of COCs, is seen less often. The occurrence of pregnancies in women using the POP or after missing pills shows that there is no long-lasting inhibition of fertility. This has been borne out by reports of the frequency of pregnancy amongst women who have discontinued the POP. Of six women in the trial of norgestrel by Eckstein et al. [30], who discontinued to become pregnant, all succeeded within 6 months. Similarly 13 of 14 women who stopped using norethisterone to become pregnant, did so within 6 months [31]. Sixteen women who had used lynoestrenol for at least 1 year and stopped in order to become pregnant conceived within 3 months [32]; all had normal pregnancies and all infants were healthy. In the Oxford/FPA study [9], 83 women discontinued the POP to become pregnant. Compared to women who had discontinued use of a diaphragm to become pregnant, rates in the POP group were less favourable but the differences were not statistically significant.

POP in lactating women

Lactation is widely regarded as being a contraindication for use of COCs, since they may reduce lactation and there is the possibility (although evidence to support it is lacking) that the transfer of the steroid to the infant in milk may have adverse effects.

In contrast, the POP is eminently suitable for use in lactating women. Progestogens when administered alone appear not to reduce the volume of milk secreted nor the duration of lactation, and some reports suggest that they may increase both [1, 33]. The proportion of the POP administered to the mother which is transferred in the milk appears to be very small and is unlikely to present a hazard to the infant. Of eight women receiving norethisterone 300 μg daily [34], four had no detectable amounts of the steroid in the milk 3–5 h after pill administration, whilst in the remaining four the concentrations were below 350 pg/ml; similar amounts were reported in another study [35], although a third study reported concentrations of 370–790 pg/ml 4 h after administration and 108–287 pg/ml at 24 h [36].

Because of the smaller dose of norgestrel used as a POP, the concentrations in milk are lower than those of norethisterone. In five women receiving 30 μg levonorgestrel daily, Nilsson et al. [37] could not detect any of the steroid even at early times after administration but others [38] have reported concentrations of 38–135 pg/ml at unspecified times after administration. Using daily doses of levonorgestrel of 50 μg, the concentration at 2–3 h after administration was 50–200 pg/ml [35] and undetectable after 4 h. It seems, therefore, that the amount of the POP being transferred to the milk of lactating women is very small – too small to have any significant effect. As expected, the highest concentration of the progestogen in milk occurs in the first 4 h after administration of the POP; if we assume, e.g. for norethisterone, a concentration of 400 pg/ml milk and the infant ingests 100 ml milk, the amount it receives is 40 000 pg. Assuming a body weight of 5 kg, and an even distribution of the steroid, the concentration would be only 8 pg/ml. This calculation assumes that no metabolism of the steroid by the infant occurs, and this concentration would be below the limit of sensitivity of present methods of estimating the progestogen. This agrees with the findings [37, 39] that no progestogen was detected in the blood of suckling infants of women using progestogens.

In a study involving 84 lactating women [40] using 350 μg norethisterone daily, 44% were still using it 6 months postpartum and it appeared to have no adverse effect on breast-feeding. In this group of women, a high proportion (68%) of those breast-feeding for over 5 months were amenorrhoeic, so that the main problem with the POP – irregular bleeding – was not important.

A number of studies have provided limited information that the POP does not affect the composition of the milk. Gupta et al. [41] studied 30 Indian women receiving 50 μg norgestrel daily over a period of 4½ months after delivery and found no change in milk volume or the quality of the milk compared to a control group. In another study [42], using 30 μg levonorgestrel daily, the drop-out rate was high but over a 3-month period there were no significant changes in milk volume or in the concentration of total nitrogen, non-protein nitrogen, a number of important proteins, and lactose. Betancourt et al. [43] compared 76 lactating women receiving 500 μg lynoestrenol daily to similar numbers of women using an IUD or a barrier method of contraception; there were no significant differences between groups in the growth pattern of the infants as measured by body weight, length, and head circumference. The quality of milk produced was not decreased by the POP and the average duration of breast-feeding did not decrease over the 6 months of the study. There was no difference between the groups in the time of starting supplementary feeds.

Unlike the COC, the POP does not affect lactation or the risk of venous thrombosis, and it is possible to start it in the immediate postpartum period. However, there is some evidence that an increase in the number of discontinuations because of abnormal bleeding (increased lochia) may result (Unpublished observation). Hence, in the UK the Family Planning Association and similar bodies now recommend delaying commencement until about 4 weeks after childbirth.

The usefulness of the POP in lactating women has recently been evaluated in two large studies, each involving 200 or more subjects [71, 72].

Metabolic effects

The POP produces few metabolic changes and those which do occur are minor ones.

Carbohydrate metabolism

The combined oral contraceptive affects the blood glucose and insulin responses to an oral glucose tolerance test, whereas a large number of early investigations showed that the POP produced little, if any, effect. These findings were confirmed [44] in a group of women using 500 μg ethynodiol diacetate daily, and this treatment also did not affect the levels of glycohaemoglobin (Hb A_1). However, in eight Cuban women treated with 350 μg norethisterone acetate daily for two months, significant deterioration of glucose tolerance occurred [45]. Spellacy et al. [46] published the results of a prospective study of 50 women studied before and after 18 months use of 75 μg norgestrel daily; they found significant increases in the fasting glucose concentration and the glucose and insulin responses to an oral glucose tolerance test. In eight women the response to an oral glucose tolerance test was classified as abnormal.

The effect of the POP in diabetic women was investigated by Radberg et al. [47, 48]. Twenty-three women with insulin-dependent diabetes were allocated randomly to a POP (lynoestrenol 500 μg daily) or a combined oral contraceptive (lynoestrenol 2.5 mg, ethinyloestradiol 50 μg daily). After 6 months treatment, the subjects had two-months without medication and this was followed by 6-months use of the other formulation. During treatment with the COC, 13 of 23 women required an increased insulin dose and there was an increase in urinary glucose excretion, although the fasting blood sugar concentration did not change; similar changes were observed during treatment with the POP except that the insulin requirement was less. In a second study using a similar crossover design, women who had had diabetes during pregnancy were investigated using an intravenous glucose tolerance test. During treatment with the COC all women showed a lower glucose tolerance compared to only one in the POP group; no significant difference occurred in either the fasting blood glucose level or the insulin response. The authors conclude that lynoestrenol alone had little effect on glucose tolerance in women predisposed to diabetes. Steel and Duncan [49] reported on the use of 350 μg norethisterone daily in 50 insulin-dependent diabetic young women over a period of 1050 woman-months of use. No increase in insulin dosage appeared necessary and the women took the pill at the time of their insulin injection. Only one pregnancy occurred – in a woman who missed taking a number of pills. Disturbance of the menstrual pattern was not a problem. No significant changes occurred in the incidence or severity of retinopathy during the period of observation. Spellacy [50] reported that of the low-dose POP formulations, norethisterone produced only mild changes in blood glucose and insulin levels, ethynodiol diacetate produced moderate changes, and norgestrel marked ones. These conclusions, however, do not appear to be supported by a consensus of the results [51].

Lipid metabolism

Early studies [2] showed that the POP had little effect on a number of aspects of lipid metabolism such as blood concentrations of cholesterol, triglycerides, free fatty acids and phospholipids. However, these studies were performed before the importance of the lipoproteins was recognized. Subsequent studies have confirmed the earlier findings and show no significant changes in high-density lipoprotein cholesterol [47, 52], although others [53] have suggested a small reduction in HDL_2.

Blood coagulation

The extensive studies of Poller [54] showed that chlormadinone acetate 500 µg daily did not affect a large number of haematological measurements, and numerous other studies [2, 55] have shown that the POP, unlike COCs, does not affect blood clotting and platelet aggregation. Ylikorkala et al. [56] measured the levels of two prostaglandins which have important effects on platelet–vascular interactions; prostacyclin (PGI_2), produced in the vascular endothelium, causes vasodilatation and is a potent inhibitor of platelet aggregation, whereas thromboxane A_2, produced in platelets, causes vasoconstriction and enhances platelet aggregation. They performed a cross-sectional comparison of a group of women using various POPs (nine using levonorgestrel 30 µg daily, nine lynoestrenol 500 µg daily, and six norethisterone 300 µg daily; mean duration of use 3.7 ± 2.0 years), with a control group and a group using various COCs. Prostacyclin concentrations were decreased in women using COCs but not in the POP group. COCs did not affect thromboxane concentrations but these were depressed in the POP group, particularly in women using levonorgestrel. This is evidence against the likelihood of an increased risk of thrombosis during the use of POPs.

Miscellaneous effects

The POP appears to have little effect on liver function whether this is assessed by bromsulphthalein excretion or by measurement of blood enzyme activity, mainly transaminases [2, 45]. The hepatic synthesis and secretion of a large number of different proteins can be stimulated by administration of oestrogens; these proteins are involved in a large range of physiological functions, e.g. transport of hormones, vitamins, and minerals, control of aldosterone secretion, and immunological processes. The stimulatory effects of oestrogen can be suppressed to varying extents by concomitant administration of a progestogen, because of its antioestrogenic activity. The extent of the suppression depends on the nature and dose of the progestogen and on the particular protein measured. However, progestogens administered alone have little if any effect on the blood concentrations of these proteins [51, 57]. Ultrastructural changes in liver-cell morphology, detectable by electron microscopy but not by light microscopy, have been observed in liver biopsies from women using the POP [2] but the significance of these results is difficult to assess.

The POP does not appear to affect thyroid or pituitary–adrenocortical function. Administration of various formulations did not affect protein-bound iodine or thyroxine concentrations, tri-iodothyronine uptake, or the free thyroxine index [2, 45]. Similarly, no changes have been detected in pituitary–adrenal function as assessed by plasma cortisol levels, cortisol secretion rate, response to ACTH or metyrapone stimulation, or dexamethasone suppression and the free cortisol index [2].

Mechanism of action

Effect on pituitary–ovarian function

The original investigations of Martinez-Manautou et al. [58] with chlormadinone acetate suggested that ovulation was not always inhibited. More detailed studies [59] in women using 50 μg norgestrel daily showed on the basis of urinary hormone estimations (LH, oestrogens, and pregnanediol) that normal ovulatory cycles occurred in about 50% of the women. In the remainder, variable effects were noted; some showed a mid-cycle peak of LH excretion whereas in others it was absent.

Pregnanediol excretion was low in most studies, suggesting a suppression of luteal activity, although less marked effects were observed on oestrogen production. This led to the suggestion that in some women there was deficient luteal function, possibly due to a suppression of LH secretion, and in others possibly due to a direct effect of the progestogen. The progestogen did not interfere with corpus luteum development, since in a study [60] of women undergoing laparotomy during treatment with norgestrel, a histologically normal corpus luteum was present in most instances. The effect of the progestogen seemed to be on corpus luteum function, since progesterone production, studied *in vitro* by these histologically normal corpora lutea, was reduced compared to synthesis of progesterone by corpora lutea from non-treated women [61]. The presence of corpora lutea histologically normal by both light and electron microscopy has been reported by a number of investigators (see [2]). The variable suppression of progesterone and LH production but with a lower effect on oestrogen production, based upon either urinary or blood estimations, has been well documented (see [2]). The main effect appears to be a direct one on the ovary, since the POP, in contrast with COCs, does not inhibit the ability of the pituitary to respond to LHRH [62].

A detailed study of hormonal changes in 43 women using 300 μg norethisterone daily, involving daily blood sampling, has been published [63–65]. A pattern of hormonal changes similar to that seen in a normal ovulation cycle was observed in 40% or ten subjects; 21% had normal follicular activity with suppressed luteal function; 23% had normal or increased follicular activity with no luteal function; and 16% showed no signs of either follicular or luteal function.

In these women, the variable suppression of the ovary was *not* related to the degree of inhibition of pituitary FSH and LH secretion. The pattern of the ovarian reaction to the POP may vary with duration of use; of a group of 21 women, eight who showed an ovulatory pattern of ovarian steroid secretion during the second cycle of use also showed a similar pattern during the sixth cycle. None of the remaining 13 women who showed absent or suppressed luteal function during the second cycle showed normal luteal activity during the sixth, although variability of their ovarian response compared to the second treatment cycle occurred. As hypothesized previously [2], the degree of suppression of progesterone synthesis will depend to a great extent on the intrinsic enzyme activity of any particular corpus luteum.

In a recent study [25], only six of 21 POP users appeared to ovulate normally, and anovulation may be associated with cyst formation in the ovary. Ovulation inhibition by the POP may be increased by concomitant administration of the dopamine antagonist sulpiride [66]. Thus, there is a wide spectrum of response of the ovary to the POP, ranging from almost no effect on ovulation to various degrees of luteal and follicular suppression and anovulation in one direction, as opposed to stimulation of oestrogen secretion in the other. Such wide variability in ovarian steroid secretion may have a marked effect on the bleeding pattern.

Effect on tubal and uterine function

The POP has a marked and variable effect on both the Fallopian tubes and the uterus. Progestogens will affect both tubal contractility and the rate of ovum transport and also affect tubal histology. They may also affect the fertilization process in the Fallopian tube and some suggest they also affect the capacitation of spermatozoa. However, as far as the human is concerned, these effects need to be confirmed with the progestogens currently used as POPs and in their present dose. There is more evidence for an effect of the POP on the endometrium, one obvious effect being the increased incidence of irregular bleeding. Many have reported changes in endometrial histology, particularly during the secretory phase. This is to be expected in view of the variable effects of the POP on ovarian steroid secretion and the administration of POP from day 1 of the cycle.

A detailed study of endometrial morphology in women taking 300 μg norethisterone daily has been reported [65]. An endometrial biopsy was taken and ovarian steroid secretion assessed during a pretreatment cycle and repeated during the second cycle of treatment. In this second cycle, biopsies were taken either between days 23 and 25 or, in those women who showed intermenstrual bleeding, within 6 hours of the onset of the bleeding. The only observable difference between biopsies from those women who had intermenstrual bleeding and those who did not was a larger glandular diameter in the latter; there was no correlation of the endometrial picture with normal or suppressed ovarian function. However, administration of norethisterone produced a number of significant changes in the endometrium: a reduced number of endometrial glands, decreased glandular diameter, a reduction in the amount of double-stranded polynucleotides and DNA per cell nucleus, and an increased number of plasmolemmal vesicles. The proliferative activity of the endometrium was suppressed. Only a minority of the subjects showed a normal secretory endometrium. The extent to which these changes would prevent implantation of the blastocyst is unclear, particularly since the normal endometrial requirements for implantation are not known.

Effect on cervical mucus and sperm penetration

Initial investigations with the POP ascribed its anti-fertility action to an effect on cervical mucus, and numerous studies have shown the amount of mucus at mid-cycle to be markedly reduced and its viscosity greatly increased. These changes are accompanied by a reduced ability of spermatozoa to penetrate the mucus under both *in vitro* and *in vivo* conditions, although a few reports suggest that the block to the passage of spermatozoa *in vivo* is not only the mucus but also some other effect at the endocervical level [1, 2]. Occasionally, mucus samples from treated women do allow sperm penetration [30]. Changes in a number of biochemical constituents of mucus, e.g. proteins and enzyme activities, as well as biophysical changes, occur under the influence of the POP.

The effect of the POP is time-dependent. It has been shown [67–69] that after administration of the POP, the penetrability of mucus by sperm decreases within 2–4 h and remains low for the next 16–20 h before it begins to increase again. These findings suggest that if one of the main sites for the anti-fertility effect of the POP is the cervical mucus, its efficiency will depend on the time at which sexual intercourse takes place in relation to the time of taking the pill. Women, therefore, should be advised to take the POP at the same time each day and to relate the time of taking to their pattern of sexual activity.

The effects of the POP, like COCs are widespread. The actions considered above are ones which can be investigated by existing methodology, and it is highly likely that effects on other processes, e.g. fertilization, which cannot be adequately examined, also occur. These widespread actions of the POP no doubt account for its high efficacy, since this does not seem explainable on the basis of any single one of the effects discussed above.

Starting, changing, and stopping the POP

Advice given to women using or about to use the POP was recently reconsidered by a joint committee representing the Medical Advisory Panel of the Family Planning Association and the National Association of Family Planning Doctors [70]. Women should start the POP preferably on the first day of the menstrual cycle and do not require to use additional contraceptive protection. The POP should be taken at the same time each day. The pills have their greatest effect on the cervical mucus from about 4–20 h after being taken, although other aspects of their contraceptive action, such as effects on ovarian activity, may not be so time-dependent and may indeed be as important in contraceptive efficacy as the action on sperm penetration of the cervical canal. Women should record any changes in menstruation. Menstrual bleeding may become irregular or may be absent altogether. If the period is overdue it is unlikely that the woman is pregnant, provided she has been taking the POP regularly and as advised. If menstruation does not occur, the POP should be continued and the doctor consulted so that the possibility of pregnancy can be excluded.

If a pill is forgotten it should be taken as soon as remembered and the next pill taken at the correct time. If the pill was more than 3 h overdue, contraceptive action may be lost and normal pill-taking should continue but with the use of another method for the next 48 h. If the woman has severe diarrhoea or vomiting, the pill may be poorly absorbed and in addition to the POP, another contraceptive method should be used for the duration of the upset and for the following 48 h.

During short-term use of an enzyme-inducing drug, another method is again advised, but should be continued for the likely duration of the enzyme-induction effect (1–4 weeks).

Women changing from COC should start the POP on the day after the last combined pill and no extra contraceptive precautions are required. When changing from the POP to a COC, the new pill should be started on the first day of bleeding. If the woman has amenorrhoea the COC could be started any time after pregnancy has been excluded.

Summary

Positive attributes of the POP

1. An acceptable efficacy.
2. A good general tolerance – it is suitable for women who complain of side-effects with other contraceptive methods, especially combined pills.

3. Avoidance of side-effects in which oestrogens are implicated.
4. Minimization of side-effects in which progestogens are implicated.
5. Body tissues exposed to lower concentrations of exogenous steroid, and hence less effect on metabolic processes.
6. No consistent inhibition of ovulation, and therefore ready return of fertility on discontinuation.
7. Particularly suitable for women over 45 years of age for whom combined oral contraceptives are contraindicated (over 35 if a cigarette smoker).
8. Particularly suitable for women with hypertension or diabetes, for breast-feeding women, and possibly for those with a risk or past history of thrombosis (in this case, keeping careful records and good counselling are essential, since the data sheets still call the latter a contraindication).
9. With adequate counselling, continuation rates are similar to those for COCs.
10. Start on day one of the menstrual cycle, with no extra contraceptive precautions required; daily administration without a break, obviating the necessity to remember when to start the next pack.
11. Can be started immediately postpartum or post-abortion.

Negative attributes of the POP

1. An efficacy lower than COCs.
2. A high incidence of disturbance of menstruation which is unacceptable to some women.
3. No large-scale epidemiological data to give indication of risk of serious side-effects such as thromboembolism, cerebrovascular disease or coronary heart disease.
4. If pregnancy occurs, there may possibly be an increased risk of an ectopic pregnancy. A past history of the latter is therefore a strong relative contraindication to the POP.
5. Regularity of pill taking is essential. Time of pill-taking in relation to time of sexual intercourse may be critical, and taking the POP before going to bed should be avoided for the 'p.m. lover'; it is better to take it at another regular time.
6. Occurrence of functional ovarian cysts, often associated with pain.

On the basis of present evidence, the POP appears to be a contraceptive method which should be more widely available. Many women will discontinue in the first few months of use because of disturbances of the menstrual pattern, but those women who do continue may find the disturbance lessens. For those who do not experience such disturbances the method is highly acceptable; a number of reports describe groups of women who have used the POP over long periods with confidence and satisfaction. There appears to be no reason why such women should not continue using the POP until they reach the menopause. Diagnosis of the latter can be facilitated by measuring gonadotrophin levels on and off treatment, as well as by noting the presence of vasomotor symptoms. In our present state of knowledge, it is not possible to decide whether any one POP has advantages over the others.

These conclusions have been borne out by two recent reports describing experience of the use of the POP in general family planning clinics in the UK [73, 74]. Many women, and not only those in the older age groups, find the POP acceptable. Both studies found the overall failure rate (Pearl Index) to be less than 1 and recommend a more widespread use of the POP. Similar conclusions have been presented in a recent mini-review of the POP [75].

References

1. RINEHART, W. The Minipill – A limited alternative for certain women. *Population Reports A* No. 3, A53–A67 (1975)
2. FOTHERBY, K. Low doses of gestogens as fertility regulating agents. In *Advances in Fertility Regulation* (ed. E. Diczfaulsy), Scriptor, Copenhagen, pp. 283–321 (1977)
3. FOTHERBY, K. The progestogen-only contraceptive pill. *British Journal of Family Planning*, **8**, 7–10 (1982)
4. GRAHAM, S. and FRASER, I. S. The progestogen-only mini-pill. *Contraception*, **26**, 373–385 (1982)
5. RUIZ-VELASCO, V., MARISCAL, J. D. O., SALGADO, H. J. *et al.* Ethynodiol diacetate as a contraceptive. *Fertility and Sterility*, **25**, 927–934 (1974)
6. POSTLETHWAITE, D. L. Pregnancy rate of a progestogen oral contraceptive. *Practitioner*, **222**, 272–275 (1979)
7. LAWSON, P. J. Experience with norethisterone 0.35 mg daily as an oral contraceptive. *British Journal of Family Planning*, **8**, 84–89 (1982)
8. WORLD HEALTH ORGANIZATION. A randomized double-blind study of two combined and two progestogen-only oral contraceptives. *Contraception*, **25**, 243–252 (1982)
9. VESSEY, M. P., LAWLESS, M., YEATES, D. and MCPHERSON, K. Progestogen-only oral contraception. *British Journal of Family Planning*, **10**, 117–121 (1985)
10. SHROFF, N. D., PEARCE, M. Y., STRATFORD, M. E. and WILKINSON, P. D. Clinical experience with ethynodiol diacetate. *Contraception*, **35**, 121–134 (1987)
11. VESSEY, M., YEATES, D. and FLAVEL, R. Progestogen-only contraceptives In *Current Fertility Control*. John Wyeth, Slough, pp. 1–5 (1979)
12. BONNAR, J. Progestogen-only contraception and tubal pregnancies. *Lancet*, **1**, 170 (1974)
13. HAWKINS, D. F. Progestogen-only contraception and tubal pregnancies. *British Medical Journal*, **1**, 387 (1974)
14. BERGSJO, P., LANGENGEN, H. and AAS, J. Tubal pregnancies in women using progestogen-only contraception. *Acta Obstetricia et Gynecologia Scandinavica*, **53**, 377–378 (1974)
15. LIUKKO, P., ERKKOLA, R. and LAAKSO, L. Ectopic pregnancies during use of low-dose progestogens for oral contraception. *Contraception*, **16**, 575–580 (1977)
16. MERIK, O. Ectopic pregnancy during 1961–78 in Uppsala County, Sweden: Impact of demographic factors on overall incidence. *Acta Obstetricia et Gynecologica Scandinavica*, **60**, 545–548 (1981)
17. ROBINSON, N. and BERAL, V. Risk of ectopic pregnancy. *Lancet*, **2**, 1247–1248 (1979)
18. VESSEY, M. P., MEARS, E., ANDOLSEK, L. and OGRINE-OVEN, M. Randomised double-blind trial of four oral progestogen-only contraceptives. *Lancet*, **1**, 915–922 (1972)
19. PAULSEN, M. L., VARADAY, A., BROWN, B. V. and KALMAN, S. M. A randomized contraceptive trial comparing a daily progestogen with a combined oral contraceptive steroid. *Contraception*, **9**, 497–506 (1974)
20. AZNAR-RAMOS, R., GINER-VELAZQUEZ, J., LARA-RICALDE, R. and MARTINEZ-MANAUTOU, J. Incidence of side effects with contraceptive placebo. *American Journal of Obstetrics and Gynecology*, **105**, 1144–1149 (1969)
21. GOLDZIEHER, J. W., MOSES, L. E., AVERKIN, E. *et al.* A placebo controlled double-blind cross over investigation of the side effects attributed to oral contraceptives. *Fertility and Sterility*, **22**, 609–623 (1971)
22. GOLDZIEHER, J. W., MOSES, L. E., AVERKIN, E. *et al.* Nervousness and depression attributed to oral contraceptives; a double-blind placebo controlled study. *American Journal of Obstetrics and Gynecology*, **111**, 1013–1020 (1971)
23. SPELLACY, W. N. and BIRK, S. A. The effects of mechanical and steroid contraceptive methods on blood pressure in hypertensive women. *Fertility and Sterility*, **25**, 467–470 (1974)
24. WILSON, E. S. B., CRUIKSHANK, J., MCMASTER, M. and WEIR, R. J. A prospective controlled study of the effect on blood pressure of contraceptive preparations. *British Journal of Obstetrics and Gynaecology*, **91**, 1254–1260 (1984)
25. TAYOB, Y., ADAMS, J., JACOBS, H. S. and GUILLEBAUD, J. Ultrasound demonstration of increased frequency of functional ovarian cysts in women using progestogen-only oral contraception. *British Journal of Obstetrics and Gynaecology*, **92**, 1003–1009 (1985)

26. FERRARI, A., MEYRELLES, J. C., SARTORETTO, J. N. and SOARES FILHO, A. The menstrual cycle in women treated with d-norgestrel in continuous administration. *International Journal of Fertility*, **18**, 133 (1973)
27. FOSS, G. L. and FOTHERBY, K. Long term use of daily administration of low doses of norgestrel as an oral contraceptive. *Journal of Biosocial Science*, **7**, 269–272 (1975)
28. WORLD HEALTH ORGANIZATION. *The Effect of Female Sex Hormones on Fetal Development and Infant Health*. Technical Report Series, No. 657 (1981)
29. HOURIHAN, H. M., SHEPPARD, B. L. and BONNER, J. Morphometric study of oral norethisterone or levonorgestrel on endometrial blood vessels. *Contraception*, **34**, 603–612 (1986)
30. ECKSTEIN, P., WHITBY, M., FOTHERBY, K. *et al*. Clinical and laboratory findings in a trial of norgestrel. *British Medical Journal*, **3**, 195–200 (1972)
31. SMITH, M., VESSEY, M. P., BOUNDS, W. and WARREN, J. Progestogen-only oral contraception and ectopic gestation. *British Medical Journal*, **4**, 104–105 (1974)
32. RAVN, J. Pregnancy and progeny after long-term contraceptive treatment with low-dose progestogens. *Current Medical Research and Opinion*, **2**, 616 (1975)
33. AREF, I., BADRAOUI, M. H. H. and HEFNAWI, F. Contraception during lactation. *Contraception Delivery Systems*, **3**, 47–51 (1982)
34. ADEY, T., BROWN, J. B. and FOTHERBY, K. Norethisterone concentrations in milk of lactating women using a progestogen-only pill. *Journal of Obstetrics and Gynaecology*, **3**, 112–113 (1982)
35. TODDYWALLA, V. S., MEHTA, S., KATAYUN, D. V. and SAXENA, B. N. Release of 19-nor-testosterone type of contraceptive steroids through different drug delivery systems into serum and breast milk of lactating women. *Contraception*, **21**, 217–223 (1980)
36. SAXENA, B. N., SHRIMANKER, K. and GRUDZINSKAS, J. G. Levels of contraceptive steroids in breast milk and plasma of lactating women. *Contraception*, **16**, 605–613 (1977)
37. NILSSON, S., NYGREN, K.-G. and JOHANSSON, E. D. B. Norgestrel concentrations in maternal plasma, milk, and child plasma during administration of oral contraceptives to nursing women. *American Journal of Obstetrics and Gynecology*, **129**, 178–184 (1977)
38. THOMAS, M. J., DANUTRA, V., READ, G. F. *et al*. The detection and measurement of norgestrel in human milk using sephadex LH 20 chromatography and radioimmunoassay. *Steroids*, **30**, 349–361 (1977)
39. MELIS, G. B., STRIGINI, F., FRUZZETTI, F. *et al*. Norethisterone enanthate as an injectable contraceptive in puerperal and non-puerperal women. *Contraception*, **23**, 77–88 (1981)
40. WEST, P. C. The acceptability of a progestogen-only contraceptive during breast-feeding. *Contraception*, **27**, 563–569 (1983)
41. GUPTA, A. N., MATHUS, V. S. and GARG, S. K. Effect of oral contraceptives on quantity and quality of milk secretion in human beings. *Indian Journal of Medical Research*, **62**, 964–970 (1974)
42. LONNERDAL, B., FORSUM, E. and HAMBRAEUS, L. Effect of oral contraceptives on composition and volume of breast milk. *American Journal of Clinical Nutrition*, **33**, 816–824 (1980)
43. DELGADO-BETANCOURT, J., SANDEVAL, J. C., SANCHEZ, F. *et al*. Influence of Exluton and the Multiload Cu-250 I.U.D. on lactation. *Contraceptive Delivery Systems*, **5**, 91–95 (1984)
44. BLUM, M., RUSECKY, Y. and GELERNTER, I. Glycohemoglobin levels in oral contraceptive users. *European Journal of Obstetrics, Gynecology, and Reproductive Biology*, **15**, 97–101 (1983)
45. ANDINO, S. Clinical trial of two contraceptive preparations, norethisterone enanthate and norethisterone acetate. *Contraception*, **23**, 141–155 (1981)
46. SPELLACY, W. M., BUHI, W. C. and BIRK, S. A. Prospective studies of carbohydrate metabolism in normal women using norgestrel for 18 months. *Fertility and Sterility*, **35**, 167–171 (1981)
47. RADBERG, T., GUSTAFSON, A., SKRYTEN, A. and KARLSSON, K. Oral contraception in diabetic women: A cross-over study on serum and high density lipoprotein lipids and diabetes control during progestogen and combined estrogen/progestogen contraception. *Hormone and Metabolic Research*, **14**, 61–65 (1982)
48. RADBERG, T., GUSTAFSON, A., SKRYTEN, A. and KARLSSON, K. Metabolic studies in gestational diabetic women during contraceptive treatment: Effects on glucose tolerance and fatty acid composition of serum lipids. *Gynecologic and Obstetric Investigation*, **13**, 17–29 (1982)
49. STEEL, M. J. and DUNCAN, L. J. P. The progestogen only contraceptive pill in insulin dependent diabetics. *British Journal of Family Planning*, **6**, 108–110 (1981)
50. SPELLACY, W. N. Carbohydrate metabolism during treatment with estrogen, progestogen, and low-dose oral contraceptives. *American Journal of Obstetrics and Gynecology*, **142**, 723–734 (1982)

51. FOTHERBY, K. A metabolic assessment of different oral contraceptives. *Journal of Obstetrics and Gynaecology*, **3** [Suppl. 2], S77–S82 (1983)
52. BLUM, M., WERCHEW, M. and GELERNTER, I. Effect of oral contraception by progesterone pill on lipids and glucose metabolism. *Contraceptive Delivery Systems*, **3**, 55–59 (1983)
53. WYNN, V. and NITHTHYANANTHAN, R. The effect of progestins in combined oral contraceptives on serum lipids with special reference to high-density lipoproteins. *American Journal of Obstetrics and Gynecology*, **142**, 766–772 (1982)
54. POLLER, L. Oral contraception, blood coagulation and platelets. In *Recent Advances in Thrombosis*, Churchill Livingstone, London, p. 181 (1973)
55. CONARD, J., SAMAMA, M., HORELLOU, M. H. *et al.* Antithrombin III and oral contraception with progestogen-only preparation. *Lancet*, **2**, 471 (1979)
56. YLIKORKALA, O., PUOLAKKA, J. and VIINIKKA, L. The effect of oral contraceptives on anti-aggregatory prostacyclin and pro-aggregatory thromboxane A in humans. *American Journal of Obstetrics and Gynecology*, **142**, 573–576 (1982)
57. YOUNG, D. L. and CHAN, P. L. Effects of oral contraceptives on lipids. *American Journal of Clinical Nutrition*, **28**, 686–691 (1975)
58. MARTINEZ-MANAUTOU, J., CORTEZ, V., GINER, J. *et al.* Low doses of progestogen as an approach to fertility control. *Fertility and Sterility*, **17**, 49–58 (1966)
59. FOTHERBY, K., SVENDSEN, B. K. and FOSS, G. L. Ovarian function in women receiving low doses of a synthetic progestin, norgestrel. *Journal of Reproduction and Fertility* [Suppl.] **5**, 155–167 (1968)
60. WRIGHT, S. W., FOTHERBY, K. and FAIRWEATHER, P. Effect of daily small doses of norgestrel on ovarian function. *Journal of Obstetrics and Gynaecology of the British Commonwealth*, **77**, 65 (1970)
61. MUKHERJEE, T. K., WRIGHT, S. W., DAVIDSON, N. T. H. and FOTHERBY, K. Effect of norgestrel on corpus luteum function. *Journal of Obstetrics and Gynaecology of the British Commonwealth*, **79**, 175–182 (1972)
62. DERICKS-TAN, J. S. E., KROG, W., AKTORIES, K. and TAUBERT, H.-D. Dose-dependent inhibitions by oral contraceptives of the pituitary to release LH and FSH in response to stimulation with LH-RH. *Contraception*, **14**, 171 (1976)
63. LANGREN, B.-M. and DICZFALUSY, E. Hormonal effects of the 300 µg norethisterone minipill. 1. Daily steroid levels in 43 subjects during a pretreatment cycle and during the second month of NET administration. *Contraception*, **21**, 87–113 (1980)
64. LANDGREN, B.-M., LAGER, S. and DICZFALUSY, E. Hormonal effects of the 300 µg norethisterone minipill. *Contraception*, **23**, 269–298 (1981)
65. JOHANNISSON, E., LANDGREN, B.-M. and DICZFALUSY, E. Endometrial morphology and peripheral steroid levels in women with and without intermenstrual bleeding during contraception with the 300 µg norethisterone minipill. *Contraception*, **25**, 13–31 (1982)
66. PAYNE, M. R., HOWIE, P. W., MCNEILLY, A. S. *et al.* Sulpiride and the potentiation of progestogen only contraception. *British Medical Journal*, **291**, 559–561 (1985)
67. WRIGHT, S., FOTHERBY, K. and DAVIES, J. E. L'effet du d- et du l-norgestrel sur la penetration du mucus cervical par le sperme. *La Revue de Medecine*, **19**, 153–155 (1978)
68. COX, H. J. E. The pre-coital use of mini-dosage progestogens. *Journal of Reproduction and Fertility* [Suppl.], **5**, 167–172 (1968)
69. LEBECH, P. E., SVENDSEN, P. A., OSTERGAARD, E. and MOCH, F. The effects of small doses of megestrol acetate on the cervical mucus. *Acta Obstetricia et Gynecologica Scandinavica*, **48** [Suppl. 3], 22–25 (1969)
70. MILLS, A. The forgotten progestogen-only pill. *British Journal of Family Planning*, **12** [Suppl.], 41–46 (1987).
71. CANTO, T. E., VERA, L., POLANCO, L. E. and COLVEN, C. E. Minipill in lactating women. *Contraception*, **39**, 589–601 (1989)
72. McCANN, M. F., MOGGIA, A. V., HIGGINS, J. E., POTTS, M. and BECKER, C. Effects of a progestogen-only oral contraceptive on breast feeding. *Contraception*, **40**, 635 (1989)
73. BROOME, M. and FOTHERBY, K. Clinical experience with the progestogen-only pill. *Contraception*, in press
74. BISSET, A. M., DINGWALL-FORDYCE, I. and HAMILTON, M. K. Efficacy of the POP as a contraceptive method. *Brit. J. Fam. Plann.* In press (1990)
75. CARDY, G. C. Progestogen-only pills. *Br. J. Sexual Med.*, 492—52 (Feb. 1990)

Chapter 7

Systemic hormonal contraception by non-oral routes

Ian S. Fraser

In practice, the topic of systemic hormonal contraception by non-oral routes covers mainly steroid hormones (oestrogens and progestogens), although the latest developments under investigation also include agents such as gonadotrophin-releasing hormone superanalogues and antiprogestogens. This review will be confined to female methods of contraception.

Steroids can be administered by almost any route including oral, subcutaneous, intramuscular, intravenous, vaginal, intrauterine, intracervical, rectal, intranasal and transdermal. At the present time, only some of these are practicable routes for contraception. The major aims of non-oral administration of contraceptive steroids include long duration of action, continuous and steady steroid blood levels and avoidance of the 'first-pass' effect through the hepatic portal system.

Long-acting hormonal contraception has had a chequered career which revolves around the remarkable injectable progestogen, depot medroxyprogesterone acetate (DMPA; Depo-Provera). A complex major controversy has developed around this contraceptive for reasons which are political and emotional rather than scientific. An understanding of this issue is of some relevance to the acceptance of the concept of prolonged duration hormonal contraception and will be discussed later.

The published literature on these agents is voluminous and interested readers are referred to several other publications for additional references [1–5].

Background: a continuing story of controversy

DMPA is the most widely used and successful non-oral hormonal contraceptive ever developed, and from almost every objective scientific standpoint thoroughly deserves this position. Why then should there be such controversy about its safety and such antagonism by narrow-interest groups to its general availability as one of a range of methods with different appeal to different individuals? The answers to this question are complex, have changed from time to time over the past 15 years, but have important implications for the development of new long-acting methods.

A brief history of the saga is appropriate. Medroxyprogesterone acetate was synthesized in the mid 1950s [6] and put into clinical trials as DMPA for the treatment of threatened abortion and endometriosis. In 1960, the United States Food and Drug Administration (USFDA) approved DMPA for general marketing for these indications on the basis of its safety. When women who were given massive doses (1–4 g) to inhibit premature labour failed to conceive for 1–1½ years postpartum, clinical contraceptive trials were initiated and reported in 1966 [7–10].

The first Upjohn contraceptive marketing application for DMPA to the USFDA was placed in 1967. The first delays occurred over questions of reversibility, the possible risk of cervical carcinoma-in-situ and the interpretation of toxicology in beagle dogs. In spite of these questions, in 1973 the USFDA announced its intention to approve Depo-Provera as a contraceptive. Extraordinary political pressure then prevented this final approval and led to withdrawal of marketing approval for threatened abortion and endometriosis because of alleged ineffectiveness and questions of safety, including the observation that other progestogens administered during pregnancy might have an occasional association with birth defects. The USFDA managed to delay making a final decision on contraceptive marketing of DMPA until 1978 when approval was finally refused. This denial was made in the face of two separate strong recommendations for approval by its own Obstetric and Gynecology Advisory Subcommittee. Following this, it took 5 years before the appeal by the Upjohn Company was finally heard by a Public Board of Inquiry. Two years later a majority recommendation against approval was made but has not been acted upon by the USFDA; an extraordinary tale of inordinate delays, political pressures, emotions and little attention to science and to the lack of real clinical and scientific evidence that DMPA is not safe.

What is so sad is that the British Minister of Health managed to do exactly the same thing after a clear recommendation in favour of contraceptive marketing from the United Kingdom Committee for the Safety of Medicine (CSM) – the first time a minister has gone against the recommendation of the CSM [11]. In the United Kingdom there were also unexplained delays in preparation of the Public Hearing report before recommendation of approval was made and marketing allowed.

In contrast it is fascinating to find that every independent scientific group that has thoroughly reviewed all the data on DMPA has recommended its wider use as a safe contraceptive. These include the Obstetrics and Gynecology and Biostatistics Advisory Committees of the USFDA, the United Kingdom CSM, the Swedish Board of Health and Welfare, the West German and New Zealand Drug Boards, an ad hoc Consultative Panel of the US Agency for International Development, the International Medical Advisory Panel of the International Planned Parenthood Federation, and several groups convened by the Special Programme of Research in Human Reproduction of the World Health Organization.

It must also be recognized that there are legitimate concerns about DMPA, many of which are not directly clinical but do have serious implications for the development of other long-acting methods:

1. '*Potential for abuse*' towards underprivileged ethnic groups and mentally retarded individuals.
2. '*Method least in control of the woman herself*'.
3. *Community suspicion of multinational corporations*, i.e. Upjohn Company, making money out of 'uninformed' people in developing countries.
4. *Interpretation of animal toxicology*. Tough long-term animal toxicology requirements for contraceptives have been applied in many countries for nearly 20 years [12]. One difficult aspect of use of animal models is the fact that many reactions will be species specific; others may result from the desired pharmacological action of a drug given at excessively high doses. Extrapolation to humans may be

difficult. There are indications that requirements for animal toxicity may soon change.

Two observations in animals have led to controversy. When treated with high-dose progestogens for several years beagle bitches will develop an increased number of benign and malignant breast nodules, while rhesus monkeys treated for 10 years with 50 times the human dose of DMPA or NET-EN will sometimes develop endometrial carcinoma. There is now extensive evidence that these observations have little relevance to women because of species differences [5, 13]. The final proof about rare effects or lack of effects in humans can only come from careful clinical studies following initial reassurance from animal studies that the drug is not toxic.

5. *Legitimate scientific concerns*. These concerns are surprisingly limited, and include the clinical and metabolic issues discussed below.

One very important issue involves the depth of safety information which should be expected for a drug before it is approved for general marketing. Much of what seems to be expected for DMPA can only be obtained by very expensive large-scale long-duration follow-up studies in populations which have had general marketing and widespread usage for years. This is exactly what is happening with DMPA. The data are coming from several of the 84 countries where it has been marketed for years, and at this stage, if anything, it looks a safer drug than the combined oestrogen-progestogen pill.

Over the past 10 years a massive effort has been invested into the development of a range of approaches to the difficult goal of simple and safe long-acting contraception.

Practical routes of administration

The current status of existing agents and of systems under development is summarized in Table 7.1. These utilize a wide range of technologies, many of which are novel and complex and many of which have proven very expensive. Numerous international agencies and pharmaceutical companies have contributed to these developments.

The more traditional intramuscular injectable methods consist of steroid acetates or esters which have been formulated in oily solutions or microcrystalline suspensions. The steroid esters in oily solution appear to be distributed to storage sites in adipose tissue from which they are slowly released into the circulation. The active steroid moiety is then cleaved from the ester after which it is able to exert its biological effect. Microcrystalline suspensions remain as a depot at the site of injection and the active steroid or ester is slowly released from the surface of the crystals.

A continuing effort is being made to develop new progestogenic steroids and new long-acting progestogen esters, which may avoid some of the disadvantages of existing methods. A massive cooperative effort involving several of the leading chemists in the field and a network of developing country centres supported by the World Health Organization has synthesized over 200 systematically selected esters of norethisterone and levonorgestrel [14]. Several of these show very prolonged biological activity and at least one is now in clinical trial. During the course of this programme it has been found that the exact pharmaceutical formulation of the microcrystals or solution of the compound is critical for maximum duration of action, and the optimum formulation varies from compound to compound.

Table 7.1 Current long-acting hormonal contraceptives (Modified from Fraser I.S. [5])

Duration of action	*Type of system*	*Existing systems in human use or trial*	*Stage of development*	*Comments*
1 month	Injectable	1. DMPA (25 mg) + EC (5 mg)	Post-phase III	Dose reduction studies under way
		2. NET–EN (50 mg) + EB (5 mg)	Phase III	
		3. NET–EN(20 mg) alone	Phase II	
		4. DHPA (150 mg) + EE (10 mg)	Post-phase III	
		5. Others	Phase I–II	
	Oral	1. Several formulations	Phase II–III	Peoples' Republic of China only
2–3 months	Injectable	1. NET–EN (200 mg)	Marketing	First-order release
		2. DMPA (150 mg)	Marketing	First-order release
		3. NET microcapsules (100 mg)	Phase II	Possible zero-order release
		4. LNG cyclobutyl carboxylate	Phase I–II	
		5. Others	Pre-phase I	
	Vaginal ring	1. LNG (300 μg) + E_2 (180 μg)	Phase III	Cyclical use 3 weeks out of 4; with ovulation inhibition
		2. LNG (20 μg)	Phase III	Continuous use; zero-order release; 'minipill' effect
		3. Others	Phase I–II	Potential for longer duration of use
6 months	Injectable	1. DMPA (450 mg)	Marketing	First-order release
		2. NET microcapsules (200 mg)	Phase II–III	Possible zero-order release
		3. Others	Pre-phase I	
	Implant –biodegradable	1. NET-cholesterol pellets	Phase I	Attenuated first-order release
		2. BIDS–LNG	Phase I (discontinued)	Single implant } Near zero-order release
	–non-biodegradable	1. NET-acetate silastic (500 μg)	Phase II	Single implant } Near zero-order release
1–2 years	Implant –biodegradable	1. Caprolactone LNG pellets (50 μg)	Phase II	Single implant } Near zero-order release
	–non-biodegradable	1. ST1435 silastic (120 μg)	Phase I–II	Single implant } Near zero-order release
		2. Others	Phase I	
	Intrauterine devices	Progesterone or progestogen releasing	Phase I to marketing	
5 years +	Implant –non-biodegradable	1. Norplant I (30–50 μg)	Marketing	6 implants } Zero-order release
		2. Norplant II (30–50 μg)	Phase III	2 implants } Zero-order release

DMPA = depot medroxyprogesterone acetate; NET–EN = norethisterone enanthate; DHPA = dihydroxyprogesterone acetophenide; LNG = levonorgestrel; EC = oestradiol cypionate; EB = oestradiol benzoate; EE = oestradiol enanthate; E_2 = oestradiol 17β; BIDS = biodegradable implantable delivery system; (parentheses) = total dose or daily release rates

Monthly injectables consisting of a range of different oestrogen–progestogen combinations have been extensively tested in small clinical trials [15–17]. Contraceptive failure has not been recorded with most of them, but dosages are probably unnecessarily high. Dose-reduction studies are under way. A major advantage of these preparations is a much lower incidence of menstrual disturbances than with other long-acting methods. Effective once-a-month oestrogen–progestogen pills are under study in the People's Republic of China [18], but face a number of metabolic and toxicological concerns.

Two highly effective 2–3 monthly injectable preparations are already marketed widely around the world. DMPA is marketed for contraception as a microcrystalline suspension of 150 mg administered once every 84–90 days in 84 countries (including many developed countries) and there are very few countries where it is not registered for other indications such as cancer or endometriosis. It is calculated that 20 million year-equivalents of Depo-Provera have been used for contraception since 1963 and approximately 4 million year-equivalents were used in 1986. DMPA has been extensively studied with mention in well over 1000 published papers, and is probably the most thoroughly investigated single hormonal contraceptive preparation in existence [19]. Over 3.2 million woman-months of surveillance have been reported in controlled trials, and approximately 20 large-scale clinical studies are currently in progress. DMPA can also be given in dosages of 300–500 mg once every 6 months, but this is not widely recommended.

Norethisterone enanthate (NET-EN) is marketed as a contraceptive in over 40 countries and is administered in doses of 200 mg in oily solution every 56–84 days [2]. World-wide usage in 1986 amounted to over 200 000 year-equivalents. Usage is rapidly increasing, and numerous large-scale trials are under way. NET EN does not face the same political pressures as DMPA, but does face the same type of metabolic, clinical and toxicology issues.

A more even release of steroid is obtained by the intramuscular injection of progestogen-containing biodegradable-polymer microcapsules [20]. This type of polymer delivery system is still in the early stages of clinical trial but can be modified to provide release of various steroids over 3–6-month periods, and holds considerable promise. Six-months is probably the practical limit of duration of action of a non-recoverable injection.

The subcutaneous route of administration provides a different range of possibilities. Although simple injections can be given by this route, the main advantage is the potential for the placement of biodegradable polymers or non-biodegradable silicone rubber steroid-releasing implants. These offer the potential for much longer durations of action (6 months to 6 years or more). These systems also permit removal if problems develop or if the subject wishes to fall pregnant. The biodegradable capsules [21] will only permit easy removal for a portion of their lifespan. Most present-day systems release levonorgestrel, but many other progestogens have been tested in the past [15, 22]. A progestogen which has potential advantages in lactating women is ST 1435 [23], because it has no oral activity and is unlikely to be absorbed by the neonate. The only currently marketed system is the Population Council's highly effective 6 year, 6 silastic capsule levonorgestrel system 'Norplant' [24].

The vagina is an excellent surface for steroid absorption and several silicone rubber vaginal ring systems of widely differing design and widely differing steroid-release rates are currently in clinical trial [25]. They can be designed to last for any duration from 1 month to 1 year, but most are changed for hygienic reasons once every 3 months. They have an excellent potential for widespread acceptability.

Several intrauterine low-dose progestogen-releasing devices have been designed to last for varying durations from 1 to 5 years (or more). These systems release progesterone or progestogens continuously at a low rate across a thin, precisely-manufactured rate-limiting membrane. They have the major advantages over other intrauterine devices that menstrual blood loss and pain are reduced, but at the expense of increased nuisance-value spotting.

A very recent approach to continuous steroid delivery is the use of steroid creams or steroid-containing skin patches with a rate-limiting membrane in contact with the skin. Some steroids are well-absorbed across the skin while others are not. These systems will probably have to be changed every 3–5 days, but will provide fairly constant blood levels. This approach still requires much development.

Pharmacology

Pharmacokinetics

This discipline involves the study of kinetics (mainly in plasma) of administered drug, and the range of methods described above provides several different kinetic profiles (Figure 7.1). Most oral and injected drugs exhibit first-order kinetics with initial high plasma levels followed by an exponential decay. The absolute levels of the peak and the rate of disappearance of the progestogen or oestrogen from the plasma depend on the dosage and formulation as well as many aspects of absorption from the injection site, blood and tissue distribution, plasma binding, metabolism, and excretion. Rapid early absorption and metabolism may be caused by excessive massaging of the injection site.

Steroids which can be formulated as microcrystals (e.g. DMPA) tend to have a slower release into the circulation than steroid esters formulated in oily solution (e.g. NET-EN and most monthly injectables). Microcrystals remain at the depot site and are gradually eroded at the surface to release the active steroid. Crystal size and method of formulation may be critical for duration of action, and may vary from ester to ester. On the other hand, esters in oily solution are absorbed from the injection site into the circulation, whence they are stored mainly in adipose tissue. Slow release then occurs over the following weeks, and hydrolysis of the ester to release the active steroid (e.g. NET from NET-EN) probably occurs mainly in the liver [26].

There are substantial individual variations in pharmacokinetics and hence in duration of action in different women. These variations have been discussed by Fotherby [27] and Fraser [5]. In some DMPA users the depot persists for many months and this can be responsible for an unpredictable delay in the return of fertility after the last injection. For this reason DMPA dosage reduction studies down to 100 mg once every 84–90 days are currently under way. Ethnic differences may be important.

New delivery systems are all aimed at reducing the initial peak and then providing more or less constant blood levels (zero-order release) for the desired period. It is hoped that this will maintain efficacy, reduce total 'body burden' of administered steroid and minimize unwanted effects. With true zero-order release systems it is possible to set the release at a high level to predictably inhibit ovulation, or at a lower level to provide a 'minipill' effect with less frequent interference with ovulation. The

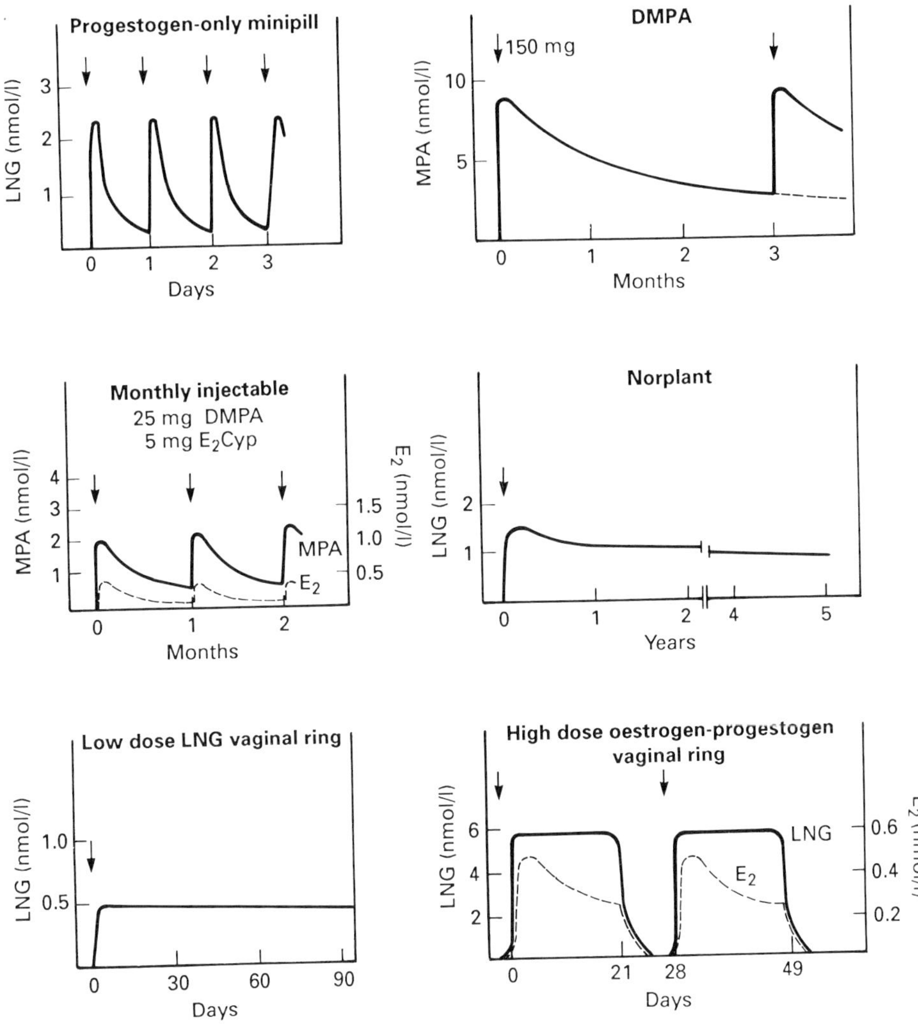

Figure 7.1 Plasma levels of contraceptive steroids achieved by different long-acting hormonal methods compared with the levonorgestrel minipill (LNG = levonorgestrel; MPA = medroxyprogesterone; E_2 = oestradiol)

best available zero-order release systems are the vaginal rings and the subcutaneous implants, especially Norplant which maintains mean plasma levonorgestrel levels of around 1 nmol/l with only gradual decline for at least 5–6 years [28].

Pharmacodynamics and mechanism of action

Pharmacodynamics are the changes in endogenous parameters, e.g. hormones, induced by administered drug, and extensive information is now available for most agents with respect to changes in LH, FSH, oestradiol and progesterone. Classical injectables (DMPA, NET-EN and monthlies) all predictably inhibit ovulation by an action predominantly at the hypothalamic level. This effect is also achieved by the oestrogen–progestogen vaginal rings and by Norplant. However, low-dose progestogen-only implants and vaginal rings may not reliably inhibit ovulation, and may produce a range of progestogen-only minipill type effects on plasma LH, FSH, oestradiol and progesterone levels [29]. Predictable ovulation inhibitors suppress cyclical release of FSH and LH, and as a consequence follicular and luteal release of oestradiol and progesterone. Progestogen-only methods appear to produce less profound suppression of basal plasma levels than oestrogen–progestogen combinations, but do provide effective inhibition of the oestrogen positive feedback mechanism. It is encouraging to see that there is no greater suppression of any of these hormone levels after 10 years of use of DMPA than after one cycle [30].

Non-ovulation inhibiting methods must act mainly by effects on cervical mucus, endometrium, tubal function and corpus luteum function. Progestogens all bind to progesterone receptors, but depending on their individual structures may also bind to other receptors at high doses (e.g. androgen or corticosteroid receptors), and may act in slightly different ways depending on their structure [31]. MPA may act partly through androgen receptors to induce gonadotrophin suppression [32], although it does not have overt androgenic activity in humans. In fact in women it can often be shown to have an anti-androgenic action. Effects of progestogens on androgen and corticosteroid receptors may be seen with progressively increasing doses, usually at a level well above the standard contraceptive range. Progestogens produce significant inhibition of regeneration of oestrogen and progestogen receptors in the endometrium and cervix [33, 34], and this is clearly part of their mechanism of action.

Clear progestogenic effects are seen in cervical mucus [35] and in the endometrium [36–38]. With injectable progestogens the endometrium becomes steadily 'suppressed', especially with DMPA where the changes become progressively more 'atrophic' with repeated injections. With other agents, the appearances of the endometrium are a reflection of the combined effects of varying amounts of endogenous and exogenous oestrogen as well as the progestogen.

Clinical aspects

Contraceptive efficacy

The major injectable preparations are highly effective contraceptives. DMPA has been very extensively studied with reported pregnancy rates between 0.01 and 1.2 per 100 woman-years [1]. In the major trials the pregnancy rates have generally been less than 0.5 per 100 woman-years, and this figure compares very favourably with the rates reported in combined oral contraceptive trials. The major advantage of the injectables over oral contraceptives is that the use-effectiveness approaches theoretical effectiveness. Factors such as disturbed absorption, missed pills and drug interactions do not contribute to the failure rate.

Norethisterone enanthate is also a highly effective contraceptive, but in general the pregnancy rates have been slightly higher than with DMPA [39, 40]. Regimens which utilize doses of 200 mg every 56–70 days exhibit pregnancy rates of about 0.5 to 1.5 per 100 woman-years. Numerous small-scale clinical trials of monthly injectables have been published and only rare pregnancies have been reported with any of the oestrogen–progestogen combinations [15–17]. This extraordinarily high contraceptive efficacy is in keeping with the indication from pharmacokinetic data that initially dosage levels were unnecessarily high [41]. New preparations have great promise.

Much less information is available about the zero-order release systems, but recent experience, particularly with 'Norplant' indicates a very high efficacy for up to 5 years of use [42]. It is anticipated that the vaginal-ring systems will also provide good contraceptive efficacy and this should certainly be the case with those releasing a combination of an oestrogen and a progestogen [43].

Menstrual disturbances

Long-acting hormonal contraceptives produce an almost invariable disturbance of the menstrual cycle and this may be a source of major concern to the woman, especially if adequate counselling had not been given before treatment started. The more extreme disturbances are produced by the progestogen-only methods, especially the higher-dose first-order release formulations like DMPA. A wide range of disturbances have been reported with these contraceptives. They include frequent amenorrhoea, frequent oligomenorrhoea, less frequent irregular or prolonged bleeding or spotting, and very occasional heavy bleeding, but the most consistent finding is the complete unpredictability of the bleeding patterns [44].

DMPA causes amenorrhoea of greater than 90 days duration in up to 40% of women by the end of 12 months of use [45, 46]. NET-EN causes less amenorrhoea than DMPA, but the incidence of other types of menstrual disturbance is similar to DMPA [47, 48]. Normal length 'cycles' are uncommon with both preparations. Of all the long-acting injectable or implantable methods, monthly injectables which contain both oestrogen and progestogen give the best approximation at the present time to a normal menstrual cycle. In a detailed study of Cycloprovera (DMPA 25 mg, oestradiol cypionate 5 mg; Upjohn Company) the incidence of amenorrhoea fluctuated around 10% during the first year but gradually increased to around 25% after 2 years [49]. Irregular bleeding, and profuse and prolonged bleeding have also occasionally been reported with these preparations.

The severity of menstrual disturbances seen with low-dose zero-order progestogen-release systems generally lies between DMPA and the monthly injectables [50].

Menstrual disturbances are the commonest medical reason for discontinuation of long-acting methods, and it seems that extreme disturbances, including amenorrhoea and prolonged or heavy bleeding, are most likely to lead to discontinuation. The frequency of discontinuation is greatly influenced by physician attitude, extent of pretreatment counselling and society expectations.

Amenorrhoea appears to be associated with development of a highly suppressed ('atrophic') endometrium but the aetiology of irregular bleeding episodes is unknown [51]. Episodes do not appear to be related to fluctuations in circulating hormone levels, but may be related to disturbances of endometrial vascular morphology. Endometrial oestrogen and progesterone receptors are greatly suppressed and there are almost certainly abnormalities of local lysosome, prostaglandin, and haemostatic function.

Management of these menstrual disturbances is a major problem [52], and pretreatment counselling is of paramount importance. Oestrogen administration for at least 10–14 days will usually stop an episode of bleeding, but a withdrawal bleed will almost always occur a few days after therapy. There is no good evidence that this will improve bleeding patterns in the long-term. However, it does give a good opportunity to maximize the effects of ongoing counselling. Cyclical oestrogen administration does improve the regularity of bleeding patterns [53], but greatly complicates the method. Experienced clinicians find that oestrogens are only indicated in 0.5 to 4 cases per 100 woman-years of use. Numerous oestrogen regimens and other therapies have been tried [52], but an acceptable approach for episodes of prolonged, frequent or heavy bleeding is the use of a single course of ethinyloestradiol 30–50 μg (or other equivalent preparation) daily for 21 days. Curettage is very rarely required to stop an episode of bleeding, but may occasionally be indicated for diagnostic purposes, especially in older women.

Delay in the return of fertility

There is clear evidence of a short delay in the return of ovulation, menstruation and fertility in women who have used DMPA. This is due to persistence of the drug in the circulation following slow removal from the injection site. Most evidence suggests that the conception rate curve is shifted to the right by 3–5 months but is similar in shape to non-contraceptive users [54–56]. Approximately 60% of women will conceive by 12 months after discontinuation and 85% by 24 months. There is no evidence that DMPA or any other injectable causes persistent amenorrhoea or permanent infertility. Return of fertility is almost certainly quicker following other existing long-acting hormonal methods.

Other side-effects and complications

Side-effects other than menstrual changes have never presented a problem in clinical trials and are not a common cause of discontinuation [1, 15]. However, mention of minor and major side-effects during the counselling session prior to commencement of treatment appears crucial to the success of long-acting contraceptives. Weight gain, headaches, dizziness, abdominal bloating, fatigue, nervousness and other mood changes have been reported with frequencies varying between 5% and 15% of users. This frequency of complaint is not dissimilar to users of oral contraceptives and intrauterine devices [57, 58].

Progestogen-only contraceptives do not usually influence blood pressure or blood coagulability. In fact these are probably the hormonal contraceptives of choice for women with a previous history of venous thromboembolism.

Progestogen-only methods may significantly reduce the incidence of vaginal moniliasis [59] and, as with combined oral contraceptives, reduce the incidence of pelvic inflammatory disease [60].

The issue of neoplasia

Much of the concern about cancer arises from animal toxicology studies, whereas direct clinical data (mainly from DMPA) are thus far reassuring. The chief areas of concern are neoplasms of breast, cervix, and endometrium.

Several clinical studies have examined the relationship between DMPA and breast cancer. None of these showed a significant increase in risk but only two included an appropriate comparison group [61]. High doses of DMPA cause breast atrophy and there are good theoretical reasons to expect that DMPA and other progestogens may actually provide a small protective effect against breast cancer in women.

Two early clinical studies using inappropriate control groups [62, 63] suggested that DMPA might predispose to cervical dysplasia or neoplasia. However, at least eight other studies have shown no difference or a reduced incidence of cervical abnormalities in DMPA users [1]. None of these studies are conclusive, and the results of extensive, ongoing studies are awaited.

Only two cases of endometrial cancer appear to have been reported in DMPA users, and one of these clearly had the cancer before starting treatment. This paucity of reported cases, taken with the protective effect of combined oral contraceptives [64] and the use of progestogens for treating established endometrial cancer, all point to a major protective effect of progestogen-only methods against development of endometrial cancer.

There is no evidence that DMPA, NET-EN, or the low-dose delivery systems influence the risk of hepatic neoplasia or pituitary adenomas, but those agents which act by the inhibition of ovulation may help to reduce the risk of ovarian carcinoma [65].

Fetal exposure

Several reports have suggested that high doses of progestogens given for pregnancy maintenance (e.g. threatened or recurrent abortion) may have a low-grade teratogenic potential. There may be an increase in risk of congenital heart disease up to twofold [66] and possibly also in central-nervous-system malformations. The authors of most studies have acknowledged that an excessive number of malformations can be expected among babies born to mothers with a history of threatened abortion [67]. On the other hand, exposure to massive doses of norethisterone (10–40 mg daily) from the 4th to the 35th week of pregnancy was associated in one study with some degree of virilization among 18% of female infants born to 82 mothers [68]. Norethisterone does appear to have a weak androgenic effect in humans, but is minimal with lower doses or shorter exposure [69]. Case reports of virilization after DMPA use are rare [70]. The incidence of hypospadias may be slightly increased, but the excess risk of this, if any, must be small [71]. Meaningful conclusions about very low potential teratogenic risks with the very much lower doses used for contraception are unlikely ever to be reached because the accidental pregnancy rate is so low.

There is very little evidence to implicate prenatal progestogen use in the modification of later reproductive or sexual development or behaviour, although the effects of the synthetic oestrogen, stilboestrol, are well known [72].

Lactation

Lactation has a very important, but in later months an unreliable, contraceptive action. Progestogens do not suppress lactation in the way that oestrogens do, and therefore have some advantages for contraception during breast feeding [73]. However, it is known that very small amounts of progestogen are transferred into the mother's milk, and concern has been expressed that these might have an adverse effect on neonatal growth or subsequent development. There is no evidence for this in humans [74], although under certain experimental conditions, exposure of neonatal animals to sex steroids (androgens and oestrogens) may exert an organizing effect on certain aspects of central-nervous-system function and responsiveness [75]. With low zero-order release contraceptives the amount of steroid transferred is so low that it is very hard to believe that it could have any biological effect in the neonate.

It is usually recommended that progestogen-only contraception be started 6–8 weeks postpartum in the lactating woman.

Metabolic effects

Effects on biochemical parameters have been clearly demonstrated with high doses of progestogens, oestrogens, and androgens, but they became progressively more difficult to demonstrate with lower-dose preparations.

Small but significant changes in carbohydrate metabolism have been reported with contraceptive doses of DMPA, NET-EN and monthly injectables. The most consistent finding is an exaggerated insulin response without hyperglycaemia during a glucose tolerance test, although a variety of individual responses have been reported [1]. Even with very high doses of DMPA used for treatment of cancer, the development of diabetes has been rare [76]. It seems fair to conclude that the diabetogenic effect of injectable progestogens is definite but slight, and is of the same order as for combined oral contraceptives, and probably less than pregnancy.

The effects on plasma lipids are even more confusing and controversial, and are certainly dose related [77]. Progestogens do not increase fasting plasma triglyceride levels, but may slightly depress high-density lipoprotein cholesterol (HDL-C) and increase low-density lipoprotein cholesterol (LDL-C). These changes in HDL-C and LDL-C might just adversely affect subsequent risk of cardiovascular disease, although the situation is quite controversial [78]. No detectable changes occur with low-dose-release devices.

Progestogens do not appear to affect liver function adversely, but oestrogen–progestogen combinations almost certainly will. Progestogens alone can probably be used safely in women with a history of recurrent obstetric cholestasis [79]. Progestogens do not influence blood coagulation or fibrinolysis, although oestrogens do [80, 81]. Progestogens do not influence other metabolic or haematological parameters [82], although very high doses of DMPA may cause adrenocortical suppression [83]. Contraceptive doses of DMPA do not interfere with the circadian rhythm or responsiveness of the adrenals [84]. Under certain experimental conditions, progesterone and most progestogens can be shown to have a weak suppressive effect on wound healing, cell-mediated immunity, and some circulating antibody responses [1]. In most cases these are of the same order as immunological changes seen in pregnancy, and no clinical evidence of immunological disturbance has been seen.

Acceptability

Acceptability implies a weighing up of the advantages and disadvantages of a particular method in terms of the individual life style and preferences of a couple. This also includes important factors relating to the enthusiasm and counselling of the physician and health care personnel, and to the attitude of the popular press.

At this point it is useful to list those aspects of various types of non-oral hormonal contraception which are usually seen as advantages (Table 7.2) and compare them with a list of disadvantages (Table 7.3). It must be recognized that these do not all apply to any one method. It must also be recognized that non-oral hormonal methods do not appeal to all women, but merely provide another range of contraceptive approaches with varying individual appeal. However, in those countries where long-acting methods are widely available, acceptability is generally excellent.

In almost all trials where continuation rates with injectables have been compared to other contraceptive methods, the continuation rates have been very similar or even better for the injectables [1]. Most of the studies have involved DMPA, and continuation rates with this injectable have generally been in the range of 50%–80%

Table 7.2 Advantages of long acting hormonal contraceptives

All methods
Long action with one treatment
Relative simplicity of administration
Independent of coitus
Freedom from 'fear of forgetting' daily pills
Safety margin for timing of successive treatments
High use-effectiveness
High acceptability and high continuation rates of use
Minimal gastrointestinal disturbance
Almost invariable reduction of menstrual blood loss
Avoidance of 'first-pass' effects through liver
Some methods
Elimination of early peak in blood levels
Zero-order release of contraceptive steroid
Low total body load of steroid to be metabolized
No oestrogenic side-effects
Amenorrhoea may be a health benefit and a convenience
No suppression of lactation
Simplification of reversibility
Regular contact with health personnel

Table 7.3 Concerns about long-acting hormonal contraceptives

All methods
Almost invariable change in menstrual pattern
'Minor' side-effects
Minor metabolic changes
Theoretical effects on fetus and breast-fed neonate
Theoretical concerns about neoplasia
Suspicion of the integrity of the Scientific community and Multinational pharmaceutical companies
Some methods
Problems of informed consent and 'potential for abuse'
Method 'least in control' of the woman herself
Cannot be rapidly reversed
Delay in return of fertility (but no permanent sterility)
Controversy about the interpretation of animal toxicology

at the end of a year. In one exceptional study they were as low as 18.3% [85] and conversely they have been as high as 70% at the end of 2 years in other studies [86]. There are clearly many factors which affect the attitude of the patient and the physician to these contraceptives in any particular centre, and physician factors may indeed make a major impact. In a multicentre World Health Organization trial [39], two centres in India had dramatically different DMPA discontinuation rates for amenorrhoea and menstrual disturbances, although the actual incidences of amenorrhoea were identical (Table 7.4). In retrospect it appears that detailed positive counselling was provided in centre A but not centre B.

Continuation rates with NET-EN, monthly injectables, subcutaneous implants, and vaginal rings are also likely to be high in most communities [17, 42, 48]. With all these preparations, menstrual disturbances are the single major medical reason for discontinuation, and the more extreme disturbances such as amenorrhoea and prolonged or heavy bleeding are responsible for the highest proportion of discontinuations. Other medical causes account for only a small proportion of the total.

Table 7.4 A comparison of termination rates and menstrual bleeding patterns with DMPA and NET–EN in two centres with different approaches to patient counselling

	One-year termination rate for amenorrhoea (per 100 women)		*% of women with amenorrhoea >90 days*	
	DMPA	*NET-EN*	*DMPA*	*NET-EN*
Centre A	24	0	24	7
Centre B	69	10	23	5
	One-year termination rate for bleeding problems (per 100 women)		*Mean number of bleeding and/or spotting days per 90 days*	
	DMPA	NET-EN	DMPA	NET-EN
Centre A	6	0	22	20
Centre B	49	53	25	24

Future advances

Advances will continue to be aimed towards the Utopian goal of simple, prolonged and easily reversible application with very high efficacy and minimal side-effects. Very high efficacy can be achieved, but side-effects still occur. Of these the menstrual disturbances constitute the major problem, and a massive research effort needs to be initiated to solve it. Over the past few years there has been an impressive proliferation of different approaches to the expensive technology of long duration of action. Some of these have widespread appeal, and it seems likely that there will be a rationalization of the large number of technologies during the next 5–10 years. Most of the presently envisaged approaches have been mentioned earlier in this article. Perhaps the most fascinating and ingenious of these involve the use of biodegradable polymer delivery systems, and these have been well described [20, 21]. In addition to using these with traditional steroids such as oestrogens and progestogens, in future it may be possible to provide prolonged release of antiprogestogens and gonadotrophin-releasing hormone superanalogues.

References

1. FRASER, I. S. and WEISBERG, E. A comprehensive review of injectable contraception with special emphasis on depot medroxyprogesterone acetate. *Medical Journal of Australia* [Suppl.], **1,** 1–19 (1981)
2. BENAGIANO, G. and PRIMIERO, F. M. Long acting contraceptives: present status. *Drugs*, **25,** 570–609 (1983)
3. POPULATION REPORTS. *Long Acting Progestins – Promise and Prospects*. Series K, Vol. 11, No. 2, Population Information Programs. Johns Hopkins University, Baltimore, pp. 17–55 (1983)
4. MISHELL, D. R. Jr. (ed.) Long acting steroid contraception. *Advances in Human Fertility and Reproductive Endocrinology*, Vol. 2, Raven Press, New York (1983)
5. FRASER, I. S. Long acting hormonal contraceptives. In *Clinical Reproductive Endocrinology* (ed. R. P. Shearman), Churchill Livingstone, London, pp. 634–655 (1985)
6. BABCOCK, J. C., GUTSELL, E. S. and HERR, M. E. Six methyl seven hydroxyprogesterone seventeen acylates: a new class of potent progestins. *American Chemical Society Journal*, **80,** 2092–2093 (1958)
7. COUTINHO, E. M. and DE SOUZA, J. C. Conception control by monthly injections of medroxyprogesterone suspension and long acting oestrogen. *Journal of Reproduction and Fertility*, **15,** 209–218 (1966)
8. CSAPO, A., DE SOUZA-FILHO, M. B., DE SOUZA, J. C. and DE SOUZA, O. The effects of massive progestational hormone treatment on the human uterus. *Fertility and Sterility*, **17,** 621–626 (1966)
9. ZANARTU, J. and ONETTO, E. Long acting injectable progestogens in fertility control. In *Proceedings of the Sixth Pan-American Congress on Endocrinology*, Mexico City, October 1965. Excerpta Medica (International Congress Series No. 112), Amsterdam, p. 134 (1965)
10. SEGAL, S. J. and CROXATTO, H. B. Single administration of hormones for long term control of

reproductive function. Paper presented at the *XXIII Meeting of the American Fertility Society*, Washington, DC, 14–16 April (1967)

11. LEADING ARTICLE. Rejecting scientific advice. *British Medical Journal*, **284**, 1426 (1982)
12. BERLINER, V. R. Food and drug administration requirements for toxicity testing of contraceptive products. In *World Health Organization Symposium on Pharmacological Models in Contraceptive Development* (eds. M. H. Briggs and E. Diczfalusy), *Acta Endocrinologica* [Suppl.], **185**, 240–253 (1974)
13. BENAGIANO, G. and FRASER, I. S. The Depo-Provera debate: Commentary on the article 'Depo-Provera. A critical analysis'. *Contraception*, **24**, 493–528 (1981)
14. CRABBÉ, P., DICZFALUSY, E. and DJERASSI, C. Injectable contraceptive synthesis: an example of international cooperation. *Science*, **209**, 992–994 (1980)
15. BENAGIANO, G. Long acting systemic contraceptives. In *Regulation of Human Fertility* (ed. E. Diczfalusy), Scriptor, Copenhagen, pp. 323–360 (1977)
16. TOPPOZADA, M. The clinical use of monthly injectable contraceptive preparations. *Obstetrical and Gynecological Survey*, **32**, 335–346 (1977)
17. HALL, P. and FRASER, I. S. Monthly injectable contraceptives. In *Advances in Human Fertility and Reproductive Endocrinology, Vol. 2: Long Acting Steroid Contraception* (ed. D. R. Mishell Jr.), Raven Press, New York, 65–88 (1983)
18. FAN, H. M. Studies on long acting oral contraceptives. In *Recent Advances in Fertility Regulation* (ed. C. F. Chang, D. Griffin and A. Woolman), Atar SA, Geneva, pp. 378–393 (1981)
19. FRASER, I. S. and HOLCK, S. Depot medroxyprogesterone acetate. In *Advances in Human Fertility and Reproductive Endocrinology, Vol. 2: Long Acting Steroid Contraception* (ed. D. R. Mishell Jr.), Raven Press, New York, pp. 1–30 (1983)
20. BECK, L. R. and TICE, T. R. Poly[lactic acid] and poly[lactic acid-Co-Glycolic acid] contraceptive delivery systems. In *Advances in Human Fertility and Reproductive Endocrinology, Vol. 2: Long acting Steroid Contraception* (ed. D. R. Mishell Jr.), Raven Press, New York, pp. 175–199 (1983)
21. GABELNICK, H. L. Biodegradable implants: alternative approaches. In *Advances in Human Fertility and Reproductive Endocrinology, Vol. 2: Long Acting Steroid Contraception* (ed. D. R. Mishell Jr.), Raven Press, New York, pp. 149–173 (1983)
22. COUTINHO, E., DA SILVA, A. R., MOTTOS, C. E. R. *et al.* Contraception with long acting subdermal implants: 1. An effective and acceptable modality in international clinical trials. *Contraception*, **18**, 315–334 (1978)
23. COUTINHO, E., DA SILVA, A. R. and KRAFT, H.-G. Fertility control with subdermal silastic capsules containing a new progestin (ST-1435). *International Journal of Fertility*, **21**, 103–108 (1976)
24. POPULATION COUNCIL. Special issue on Norplant. *Studies in Family Planning*, **14**, 159–193 (1983)
25. DICZFALUSY, E. and LANDGREN, B.-M. New delivery systems: vaginal rings. In *Recent Advances in Fertility Regulation* (ed. C. F. Chang, D. Griffin and A. Woolman), Atar SA, Geneva, pp. 43–69 (1981)
26. BACK, D. J., BRECKENRIDGE, A. M. and CHAPMAN, C. R. Studies on enzymatic cleavage of norethisterone oenanthate. *Contraception*, **23**, 125–136 (1981)
27. FOTHERBY, K. Factors affecting the duration of action of the injectable contraceptive norethisterone enanthate. *Contraception Delivery Systems*, **2**, 249–257 (1981)
28. CROXATTO, H. B., DIAZ, S. and MIRANDA, P. Plasma levels of levonorgestrel in women during long term use of Norplant. *Contraception*, **23**, 197–209 (1981)
29. LANDGREN, B. M. and DICZFALUSY, E. Hormonal effects of the 300 μg norethisterone minipill. *Contraception*, **21**, 87–99 (1980)
30. JEPPSSON, S., GERSHAGEN, S., JOHANSSON, E. D. B. and RANNEVIK, G. Plasma levels of medroxyprogesterone acetate (MPA), sex hormone-binding globulin, gonadal steroids, gonadotrophins and prolactin in women during long term use of depo-MPA (Depo-Provera) as a contraceptive agent. *Acta Endocrinologica*, **99**, 339–343 (1982)
31. ROZENBAUM, H. Relationships between chemical structure and biological properties of progestogens. *American Journal of Obstetrics and Gynecology*, **142**, 719–724 (1982)
32. PEREZ-PALACIOS, G., FERNANDEZ-APARICIO, M. A. and MEDINA, M. On the mechanism of action of progestins. *Acta Endocrinologica*, **97**, 320–328 (1981)
33. TSENG, L. and GURPIDE, E. Effects of progestins on estradiol receptor levels in human endometrium. *Journal of Clinical Endocrinology and Metabolism*, **41**, 402–409 (1975)
34. RALL, M. J., SOTO FERREIRA, G. and HANSSENS, K. Y. Effect of medroxyprogesterone acetate contraception on cytoplasmic estrogen receptor content of the human cervix uteri. *International Journal of Fertility*, **23**, 51–56 (1978)

35. KESSERU-KOOS, E. Influence of various hormonal contraceptives on sperm migration in vivo. *Fertility and Sterility*, **22,** 584–588 (1971)
36. LEE, R. A. Contraceptive and endometrial effects of medroxyprogesterone acetate. *American Journal of Obstetrics and Gynecology*, **104,** 130–134 (1968)
37. KHOO, S. K., MACKAY, E. V. and ADAM, R. R. Contraception with a six monthly injection of progestogen: 3. Effects on the endometrium. *Australian and New Zealand Journal of Obstetrics and Gynaecology*, **11,** 226–232 (1971)
38. ROBERTS, D. K., MORBELT, D. V. and POWELL, L. C. The ultrastructural response of human endometrium to medroxyprogesterone acetate. *American Journal of Obstetrics and Gynecology*, **123,** 811–818 (1975)
39. WORLD HEALTH ORGANIZATION. Expanded Program of Research Development and Research Training in Human Reproduction (Task Force on long-acting systemic agents for the regulation of fertility). Multinational comparative clinical evaluation of two long-acting injectable contraceptive steroids: Norethisterone enanthenate and medroxyprogesterone acetate: 1. Use effectiveness. *Contraception*, **15,** 513–533 (1977)
40. WORLD HEALTH ORGANIZATION. Multinational comparative clinical trial of long acting injectable contraceptives: Norethisterone enanthate given in two dosage regimens and depot medroxyprogesterone acetate. A preliminary report. *Contraception*, **25,** 1–11 (1982)
41. GUAL, C., PEREZ-PALACIOS, G. and PEREZ, A. E. Metabolic fate of a long acting injectable estrogen-progestogen contraceptive. *Contraception*, **7,** 271–279 (1973)
42. DIAZ, S., PAVEZ, M., MIRANDA, P. *et al.* A five-year clinical trial of levonorgestrel silastic implants (Norplant™). *Contraception*, **25,** 447–456 (1982)
43. POPULATION COUNCIL. An international comparative trial. A multicentre study of levonorgestrel-estradiol contraceptive vaginal rings: 1. Use-effectiveness. *Contraception*, **24,** 341–358 (1981)
44. FRASER, I. S. Abnormal uterine bleeding due to hormonal steroids and intrauterine devices. In *Recent Advances in Fertility Regulation* (ed. D. Griffin and A. Woolman), Atar SA, Geneva, pp. 265–300 (1981)
45. SCHWALLIE, P. C. and ASSENZO, J. R. Contraceptive use-efficacy study utilising Depo-Provera administered as an injection every 90 days. *Fertility and Sterility*, **24,** 331–342 (1973)
46. GRAY, R. H. Patterns of bleeding associated with the use of steroidal contraceptives. In *Endometrial Bleeding and Steroid Contraception* (ed. E. Diczfalusy, I. S. Fraser and F. T. G. Webb), Pitman, Bath, pp. 14–49 (1980)
47. WORLD HEALTH ORGANIZATION. Expanded Program of Research, Development and Research Training in Human Reproduction (Task Force on long acting systemic agents for the regulation of fertility). Multinational comparative clinical evaluation of two long-acting injectable contraceptive steroids: Norethisterone enanthate and medroxyprogesterone acetate: 2. Bleeding patterns and side effects. *Contraception*, **17,** 395–407 (1978)
48. HOWARD, G., BLAIR, M., CHEN, J. K. *et al.* A clinical trial of norethisterone oenanthate (Norigest) injected every two months. *Contraception*, **25,** 333–343 (1982)
49. KOETSAWANG, S., SRISUPANDIT, S., KIRIWAT, O. and KOETSAWANG, A. Monthly injectable contraceptive: A two year clinical trial. *International Journal of Gynaecology and Obstetrics*, **16,** 61–64 (1978)
50. FAUNDES, A., SIVIN, I. and STERN, J. Long acting contraceptive implants: An analysis of menstrual bleeding patterns. *Contraception*, **18,** 355–366 (1978)
51. DICZFALUSY, E., FRASER, I. S. and WEBB, F. T. G. (ED.) *Endometrial Bleeding and Steroidal Contraception.* Pitman Press, Bath (1980)
52. FRASER, I. S. A survey of different approaches to management of menstrual disturbances in women using injectable contraceptives. *Contraception* **28,** 385–397 (1983)
53. EL-HABASHY, M. A., MISHELL, D. R. and MOYER, D. L. Effect of supplemental oral estrogen on long acting injectable progestogen contraception. *Obstetrics and Gynecology*, **35,** 51–54 (1970)
54. SCHWALLIE, P. C. and ASSENZO, J. R. The effect of depot medroxyprogesterone acetate on pituitary and ovarian function and the return of fertility following discontinuation. *Contraception*, **10,** 81–89 (1974)
55. PARDTHAISONG, T., GRAY, R. H. and MCDANIEL, E. B. Return of fertility after discontinuation of depot medroxyprogesterone acetate and intrauterine devices in Northern Thailand. *Lancet*, **1,** 509–511 (1980)
56. PARDTHAISONG, T. Return of fertility and outcome of pregnancy after discontinuation of the injectable contraceptive, depot medroxyprogesterone acetate. *PhD Thesis*, University of London (1981)
57. SCUTCHFIELD, F. D., LONG, W. M., CORREY, B. and TYLER, W. Medroxyprogesterone acetate as an injectable female contraceptive. *Contraception*, **3,** 21–32 (1971)
58. SCHWALLIE, P. C. and ASSENZO, J. R. Contraceptive use-efficacy study utilizing Depo-Provera administered as an injection once every six months. *Contraception*, **6,** 315–322 (1972)

59. TOPPOZADA, M., ONSEY, A. F. and FARES, E. The protective influence of progestogen-only contraception against moniliasis. *Contraception*, **20,** 99–206 (1979)
60. SENANAYAKE, P. and KRAMER, D. G. Contraception and the etiology of pelvic inflammatory disease: new perspectives. *American Journal of Obstetrics and Gynecology*, **138,** 852–864 (1980)
61. GREENSPAN, A. R., HATCHER, R. A., MOORE, M. *et al.* The association of depot medroxyprogesterone acetate and breast cancer. *Contraception*, **21,** 563–569 (1980)
62. POWELL, L. C. and SEYMOUR, R. J. Effects of depot medroxyprogesterone acetate as a contraceptive agent. *American Journal of Obstetrics and Gynecology*, **119,** 36–48 (1971)
63. LITT, B. D. Statistical review of carcinoma-in-situ reported among contraceptive users of Depo-Provera. Memorandum dated 17 June 1974. Submitted at FDA Hearing, 7 May 1975
64. WEISS, N. N. and SAYVETZ, T. A. Oral contraceptive use and endometrial carcinoma. *New England Journal of Medicine*, **302,** 511–514 (1980)
65. CASAGRANDE, J. T., LOUIE, E. W. and PIKE, M. C. 'Incessant ovulation' and ovarian cancer. *Lancet*, **2,** 170–173 (1979)
66. HEINONEN, O. P., SLOANE, D., MANSON, R. R. *et al.* Cardiovascular birth defects and antenatal exposure to female sex hormones. *New England Journal of Medicine*, **296,** 67–69 (1977)
67. HARLAP, S., PRYWES, R. and DAVIES, A. M. Birth defects and oestrogens and progestogens in pregnancy. *Lancet*, **1,** 682–684 (1975)
68. JACOBSON, B. D., Hazards of norethindrone therapy during pregnancy. *American Journal of Obstetrics and Gynecology*, **84,** 962–967 (1962)
69. KEITH, L. and BERGER, G. The relationship between congenital defects and the use of exogenous progestational 'contraceptive' hormones during pregnancy – a 20 year review. *International Journal of Gynaecology and Obstetrics*, **15,** 115–124 (1977)
70. BURSTEIN, R. and WASSERMAN, H. C. The effect of Provera on the fetus. *Obstetrics and Gynecology*, **23,** 931–934 (1964)
71. GRAY, R. Teratogenesis. In *Progestogens In Therapy* (ed. G. Benagiano, P. Zulli and E. Diczfalusy), Serona Symposia, Raven Press, New York, pp. 109–125 (1983)
72. EDITORIAL. Prenatal determination of adult sexual behaviour. *Lancet*, **2,** 1149–1150 (1981)
73. HULL, V. The effect of hormonal contraceptives on lactation: current findings, methodological considerations and future priorities. *Studies in Family Planning*, **12,** 134–163 (1981)
74. SCHWALLIE, P. C. Effect of depot medroxyprogesterone acetate on the fetus and nursing infant. *Contraception*, **23,** 375–386 (1981)
75. RUBIN, R. T., REINISCH, J. M. and HASKETT, R. F. Post natal gonadal steroid effects on human behavior. *Science*, **211,** 1318–1324 (1981)
76. VECCHIO, T. J. Injectable medroxyprogesterone acetate contraception: metabolic and endocrine effects. *Journal of Reproductive Medicine*, **10,** 193–196 (1972)
77. FRASER, I. S. Lipid changes and medroxyprogesterone acetate. *Contraception Delivery Systems*, **3,** 1–7 (1983)
78. LEES, R. S. and LEES, A. M. High density lipoproteins and the risk of atherosclerosis. *New England Journal of Medicine*, **306,** 1546–1548 (1982)
79. KREEK, M. J. and SLEISENGER, M. H. Estrogen induced cholestasis due to endogenous and exogenous hormones. *Scandinavian Journal of Gastroenterology* [Suppl.] **7,** 123–131 (1970)
80. WHIGHAM, K. A. and HOWIE, P. W. The effect of an injectable progestogen contraceptive on blood coagulation and fibrinolysis. *British Journal of Obstetrics and Gynaecology*, **86,** 806–816 (1979)
81. HOWARD, G., BLAIR, M., FOTHERBY, K. *et al.* Some metabolic effects of long term use of the injectable contraceptive norethisterone oenanthate. *Lancet*, **1,** 423–425 (1982)
82. AMATAYAKUL, K. Safety and hazards of injectable hormonal contraceptives. *Singapore Journal of Obstetrics and Gynecology*, **9,** 57–67 (1979)
83. HELLMAN, L., YOSHIDA, K., ZUMOFF, B. *et al.* The effect of medroxyprogesterone acetate on the pituitary-adrenal axis. *Journal of Clinical Endocrinology and Metabolism*, **42,** 912–917 (1976)
84. AEDO, A.-R., LANDGREN, B.-M. and DICZFALUSY, E. Studies on ovarian and adrenal steroids at different phases of the menstrual cycle. III. Steroid and lutropin levels before and after the administration of a single contraceptive dose of a depot medroxyprogesterone acetate. *Contraception*, **24,** 117–128 (1981)
85. BLOCH, B. Depot medroxyprogesterone acetate (Depo-Provera) as a contraceptive preparation. *South African Medical Journal*, **45,** 777–781 (1971)
86. MCDANIEL, E. B. and PARDTHAISONG, T. Use effectiveness of six-month injections of DMPA as a contraceptive. *American Journal of Obstetrics and Gynecology*, **119,** 175–180 (1974)

Chapter 8

Postcoital contraception

A. Yuzpe and A. Kubba

Sexual intercourse is a spontaneous, pleasurable, instinctive, physiological act. It is often unpremeditated and in many instances unprotected. Methods which aim to control the timing of pregnancy have been in use since time immemorial. Ideally, they should not interfere with the spontaneity or pleasure of the sexual act but at the same time should operate when the need arises. Numerous contraceptive techniques ranging from the primitive to the highly sophisticated have tried to achieve this goal. As yet, none has been totally successful; systemic methods of contraception aim mainly at inhibiting ovulation and need to be taken for substantial periods of time regardless of the frequency of sexual activity of the woman concerned; methods linked to coitus, i.e. barriers, by their nature need planning and premeditation.

The need for a *post hoc* method of contraception exists in cases such as failures, both method and user, of conventional forms of fertility control, especially in the field of barrier contraceptives and where the use of an effective contraceptive is omitted in an isolated episode. Sexual assault and incest are numerically smaller, but very important, categories where postcoital interception is indicated.

First coital encounters are notorious for being unprotected through complete omission or inadequate use of contraception [1,2]. The other contraceptive emergency where back-up is essential is when method failure such as condom rupture, diaphragm displacement, or pill omission (especially around the pill-free week) occurs. The emergency postcoital consultation is a suitable opportunity to introduce and discuss with the woman the different contraceptive options available, allowing her to make an informed choice.

Since the mid-sixties, research in the field of postcoital contraception has followed two parallel lines. Firstly, in developed countries, postcoital agents have been seen as non-recurrent emergency methods of contraception employed to prevent pregnancies after single coital exposures. As contraceptive technology advances, consumers' expectations rise and their tolerance of accidental pregnancy declines. As contraceptive choice widens and the risks and drawbacks of the various methods become apparent there will be an increase in frequency of method changes by users. This carries an inherent risk of incorrect use and 'accidents'.

The second application of postcoital techniques has been evaluated mainly in developing countries. Its application has aimed to simplify contraceptive use by timing administration of the steroid contraceptive agent to coincide with the coital act, thereby achieving a reduction in the total dosage and increasing safety. This requires a regimen which would be equally safe and effective if used to prevent a pregnancy following a single exposure in a cycle, or after as many as 20 or more exposures per cycle.

Medical folklore has an abundance of postcoital methods – very elaborate but rather ineffective and at times dangerous – that have been used through the ages. Modern postcoital technology has until now been based on the use of either steroid hormones or the intrauterine contraceptive device.

Until recently no drug has been marketed for sole use as a postcoital agent. In Hungary a preparation containing 0.75 mg d-norgestrel (Postinor) has been available on prescription since 1981 [3]. Drug regulatory agencies in North America have not given marketing approval to postcoital agents. In the UK, the Committee on Safety of Medicines has ruled that the combined oestrogen–progestogen regimen is safe. The combined oestrogen–progestogen regimen is now licensed as an emergency contraceptive in the UK under the name PC4, and in Germany as Tetragynon (Schering Pharmaceutical). In this chapter we will review the currently available postcoital methods, potential for research in this field, and the use of non-steroidal agents for this purpose.

The 'morning-after' pill

This somewhat inaccurate term is used to describe emergency postcoital agents taken in various dosage regimens after a single unprotected exposure. High-dose steroidal and non-steroidal oestrogens, and lower-dose oestrogen–progestogen combinations, have been employed. Varying efficacy figures have been quoted by different authors, with failure rates ranging between 0 and 5%. The main side-effects of these regimens are nausea and vomiting. Anxieties about the possible teratogenic potential of such agents in the case of treatment failure have not been confirmed. The risk is likely to be small, but it is still a major cause of unease to both the pharmaceutical industry and the prescribing physician, because of both human and medicolegal implications. Although called the 'morning-after' pill, these agents can be used up to 48–72 h after exposure. Various regimens exist with varying dosages and duration of treatment.

Oestrogens only

Since the pioneering work of Morris and van Wagenen [4], both synthetic and conjugated natural oestrogens, have been used as emergency postcoital contraceptive agents. Most regimens employ rather high doses of oestrogen to achieve maximum efficacy. The period of administration varies from 3 to 5 days, with the inevitable side-effects of nausea and vomiting occurring frequently.

Diethylstilboestrol (DES)

The first oestrogen to be used postcoitally was diethylstilboestrol and its diphosphate derivative. The association of vaginal adenosis and adenocarcinoma in female offspring, and genital abnormalities and sexual dysfunction in male offspring, of women exposed to DES in early pregnancy [5] meant that use of DES in such a way was halted. However, these effects of DES on embryogenesis have not been demonstrated in postcoital therapy. This is to be expected, since the period of any possible exposure to postcoital agents is limited to the peri-implantation phase, i.e.

the blastocyst stage of embryogenesis. Noxious agents at this stage would have an 'all or none' effect on the early embryo.

The dose of DES used was 50 mg per day for 5 days, though 25 mg per day regimens have been used with varying success. [6–9]. Regimens of 10 mg per day for 5 days proved inadequate [10]. A dosage of 50 mg DES per day for 5 days was ultimately recommended for postcoital contraception [7].

Conjugated equine oestrogens (CEE)

These so-called natural oestrogens are derivatives of equine urinary extracts. Only a few studies report their use. The largest series of oral CEE was reported by Crist and Farrington [11]. The dosage employed was 30 mg per day for 5 days with no reported failures. CEE at a dosage of 50 mg was used intravenously on each of 2 consecutive days to treat 200 rape victims. The treatment usually began within 24 h. Follow-up was difficult, although no failures were reported [12].

Ethinyloestradiol (EE)

Ethinyloestradiol was probably the most widely used and popular postcoital agent until the mid 1970s. Its wider use in combined oral contraceptive preparations reduced the anxieties about its use postcoitally. Doses ranging from 1 to 5 mg per day, initiated usually within 48 h following exposure and continued for 3 to 5 days, have been described. Lower-dosage and shorter-duration regimens resulted in higher failures. Most workers now agree that a dosage of 5 mg per day for 5 days is the most effective.

Depot oestrogens

Coutinho (in a personal communication to Blye [12]), reported the use of depot oestradiol propionate intramuscularly as a postcoital agent. Of 12 women, two failures resulted, both of which were ectopic pregnancies. The explanation given was that the slow release of this depot oestrogen may have retarded zygote transport in the fallopian tube, with resultant tubal implantation. Schindler *et al.* employed oestradiol-benzoate 12.5 mg combined with 10 mg oestradiol-phenylpropionate. In 100 treatment cycles the failure rate was 3% [13].

The combination of a subluteolytic dose of depot oestradiol cypionate and bromocriptine given in mid- to late luteal phase can produce luteolysis, and has potential as an interceptive preparation. The main drawback are the side-effects associated with bromocriptine [14].

The paucity of clinical trials employing intramuscular depot oestrogens for postcoital contraception reflects their record of impracticality and poor efficacy compared to the oral regimens.

Efficacy of oestrogen-only regimens

Comparison of failure rates of the different oestrogen regimens is almost impossible because of the variable conditions under which the studies were carried out. A dosage high enough to achieve maximum efficacy is often traded off against a higher incidence of side-effects. With diethylstilboestrol, failure rates varied from 0 in the 50 mg regimens to 0.8% in those under 50 mg. Ethinyloestradiol proved to be the most effective oestrogen-only postcoital contraceptive, with failures ranging from 0 to 0.6 [15, 16].

Conjugated equine oestrogens were compared to the 5 mg ethinyloestradiol regimen and found to be inferior [15]. The failure rate in the aforementioned comparative study, was 1.4%.

Side-effects of postcoital oestrogens

Numerous side-effects have been reported with high-dose oestrogen regimens. The commonest of these are nausea and vomiting. Others include breast tenderness, headache, lack of concentration, dizziness, menorrhagia, and abdominal pain. The only serious complication ever reported with oral postcoital agents is a case of pulmonary oedema after three doses of stilboestrol [17]. The incidence of nausea and vomiting varies in the different studies but is usually in excess of 50%. However, there is a suggestion that CEE produces milder and less frequent side-effects than DES or EE [18].

Disruption of the menstrual pattern in the treatment has been reported with the various oestrogens. After DES administration 12%–13% of cases experienced a delay in the onset of the next period, whereas up to 11% of those treated had a shorter cycle [7,19]. Approximately 50% of those treated reported lighter or heavier menses [19]. Menstrual patterns following EE treatment are similar to those with DES [7]. Similarly, CEE therapy results in menstrual delay in 13% and a shorter cycle in 19% of cases. Of those treated, 70% reported a change in the character of their subsequent menses [18].

In cases of treatment failure, 10% of the resultant pregnancies are likely to be ectopic. This figure suggests that postcoital contraception plays a permissive rather than a causative role in the aetiology of ectopic pregnancy. As is argued with normal IUD use, methods preventing uterine implantation while having less or no effect on tubal implantation will decrease the number of intrauterine pregnancies and hence produce an apparent proportional increase in tubal pregnancies. Morris and van Wagenen agree with this view that the expected number of ectopic pregnancies is occurring against a drop in the incidence of intrauterine pregnancies [17].

Oestrogen–progestogen combination

This is currently the most popular and most acceptable form of morning-after treatment. A combination of ethinyloestradiol and norgestrel has been in use since the early seventies [20]. Since then several reports of the use of this emergency postcoital combination have been published [21–28, 32]. The recommended regimen employs two doses each of 1 mg of dl-norgestrel and 100 μg of ethinyloestradiol 12 h apart. The treatment must be initiated within 72 h of exposure to the risk of pregnancy. One other combination postcoital regimen using the non-steroidal oestrogen dienoestrol with ethynodiol diacetate was described, with a failure rate under 1% [29].

Failure rates with ethinyloestradiol–norgestrel range between 0 and 2%. A recent report by Tully [30] suggested a failure rate of 5% in regularly cycling women exposed at mid-cycle; this failure rate is higher than those with oestrogen-only regimens.

The only randomized comparative study of ethinyloestradiol vs an ethinyloestradiol–norgestrel combination was carried out by van Santen and Haspels in a randomized double-blind trial [26]. In that study, 493 cases were recruited with 94.3% follow-up. Two pregnancies occurred in the oestrogen-only group (n = 226) and one in the EE–norgestrel group (n = 239), giving a pregnancy rate of 0.9% and 0.4% respectively. Analysis of efficacy by calculating the expected number of pregnancies by day of coitus revealed an expected number of 11.9 in the EE group and of 11 in the EE–norgestrel group. Therefore the combined regimen achieved efficacy comparable to the 5-day EE regimen. The difference between the observed and expected number of pregnancies was very statistically significant ($P < 0.0005$). In both groups, most women were treated within 24 h of coitus. No statistically significant difference in nausea and vomiting between the two regimens was noted. More protocol uniformity is needed to overcome methodological differences between such studies, particularly larger number of subjects (in view of the fact that no pregnancy would have resulted even without treatment in the majority of subjects).

Most but not all studies confined treatment to women reporting a single unprotected intercourse. In most studies the exposure occurred at mid-cycle, although treatment was not withheld when exposure was reported at other times of the cycle, especially in the preovulatory phase. This takes account of the physiological fact that sperm survival in the female genital tract is unpredictable, and that early ovulation in the cycle of treatment is a possibility. This more liberal attitude to the combined regimen reflects its perceived safety and the shorter duration of treatment, compared to the oestrogen-only regimens where treatment was limited in some studies to women at mid-cycle or those who showed evidence of sperm in cervical mucus.

The timing of onset of the next period is more predictable with the combined therapy as compared to the oestrogen-only regimens. In 98% of women treated, menses began within 21 days of the treatment [27,28]. The remaining group constituted under 2% of those treated, and in such women treatment failure has to be excluded. This can be done using a sensitive pregnancy test at the follow-up visit 21 days after treatment. In general, menses were delayed in approximately 7% of cases, whereas 20% of those treated reported a shorter cycle [27]. Other researchers found shorter cycles to be even more common [31]. This is one of the attractive features of the combined therapy when compared to oestrogens alone, where subjects are 2–3 times more likely to experience a delay in menses. The sooner the menses arrive, the shorter the period of anxiety about the outcome of treatment.

The major side-effects reported with the combined method were nausea and vomiting. Nausea has been reported at rates ranging from 25% to 66%, and vomiting in 5%–24% of cases [22,24,27,28]. There was no difference between the use of the steroid in tablet or capsule form [33]. Concomitant antiemetic administration was shown in some studies to reduce the frequency and severity of these symptoms, after either combined or oestrogen-only treatment [33,34]. However, antiemetics may exacerbate mastalgia by potentiating the increase in prolactin production caused by the steroidal agents. When they occur, side-effects last only one day in the majority of users.

A rare complication of the combined regimen is ectopic gestation. One such case was reported [35] but a causal link cannot be assumed (see above).

Since its introduction in the early seventies, the combined regimen has overtaken other postcoital agents as the preferred morning-after treatment. With an efficacy comparable to other agents, coupled with the reduced incidence of side-effects and serious complications, it is the safest, cheapest and simplest form of postcoital therapy. The total dose of ethinyloestradiol administered as a single postcoital agent is 25 mg (2.5 mg b.i.d. × 5 days). This is equivalent to the oestrogen in a 30 μg cyclic combined oral contraceptive taken for 3 years or a 50 μg preparation taken for 2 years! In contrast, the combined therapy is equivalent to less than one week's intake of the 30 μg or 4 days of a 50 μg oral contraceptive preparation. Not only is the dose reduced, but the duration of the course of treatment with the combined regimen is one-fifth that of the oestrogen-only formulations. This reduces the duration of side-effects such as nausea and/or vomiting, and hence improves patient compliance.

Progestogens as postcoital agents

Progestogen-only postcoital contraception has been employed primarily as a continuing or ongoing method of fertility control. Used in this way, the total dose of a drug ingested per cycle would be proportional to coital frequency, limiting the amount of drug taken by the less sexually active. Paradoxically, however, the failure rate is higher when coital frequency and hence total dose ingested per cycle is lowest [36]. The advantage of a coitally associated oral contraceptive is that it promotes compliance in the less motivated and the forgetful. Progestogens such as quingestanol acetate [37,38] and d-norgestrel [3,36,39–41a] have been evaluated as ongoing postcoital contraceptives. The only such drug marketed is levonorgestrel, which is available in Hungary under the trade name Postinor [3]. The maximum recommended dosage of Postinor is 3 mg per cycle (i.e. four tablets each of 0.75 mg of levonorgestrel). It is recommended that Postinor be taken immediately after intercourse. If multiple intercourse takes place, a second dose 8 h later is advised. In 1983, 303 000 packets of this postcoital agent were sold in Hungary. The limitation of the total monthly doses to four means that this method is only useful for relatively sexually inactive women. Multiple doses have resulted in a high incidence of breakthrough bleeding.

In a recent study of 259 women using postcoital levonorgestrel repeatedly during the periovulatory period of one cycle, the method failure rate was 0.8% per cycle. However, because of the side-effects of menstrual disturbance (21%), nausea and headaches (20%), the investigators were not very optimistic about the viability of this approach to fertility regulation [41b].

The main drawback to progestogen-only therapy is that high doses are required. Such dosages, in turn, cause menstrual disruption and cycle irregularity as well as other side-effects including nausea, vomiting, and breast tenderness. In many cultures where a coitally associated contraceptive is desirable, menstrual irregularities are totally unacceptable, and therefore the compliance that these regimens were hoped to engender may in truth be reduced.

Levonorgestrel has also been used as an emergency postcoital agent [42]. The regimen employed is a single dose of 0.6 mg of levonorgestrel given within 12 h of coitus. A comparison between 205 cases using this regimen, and 525 cases using the combined ethinyloestradiol–norgestrel treatment showed a pregnancy rate of 2.9% for the former and 1.9% for the latter [42].

Failures of postcoital hormonal contraception

In evaluating the efficacy of a postcoital agent a number of variables must be considered. These include the fertility status of both the female and the male subjects, the regularity of the cycle, and the degree of contraceptive cover offered by dubiously effective methods such as douching. In addition one has to accept the patient's account of the timing and number of exposures in that cycle at face value, with possible omissions in order to ensure obtaining treatment. This is especially true in the average clinical situation vs the clinical-trial atmosphere. The lack of a control group in such postcoital trials, the provision of which is almost impossible because of ethical considerations, is also a significant drawback. Epidemiologists and statisticians have provided us with some answers regarding the risk of pregnancy in the untreated exposed population. Probability tables have been produced giving the chance of conception on various days of the menstrual cycle resulting from one act of intercourse on that particular day. Barrett and Marshall, in an elegant study of almost 2000 cycles, calculated the chance of conception at mid-cycle to vary between 10% and 30% [43]. They used the first day of the significant rise in basal body temperature as a reference point. The cycle point most likely to result in pregnancy following coitus was day minus 2, where the chance of conception was 30%. Other workers have confirmed these estimates [44,45].

A WHO prospective study attempted to evaluate conception rates at various times in the menstrual cycle [46]. In the study, cervical mucus changes were used as indicators of impending ovulation. The last day of fertile type mucus (Peak Day or PD) has been shown by several authors to be a reasonably accurate indicator of ovulation [47–49]. The first day of the fertile period is supposed to coincide with the first day of recognizable mucus, the so-called first wet day. The last day of the fertile period is the 4th day after the PD. Intercourse outside the fertile period resulted in low conception rates (0.004) [46], whereas the probability is highest on the peak day being 0.667. During the 3 days preceding the peak day, the probability is 0.55. (The probability of pregnancy on the peak day was calculated from a rather small number of cycles.)

Studies of the efficacy of postcoital drugs express their failure rates as percentages of those treated, i.e. per cent of cycles. The failure rate is therefore calculated per 100 woman-months or cycles, rather than per 100 woman-years (Pearl Index). Comparisons between failure rates of postcoital therapies and failures of conventional ongoing contraceptives are thus impossible. Comparisons of the pregnancies resulting after postcoital treatment to those expected (according to the different calculated risks mentioned previously), lead to the conclusion that emergency postcoital oestrogens and the ethinyloestradiol–norgestrel combination are both effective methods, preventing between 80% and 90% of expected pregnancies.

The role of postcoital contraception

As methods to detect and predict ovulation become more accurate, easier to use, and hence more accessible to the general public, the concept of regular postcoital contraception becomes a more rational choice.

Until this future role for postcoital agents is achieved, the methods remain primarily as emergency therapies, aiming to prevent unwanted pregnancies with their associated physical and psychological traumas. Postcoital contraceptives play a major back-up role in cases of barrier-method failures or misuse. Indeed, they may make barrier methods more acceptable and allow couples to use them with more confidence and less anxiety, thus enhancing relationships.

The main anxiety about postcoital agents arises when they fail and the doctor is faced with the problem of managing the unplanned pregnancy. In the majority of cases the patient elects for pregnancy termination [1,50,51]. However, a minority of couples would choose to continue the pregnancy. The possibility of a teratogenic effect of these agents can be neither confirmed nor excluded. The fact that the literature contains no reports of pregnancies being harmed by postcoital treatment is reassuring. The 'all-or-none' effect of noxious agents means that these agents either prevent implantation completely or fail to do so at all, and in the latter case the embryo develops normally. The short duration of administration of the combined regimen (12 h between first and last dose) ensures minimal exposure of the blastocyst *before* implantation takes place. The longer the course of postcoital therapy, the higher is the theoretical risk. This is greatest with failure of an ongoing (i.e. regular postcoital) regimen. In practice, the latter situation is comparable to ingestion of either the combined contraceptive or the progestogen-only pill in a patient with an early unrecognized gestation. Evidence about teratogenicity in these cases is fairly reassuring as well. (See pages 86–87.)

Another difficult area is the moral and ethical implications of postcoital contraception. A couple may accept a method which works pre-fertilization but may reject a post-fertilization form of therapy. It is desirable, therefore, to discuss the mode of action of these agents with the patient beforehand. There is a general consensus that postcoital agents are contraceptive (acting postovulation but preimplantation) rather than abortifacient, but this definition has not been tested in court.

Another anxiety on the part of the medical profession is that the existing postcoital drugs can be misused as a regular rather than an emergency method of fertility control. This is unlikely to be acceptable to the patient, as the total dose of hormones taken by a sexually active woman will be much higher than a conventional contraceptive pill. In addition, the efficacy of postcoital drugs is inferior to the conventional pill. As the quoted risk of 2% for failure applies for each cycle, after 13 cycles the annual rate could be 26 per 100 women regularly exposed. Furthermore, side-effects in the form of nausea and vomiting or menstrual irregularities would make regular use of these agents unacceptable to the majority of women.

Future refinement is postcoital technology would target selected reproductive events without disrupting the intrinsic rhythm of the menstrual cycle (i.e. at the level of the ovulation process, oöcyte maturation, or at the corpus luteum). This may lead to the development of a 'once a month' drug which will reliably prevent pregnancy when taken over a brief period at specific stages of the cycle.

Mechanism of action of hormones used postcoitally

Fertilization is known to take place in the outer one-third of the fallopian tube. After fertilization the ovum is propelled by various tubal mechanisms and reaches the endometrial cavity in an average time of 3 days. Two days later implantation starts and the process is completed on the 8th postovulation day.

Interception is any process by which ovulation, fertilization or implantation is prevented. Postcoital agents may therefore act at an ovarian, salpingeal, or endometrial level. An agent is more likely to affect several but not all of the target organs, producing changes of varying magnitudes. The main sites of action are the endometrium and the corpus luteum, though all stages of the fertilization-implantation cycle can potentially be affected, including sperm migration, tubal motility, and embryonic viability. Evidence for interference with sperm migration or capacitation is lacking in humans. The embryo toxicity of oestrogens has been demonstrated in animal models but not in humans. Failure to demonstrate βhCG in the post-treatment period of the cycle confirms the interceptive rather than abortifacient role of the postcoital agents [51a]. Furthermore once implantation has occurred the implanted embryo is resistant to large doses of exogenous ethinyloestradiol or DES [52–54].

Mechanisms involving the ovary

Administration of oestrogen or an oestrogen–progestogen combination immediately prior to the LH surge would result in ovulation suppression. The LH surge is delayed for approximately 7 days and the treatment cycle is therefore prolonged. The effect of progestogen-only regimens on ovulation is highly variable, depending on the frequency of administration of the drug and the stage in the cycle. Ovulation can be inhibited with frequent high doses of progestogens [55].

Once ovulation has occurred, the corpus luteum can be affected by several agents. With oestrogen-only regimens there is a reduction in plasma progesterone following administration of DES and ethinyloestradiol on the day of the basal body temperature rise or 3 days later [12]. This is probably a direct effect on the corpus luteum. Luteal function can also be inhibited by progestogens alone. There is a positive correlation between progestogens and $PGF_{2\alpha}$, the latter being involved in luteal regression.

Oestrogen–progestogen combinations also demonstrate a disruptive effect on the corpus luteum. Ling *et al.* studied the endocrine and endometrial changes following the administration of 2 mg norgestrel combined with 200 μg of ethinyloestradiol given at different times in the cycle [56–58]. As with progestogens only, the effects were variable. The endocrine changes may be grouped into four categories, (a) no change in the post-treatment levels of oestradiol–17β and progesterone compared to pre-treatment control cycles (b) a reduction in both oestradiol–17β and progesterone, (c) a reduction in oestradiol only, and (d) a reduction in progesterone or a fluctuation of oestradiol levels. Thus varying types of luteal response may occur. In the majority of cases, these responses are manifested by a shortened luteal phase which is the result of the reduced progesterone or oestradiol levels.

Mechanisms involving the uterus

High doses of oestrogens have been shown to interfere with implantation in humans [4]. This is the basis for the term 'interception', introduced by Naqvi and Warren to describe the mechanism of action of postcoital agents [2].

Progestogens used as ongoing postcoital contraceptives, especially if used frequently, would result in the transformation of cervical mucus to a secretory-type mucus which is thick, scanty, with poor spinnbarkeit, and thus hostile to sperm penetration. This effect will only be operative if progestogens were used frequently to maintain an effect on cervical mucus. If used only as an emergency postcoital agent, the cervical mucus effect would probably be too late to prevent a pregnancy. The more likely mechanism of action would be an endometrial one. This could vary, depending on the type and dosage of the progestogen used. Histologically the picture is one of inactivity. On a cellular level, progestogens stimulate acid phosphatases, which inactivate nuclear oestrogen receptors. The available information suggests the combination of a disruptive effect on the pituitary–ovarian axis, and direct action at ovarian and endometrial levels [59]. In addition, progestogens retard tubal motility and may predispose to ectopic pregnancy.

The combined regimen was shown by Ling *et al.* to produce asynchronous development of the glandular and stromal elements of the endometrium, with the glands lagging behind the stroma [56]; this has been confirmed by others [20]. At a cellular level, following combined therapy, a significant reduction in endometrial oestrogen and progesterone receptors is demonstrated [60,61]. Both nuclear and cytoplasmic components are affected. The activity of the enzyme isocitrate dehydrogenase, a progestogen-sensitive enzyme, was also increased, suggesting a progestational effect. Changes in endometrial biochemistry have also been demonstrated with oestrogens used alone. The biochemical changes produced in the endometrium seem to be the most consistent changes produced by postcoital hormonal contraception and are likely to prove the most important.

Postcoital IUD insertion

Lippes *et al.* [62] reported no pregnancies following the insertion of Copper-T IUDs in 97 women after unprotected intercourse within the previous 5 days. They later reported a further 202 insertions of Copper 7 IUDs [63]. In five of these cases the IUDs were inserted 6 or 7 days after intercourse, with no pregnancies resulting. Since then over 1300 postcoital IUD insertions *in situ* were reported [60,64,66] with only one failure [67]. This makes the IUD the most efficient postcoital contraceptive. This method seems to apply particularly to multiple coital exposures, where an IUD can be inserted with every chance of success up to 5 days after the calculated day of ovulation. Other instances where an IUD may be used are when oestrogens are contraindicated, when treatment is delayed beyond 72 h, or for the multiparous patient who wishes to use the IUD as an ongoing method of contraception. It is less than ideal for the young nullipara, especially one with multiple sexual partners. In the latter case, IUD use may predispose to serious complications such as the development of pelvic inflammatory disease. The IUD may increase the risk of exacerbating quiescent PID or predispose to its development. Careful selection of patients helps reduce complications, thus encouraging the user to keep the IUD as an ongoing method of contraception. On the other hand, removal with the next menstruation may minimize the risk and be acceptable to an otherwise anxious patient. The Cu-7, Cu-T 200, the ML-Cu 250 and the ML-Cu 375 have all been used for this purpose.

An immediate problem with IUDs is the pain associated with insertion. This is especially important if the patient is young, nulliparous and unprepared for an operative procedure. In such cases topical uterine anaesthesia using lignocaine may help [68]. A paracervical block or infiltration anaesthesia may also be used; but in general, IUD insertion in the nulliparous woman requesting postcoital contraception is *not* advisable (for medicolegal reasons, at least in North America).

A major problem which might result from the use of the IUD as a postcoital agent is the masking of an early gestation. This may occur, since IUD insertion is often associated with varying degrees of irregular bleeding. This is in contrast to the hormonal postcoital regimens where irregular bleeding is not a feature. Irregular bleeding masking an early pregnancy can cause a delay in the diagnosis and management of the pregnancy, whether by pregnancy termination or, if the patient wishes to continue the pregnancy, by removal of the IUD.

In a recent study [69] the continuing use of IUDs inserted postcoitally was assessed. Ninety-eight cases were followed up for 2 years and compared to controls choosing IUDs in non-emergency situations. No differences were demonstrated in efficacy, expulsions or removals for medical reasons. Removals for 'personal reasons' were statistically higher in the postcoital group and occurred early in the study period.

The mechanism of action of postcoital IUDs is by the combination of a foreign-body inflammatory response in the endometrium, an increase in local prostaglandin production, the competitive inhibitory effect of copper ions on endometrial enzymes and the possible blastocidal action of copper.

Future developments in postcoital contraception

Several agents have been used in experimental situations as interceptive agents. A number of established drugs have the potential for postcoital use.

Chinese home visiting or vacation pills

Nine 'vacation pills' have been developed in the People's Republic of China. These are mainly *progestogens* or progestogen combinations, but include one non-progestogen as listed in Table 8.1. These pills are used to cover periods of high sexual activity encountered when couples working in different parts of China visit each other and spend short periods of time together, usually 2 weeks during the course of a year. These agents are not strictly postcoital drugs; they are administered one or two days before the start of the 'vacation' and are taken daily during the period of sexual

Table 8.1 Chinese home visiting or vacation pills

Name	*Dosage (mg)*	*Efficacy (% of cycles)**	*Mode of administration*
Simple progestogens			
Norethisterone	5	99.5	In case of vacation, one pill in the evening, then one pill each day for 10–14 days; change to pill No. 1 (norethisterone-ethinyl-oestradiol combination pill–various doses) or No. 2 (megestrol + ethinyloestradiol combination pill – various doses) if vacation longer than 2 weeks
Megestrol	2	99.6	One pill at midday before vacation and then in the evening. Afterwards, one pill each day until the next day after vacation
Quingestanol	80	98.8	One pill daily for 2 weeks
Norgestrel	3	99.9	One pill 1–2 days before vacation, then one pill every day. Change to pill No. 1 or No. 2 if vacation longer than 2 weeks
R-2323	2.5	99.5	Similar to Norgestrel
Norethisterone acetate-3-oxime	1	99.3	Similar to Norgestrel
Progestogen combinations			
Mequingestanol	Megestrol 0.55 Quingestanol 0.88	98.2	One pill at midday before vacation, then one pill postcoitally
Chlorquingestanol	Chlormadinone 0.25 Quingestanol 0.85	99.5	One pill at midday before vacation, then one pill every evening
Non-progestogen			
Anordrin	7.5	99.5	Was used as a postcoital agent. Results were equivocal

* Woman-cycles, not woman-years

activity. Evidence about their efficacy in controlled trials is lacking, which is why they have not gained much popularity outside China.

An example is the use of norethisterone in a dose of 5 mg/day for 2 weeks. If given early in the cycle the above regimen suppresses ovulation. Its efficacy is quoted by workers in Shanghai as 99.5%. Long-term use of progestogens on a regular basis raises anxieties about their effect on lipoproteins.

Piperine

This alkaloid is present in various species of *Piperaceae* and exhibits profound antifertility activity pre- and postimplantation in animal models [70]. It is believed to be the main agent in indigenous preparations used for menses induction in Asia.

STS 557

This synthetic progestogen has undergone clinical trials in a WHO programme. Two dose regimens have been in use in the German Democratic Republic. STS 557 exhibits an anti-implantation effect in baboons with a single dose of 0.4 mg administered 3–6 h after the onset of mating [71]. Anxiety about its toxicity has to be allayed by further research.

Progestogens and antiprogesterones

Progesterone is the hormone of the luteal phase and of pregnancy; its role in both phases can be interfered with by inhibiting its synthesis, release, or its action on target organs [72]. Antiprogesterones are called anti-implantation agents if given postcoitally, menses inducers if used in the luteal phase, and abortifacients if administered in early pregnancy. Earlier compounds including gestrinone (R-2323), anordrin, and ORF 9371 were clinically unacceptable because of low efficacy and/or androgenic side-effects [72]. Danazol was disappointing in an early study [31,60–61] but appears in a recent study from Milan, Italy, to be comparable in efficacy to the Yuzpe regimen (G. Zuliani, 1988, personal communication).

Such compounds as RU 486 [73] and trilostane [74] have been investigated as medical abortifacients, but have the potential for use as postcoital agents. WIN 24540 (trilostane) and WIN 32729 (epostane) inhibit the 3-beta-hydroxysteroid dehydrogenase enzyme system, leading to a consistent fall in plasma progesterone in early human pregnancy.

RU 486 (mifepristone) is the antiprogesterone most likely to become commercially available in the forseeable future [12, 75]. It is a steroid derivative of the progestogen norethisterone. It is active orally, vaginally, and by injection. It works by competitive inhibition of progesterone. The mode of action of RU 486 depends on the circumstances of its use. If administered at the time of ovulation it will disrupt the process. If used postcoitally it prevents implantation. When administered in the luteal phase, usually from day 24 to day 26 (before a period is missed and regardless of whether conception has occurred) RU 486 can induce menstruation.

However, until now the main use of antiprogesterones in general and of RU 486 in particular has been in the interruption of early pregnancies. The efficacy of RU 486 depends on the duration of gestation. Prior to 5 weeks, it produces complete abortion in 90% of cases [76]. In pregnancies over 5 weeks the complete expulsion rate is lower but can be improved by the concomitant use of a prostaglandin. Side-effects of

RU 486 include nausea and vomiting but these are minimal. Its antiglucocorticoid activity does not manifest itself in the doses currently used.

Antiprogesterone monoclonal antibodies have been used in animal experiments to block implantation or interfere with early embryonic development [77]. They again have the potential for postcoital use.

Anxieties about the repetitive use of antiprogesterones are due to possible antiglucocorticold effects and their long-term effects on endometrial and mammary tissue.

Antioestrogens

Centchromen is an antioestrogen which exhibits no progestational, androgenic or antiandrogenic effect [78]. It is weakly oestrogenic but has a main side-effect of causing ovarian stimulation and enlargement. Although it is already in phase 2 clinical trials it is unlikely to make an impact as a postcoital agent. All other antioestrogens, such as tamoxifen, have the potential for use as postcoital agents, mainly in combination with antiprogestational agents. This may allow a reduction in the dose and thereby increase the safety margin.

LHRH analogues

Several analogues have been evaluated as postcoital and/or postconceptional agents [79].

Luteinizing hormone releasing hormone (LHRH) is secreted by the hypothalamus in a pulsatile fashion. It stimulates the pituitary to release FSH and LH. The pulsatile release of LHRH is important as it allows for recovery of the pituitary cells. Analogues either enhance the release of LHRH (agonists) or inhibit it (antagonists). Both are much more potent than natural LHRH. Taken orally, these peptides are destroyed by proteolytic digestion. Thus, routes of administration must be by nasal spray, subcutaneous infusion, or injection. Frequent self-administration is a draw-back. To overcome this problem, slow-release polymer biodegradable implants are being tested.

'Peptide' contraception is a safe and effective alternative to steroid contraception. The peptides' rapid degradation means that reversibility is speedy. Used daily, these analogues inhibit ovulation after an initial ovarian stimulation phase with possible unopposed oestrogen production. Used for shorter periods but in higher doses LHRH analogues disrupt ovulation or produce luteolysis [80] and have the potential for use as postcoital contraceptives. Precise timing of the administration in relation to ovulation is essential for a successful outcome. The main disadvantage is the high cost of these analogues, and the problems of menstrual irregularity in long-term users.

ORF 13811

This is a synthetic analogue of zoapatanol, which is the active constituent in a herbal tea extracted from the Mexican plant zoapatle. For centuries this has been used as an antifertility agent. ORF 13811 was shown in biological test systems to be a potent antifertility agent, acting primarily by stimulating uterine muscle contractility [81].

Conclusions

Existing postcoital agents are practical and safe forms of emergency fertility control. (For guidelines regarding use, see Appendix below). Future research in postcoital contraception should concentrate not only on safer and more effective methods but also on combining the knowledge accumulated so far with methods for detection of ovulation, so that fertility control may be achieved by disrupting the periovulatory mechanisms at ovarian or endometrial levels. This will enable us to achieve the efficacy of the contraceptive pill with fewer systemic effects.

Prostaglandins, antiprogesterones, LHRH agonists and antagonists, and hCG antagonists are all currently being evaluated as postcoital contraceptives. Alone or in combination they may one day lead to a single monthly treatment that will enable couples to control their fertility and prevent unplanned pregnancies. To achieve these goals, a task force to develop and evaluate postovulatory agents has been set up under the auspices of the World Health Organization. Their contribution to the field of postcoital contraception is eagerly awaited.

Appendix

Guidelines on practical prescribing

The following are short notes to guide the clinician in counselling clients requesting postcoital contraception.

The methods. The two methods in common use are the combined ethinyloestradiol–levonorgestrel regimen as described previously, or the immediate insertion of a copper intrauterine contraceptive device.

When can they be used? The hormonal method is effective up to 72 h after the earliest coital exposure in the cycle in question. The IUD can be used up to 5 days after the estimated day of *ovulation.*

Efficacy. The reported failure rate of the hormonal method varies between 1% and 3%. The failure rate of the IUD method is even lower.

Mechanism of action. Both methods work primarily by blocking implantation. Postcoital contraception therefore has exactly the same ethical implications as the use of an IUD. The hormonal method, if given early in the cycle, could delay ovulation; therefore patients should abstain or use a recognized barrier method up to the next menstruation. The IUD provides cover for the rest of the cycle but can be removed at the next menstruation if the patient wishes.

Side-effects. These are mainly nausea and vomiting with the hormonal method, and the risk of pelvic inflammatory disease with use of the IUD. The latter is of special significance, since a substantial number of clients requesting postcoital contraception are having intercourse either for the first time ever, the first time with a new partner, or the first time with a previous partner after a period of abstinence.

When is the IUD the preferred choice? 1. Contraindications to oral contraception. 2. Exposure beyond the 72 h limit. 3. Multiple exposures, provided the IUD is inserted in good faith, no more than 120 h after the most probable calculated ovulation date. 4. Woman's desire for the most effective method. 5. Woman's desire to use the IUD as her long-term method. 6. After vomiting of either dose of the hormonal method in a high pregnancy-risk case.

What if the treatment fails? The most important aspect of counselling is to discuss the implication of failure of the postcoital contraceptive. Ectopic pregnancy should be mentioned and the woman warned to seek advice if she experiences pelvic pain. If the pregnancy is intrauterine, the woman should be counselled on the lines that 'the possibility of a pregnancy being harmed cannot be ruled out'. The teratogenic risk is thought to be extremely small and is probably less than the risk of taking the ordinary combined pill in early pregnancy. If a woman wishes to continue to full term, detailed records should be kept of the original consultation and of the outcome.

Follow-up. Future use of a more regular method of birth control should be discussed with any woman requesting postcoital contraception. If she selects a pill (combined or progestogen-only), she must be sure her next period is normal, so it is helpful to advise starting on day 3. This is early enough for supplementary contraception to be unnecessary in that cycle (page 76). A follow-up visit 3–4 weeks later is essential to confirm success of the treatment, to allay any anxieties and to ensure that she is using her new method correctly.

References

1. MUNZ, D., CARSON, S., BROCK, B *et al.* Contraception knowledge and practice among undergraduates at a Canadian university. *American Journal of Obstetrics and Gynecology*, **124**, 499–505 (1976)
2. NAQVI, R. H. and WARREN, J. C. Interceptive: drugs interrupting pregnancy after implantation. *Steroids*, **18**, 731–739 (1971)
3. FARKAS, M. Postcoital contraception with Prostinor, a preparation containing 0.75 mg d-norgestrel. *Magyar Noorvosok Lapia*, **41**, 474 (1978)
4. MORRIS, J. M. and VAN WAGENEN, G. Compounds interfering with ovum implantation and development. III. Role of estrogen. *American Journal of Obstetrics and Gynecology*, **96**, 804–815 (1966)
5. HERBST, A. L., ULFELDER, H. and POSKANZER, D. C. Adenocarcinoma of the vagina: association of maternal stilbestrol therapy with tumor appearance in young women. *New England Journal of Medicine*, **284**, 878–881 (1971)
6. HASPELS, A. A. and ANDRIESSE, R. The effects of large doses of estrogens post coitum in 2000 women. *European Journal of Obstetrics, Gynecology and Reproductive Biology*, **3**, 113–117 (1973)
7. HASPELS, A. A. Interception: post-coital estrogens in 3016 women. *Contraception*, **14**, 375–381 (1976)
8. KUCHERA, L. K. Postcoital contraception with diethylstilbestrol. *Journal of the American Medical Association*, **218**, 562–563 (1971)
9. MORRIS, J. M. and VAN WAGENEN, G. Postcoital oral contraception. *Advances in Planned Parenthood*, **4**, 125–128 (1969)
10. MEARS, E. In *Proceedings of the Eighth International Conference of the IPPF* (ed. R. K. B. Hankinson *et al.*), IPPF, London, p.256 (1967)
11. CRIST, T. and FARRINGTON, C. The use of estrogen as a postcoital contraceptive in North Carolina – trick or treatment. *North Carolina Medical Journal*, **34**, 792–795 (1973)
12. BLYE, R. P. The use of estrogens as postcoital contraceptive agents. *American Journal of Obstetrics and Gynecology*, **116**, 1044–1050 (1973)
13. SCHINDLER, A. E., LADANYI, S., GOSER, R. and KELLER, E. Postcoital contraception with an injectable estrogen preparation (ORG 369–2) *Contraception*, **22**, 165–172 (1980)
14. BLACKWELL, R. E., BOOTS, L. R. and DOWNING POTTER, H., JR. Evaluation of Delestrogen and Parlodel as a luteolytic agent in humans. *Fertility and Sterility*, **37**, 213–217 (1982)
15. DIXON, G. W., SCHLESSELMAN, J. J., ORY, J. W. and BLYE, R. P. Ethinyl estradiol and conjugated estrogens as postcoital contraceptives. *Journal of the American Medical Association*, **244**, 1336–1339 (1980)
16. LEHFELDT, H. Choice of ethinyl estradiol as a postcoital pill. *American Journal of Obstetrics and Gynecology*, **116**, 892–893 (1973)
17. MORRIS, J. M. and VAN WAGENEN, G. Interception: the use of postovulatory estrogens to prevent implantation. *American Journal of Obstetrics and Gynecology*, **115**, 101–106 (1973)
18. NOTELOVITZ, M. and BARD, D. S. Conjugated estrogen as a post-ovulatory interceptive. *Contraception*, **17**, 443–454 (1978)
19. KUCHERA, L. K. Postcoital contraception with diethylstilbestrol updated. *Contraception* **10**, 47–54 (1974)

20. YUZPE, A. A., THURLOW, H. J., RAMZY, I. and LEYSHON, J. I. Postcoital contraception – a pilot study. *Journal of Reproductive Medicine*, **13**, 53–58 (1974)

21. GRILLO, T. A. and HATCHER, R. The use of ethinyl estradiol and norgestrel pills as a morning after contraceptive. *Bulletin of the Woodruff Medical Center*, **11**, 183 (1980)

22. HUTCHINSON, F. Experience at London Brook Street Advisory Centres. Presented at a *Symposium of the Pregnancy Advisory Service*, London, England, PAS, London, p. 40 (1983)

23. PERCIVAL-SMITH, R. and DROSS, A. Ethinyl estradiol dl-norgestrel combination as a morning-after pill: preliminary report. *British Columbia Medical Journal*, **18,** 240–241 (1976)

24. PERCIVAL-SMITH, R. Post-coital contraception using dl-norgestrel/ethinyl estradiol combination. *Contraception*, **17,** 247–252 (1978)

25. SCHILLING, L. H. An alternative to the use of high-dose estrogens for post-coital contraception. *Journal of the American College Health Association*, **27**, 247–249 (1979)

26. VAN SANTEN, M. R. and HASPEL, A. A. A comparison of high-dose estrogens versus low-dose ethinylestradiol and norgestrel combination in postcoital interception: A study in 493 women. *Fertility and Sterility*, **43**, 206–213 (1985)

27. YUZPE, A. A. and LANCEE, W. J. Ethinyl estradiol and dl–norgestrel as a postcoital contraceptive. *Fertility and Sterility*, **28**, 932–936 (1977)

28. YUZPE, A. A., PERCIVAL-SMITH, R. and RADEMAKER, A. W. A multi-center clinical investigation employing ethinyl estradiol combined with dl-norgestrel as a postcoital contraceptive agent. *Fertility and Sterility*, **37,** 508–513 (1982)

29. SZONTAGH, F. E. and KOVACS, L. Post-coital contraception with dienestrol. *Medical Gynaecology and Sociology*, **4,** 36–37 (1969)

30. TULLY, B. Postcoital contraception – a study. *British Journal of Family Planning*, **8**, 119–124 (1983)

31. ROWLANDS, S., GUILLEBAUD, J., BOUNDS, W. and BOOTH, M. Side effects of Danazol compared with an ethinylestradiol/norgestrel combination when used for postcoital contraception. *Contraception*, **27**, 39–49 (1983)

32. PARSONS, A. D. The provision of a postcoital contraception service. Presented at a *Symposium of the Pregnancy Advisory Service*, London, England, PAS, London, p. 8 (1983)

33. VAN SANTEN, M. R. and HASPELS, A. A. Interception II. Postcoital low-dose estrogen and norgestrel gestrel only. *Proceedings of the XIth World Congress of Fertility and Sterility, Dublin (1983)*

34. MORRIS, J. M. and VAN WAGNEN, G. Postcoital oral contraception. In *Proceedings of the Eighth International Conference of the IPPF* (ed. Hankinson R. K. B. *et al.*). IPPF, London, pp. 256–259 (1967)

35. KUBBA, A. A. and GUILLEBAUD, J. Case of ectopic pregnancy after postcoital contraception with ethinyloestradiol – levonorgestrel *British Medical Journal*, **287**, 1343–1344 (1983)

36. KESSERU, E., LARRANAGA, A. and PARADA, J. Postcoital contraception with d-norgestrel. *Contraception*, **7**, 367–379 (1973)

37. MISCHLER, T. W., BERMAN, E., RUBIO, E. *et al.* Further experience with quingestanol acetate as a postcoital oral contraceptive. *Contraception*, **9**, 221–225 (1974)

38. RUBIO, B., BERMAN, E., LARRANAGA, A. *et al.* A new postcoital oral contraceptive. *Contraception*, **1**, 303–314 (1970)

39. KOVACS, L. and SEREGELY, G. D-norgestrel as postcoital anticoncipient in young women. *Proceedings of the International Congress of Pediatric Gynecology*, (Abstract) Tokyo (1979)

40. LARRANAGA, A., WINTERHATTEL, M. and SARTORETTO, J. N. Evaluation of d-norgestrel 1.0 mg as postcoital contraception. *International Journal of Fertility*, **20**, 156–160 (1975)

41a. SPONA, J., MATT, K. and SCHNEIDER, W. H. F. Studies on the action of d-norgestrel as a postcoital contraceptive agent. *Contraception*, **11**, 31 (1975)

41b. WORLD HEALTH ORGANIZATION. Task Force on Post-Ovulatory Methods for Fertility Regulation. (Special Programme for Research, Development and Research Training in Human Reproduction.) Post coital contraception with levonorgestrel during the peri-ovulatory phase of the menstrual cycle. *Contraception*, **36,** 257–286 (1987)

42. HOFFMAN, K. O. K. Postcoital contraception: experiences with ethinyloestradiol/norgestrel and levonorgestrel only. *Proceedings of the XIth World Congress of Fertility and Sterility*, Dublin (1983)

43. BARRETT, J. C. and MARSHALL, J. The risk of conception on different days of the menstrual cycle. *Population Studies*, **23**, 455–461 (1969)

44. ROYSTON, J. P. Basal body temperature, ovulation and the risk of conception, with special reference to the lifetimes of sperm and egg. *Biometrics*, **38**, 397–406 (1982)

45. SCHWARTZ, D., MACDONALD, P. D. M. and HEUCHEL, V. Fecundability, and coital frequency and the viability of ova. *Population Studies*, **34**, 397–400 (1980)

46. WORLD HEALTH ORGANIZATION. Task Force on Methods for the Determination of the Fertile Period. (Special Programme of Research, Development and Research Training in Human Reproduction). World Health Organization, Geneva, Switzerland. A prospective multicenter trial of the ovulation method of natural family planning. III. Characteristics of the menstrual cycle and of the fertile phase. *Fertility and Sterility*, **40,** 773–778 (1983)

47. BILLINGS, E. L., BILLINGS, J. J., BROWN, J. B. and BURGER, H. G. Symptoms and hormonal changes accompanying ovulation. *Lancet*, **1**, 282–284 (1972)

48. FLYNN, A. M. and LYNCH, S. S. Cervical mucus and identification of the fertile phase of the menstrual cycle. *British Journal of Obstetrics and Gynaecology*, **83**, 656 (1976)

49. HILGERS, T. W., ABRAHAM, G. E. and CAVANAGH, D. Natural family planning. I. The peak symptom and estimated time of ovulation. *Obstetrics and Gynecology*, **52**, 575 (1978)

50. BAUMAN, K. E. Selected aspects of the contraceptive practices of unmarried university students. *American Journal of Obstetrics and Gynecology*, **108**, 203–209 (1970)

51. NEEDLE, R. H. The relationship between first sexual intercourse and ways of handling contraception among college students. *Journal of the American College Health Association*, **24** (2), 106–111 (1975)

51a. ROWLANDS, S., KUBBA, A. A., GUILLEBAUD, J. and BOUNDS, W. A. A possible mechanism of action of danazol and an ethinylestradiol-norgestrel combination used as postcoital contraceptive agents. *Contraception*, **33,** 539–545, (1986)

52. BACIC, M., DE CASPARIS, A. W. and DICZFALUSY, E. Failure of large doses of ethinyl estradiol to interfere with early embryonic development in the human species. *American Journal of Obstetrics and Gynecology*. **107**, 531–534. (1970)

53. KARNAKY, K. J. Prolonged administration of diethylstilbestrol. *Journal of Clinical Endocrinology and Metabolism*, **5**, 279–284 (1945)

54. KARNAKY, K. J. Estrogenic tolerance in pregnant women. *American Journal of Obstetrics and Gynecology*, **53**, 312–316 (1947)

55. CRAFT, I,. FOSS, G. L., WARREN, R. J. and FOTHERBY, K. Effect of norgestrel administered intermittently on pituitary ovarian function. *Contraception*, **12**, 589–598 (1975)

56. LING, W. Y., ROBICHAUD, A., ZAYID, I. *et al.* Mode of action of dl-norgestrel and ethinyl estradiol combination in postcoital contraception. *Fertility and Sterility*, **32**, 297–302 (1979)

57. LING, W. Y., WRIXON, W., ZAYID, I. *et al.* Mode of action of dl-norgestrel and ethinyl estradiol combination in postcoital contraception. II. Effect of postovulatory administration on ovarian function and endometrium. *Fertility and Sterility*, **39**, 292–297 (1983)

58. LING, W. Y., WRIXON W., ACORN, T *et al.* Mode of action of dl-norgestrel and ethinylestradiol combination in postcoital contraception. III. Effect of preovulatory administration following the luteinizing hormone surge on ovarian steroidogenesis. *Fertility and Sterility*, **40**, 631–636 (1983)

59. GARMENDIA, F., KESSERU, E., URDANIVIA, E. and VALENCIA, M. Luteinizing hormone and progesterone in women under postcoital contraception with d-norgestrel. *Fertility and Sterility*, **27**, 1250–1255 (1976)

60. GUILLEBAUD, J., KUBBA, A. A., ROWLANDS, S. *et al.* Postcoital contraception with danazol compared with an ethinyloestradiol – norgestrel combination or insertion of an intrauterine device. *Journal of Obstetrics and Gynaecology*, **3**, (Suppl 2), S64–S68 (1983)

61. KUBBA, A. A., WHITE, J. O., GUILLEBAUD, J. and ELDER, M. G. The biochemistry of human endometrium after two regimens of postcoital contraception; A dl-norgestrel/ethinylestradiol combination or danazol. *Fertility and Sterility*, **45,** 512–516 (1986)

62. LIPPES, J., MALIK, T. and TATUM, H. J. The postcoital copper-T. *Advances in Planned Parenthood*, **11,** 24–29 (1976)

63. LIPPES. J., TATUM, H. J., MAULID, D. and ZICLEZNY, M. A. Continuation of the study of postcoital IUDs. *Family Planning Perspectives*, **11**, 195 (1979)

64. BLACK, T. R. L., GOLDSTUCK, N. D. and SPENCE, A. Postcoital intrauterine device insertion – a further evaluation. *Contraception*, **22**, 653–658 (1980)

65. TYRER, L. The Copper-7 and postcoital contraception. *Advances in Planned Parenthood*, **15**, 111–117 (1980)

66. VAN SANTEN, M. R. and HASPELS, A. A. Interception by postcoital IUD insertion. *Contraception Delivery Systems*, **2**, 189–200 (1981)
67. KUBBA, A. A. and GUILLEBAUD, J. Failure of postcoital contraception after insertion of an intrauterine device. Case report. *British Journal of Obstetrics and Gynaecology*, **91**, 596–597 (1984)
68. HASSON, H. M. Topical uterine anaesthesia: preliminary report. *International Journal of Gynaecology and Obstetrics*, **15**, 238–240 (1977)
69. GOTTARDI, G., SPREAFICO, A. and DE ORCHI, L. The postcoital IUD as an effective continuing contraceptive method. *Contraception*, **34**, 549–558 (1986)
70. PIYACHATNRAWAT, P., GLINSUKON, T. and PEUGVICHA, P. Postcoital antifertility effect of piperine. *Contraception*, **26**, 625–632 (1982)
71. OETTEL, M., KOMOR, A., GONCHAROV, N. P. and SCHUBERT, K. STS–557 as an interceptive in rodents and baboons. *Contraception*, **21**, 537–549 (1980)
72. HEALY, D. L. and FRASER, H. M. The antiprogesterones are coming: menses induction, abortion, and labour? *British Medical Journal*, **290**, 580–581 (1985)
73. HEALY, D. L., BAULIEU, E. E. and HODGEN, G. D. Induction of menstruation by an antiprogesterone steroid (Ru486) in primates: site of action, dose-response relationships, and hormonal effects. *Fertility and Sterility*, **40**, 253–257 (1983)
74. VAN DER SPUY, Z. M., JONES, D. L., WRIGHT, C. S. W. *et al.* Inhibition of 3-beta-hydroxy steroid dehydrogenase activity in first trimester human pregnancy with trilostane and WIN 32729. *Clinical Endocrinology*, **19**, 521–532 (1983)
75. ELIA, D. Uses of RU 486: a clinical update. *IPPF Medical Bulletin*, **20**, (5), 1–2 (1986)
76. KOVACS, L., SAS, M., REECH, B. A. *et al.* Termination of very early pregnancy with RU 486 – an anti-progestational compound. *Contraception*, **29**, 339–410 (1984)
77. WANG, M. Y., RIDER, V., HEAP, R. B. and FEINSTEIN, A. Action of anti-progesterone monoclonal antibody in blocking pregnancy after postcoital administration in mice. *Journal of Endocrinology*, **101**, 95–100 (1984)
78. KAMBOJ, V. P., SETTY, B. S., HARISHCHANDRA, ROY, S. K. and KAR, A. B. Biological profile of centchromen – a new postcoital contraceptive. *Indian Journal of Experimental Biology*, **15**, 1144 (1977)
79. CORBIN, A., BEATTIE, C. W., REES, R. *et al.* Postcoital contraceptive effects of agonist analogs of luteinizing hormone-releasing hormone. *Fertility and Sterility*, **29**, 471–475 (1977)
80. SHEEHAN, K. L., CASPER, R. F. and YEN, S. S. C. Induction of luteolysis by luteinizing hormone-releasing factor (LRF) agonist: Sensitivity, reproducibility and reversibility. *Fertility and Sterility*, **37**, 209–212 (1982)
81. HAHN, D. W., TOBIA, A. J., ROSENTHALE, M. E. and MCGUIRE, J. L. Antifertility activity and general pharmacological properties of ORF 13811: a synthetic analog of zoapatanol. *Contraception*, **30**, 39–53 (1984)

Chapter 9

Intrauterine contraceptive devices

Howard J. Tatum and Elizabeth B. Connell

According to the history of contraception, the first intrauterine devices (IUDs) were inserted into female camels. Although we do not know how they arrived at the correct conclusion, we do know that centuries ago Turks and Arabs learned that inserting pebbles through hollow tubes into the uteri of their female camels would prevent them from conceiving during long trips across the desert [1]. The first reference to use in the human female came from Hippocrates who wrote about the contraceptive possibilities of placing foreign bodies in the uterus. The first documented use by women apparently occurred in the eleventh century as recorded by Avicenna, an Islamic scientist.

Numerous types of materials have been used in the fashioning of intrauterine devices, including such things as wood, glass, pewter, ivory, ebony, gold and wool [2]. Probably the most elaborate were IUDs made out of platinum and then studded with diamonds. Many of the earlier devices had stems which extended through the endocervical canal to the external cervical os. They were reportedly used, not only for contraceptive purposes, but also for the treatment of uterine descensus and malposition and for the induction of abortions.

An IUD which was deployed totally within the uterine cavity was first developed by Richter in 1909 [3]. He fashioned a ring-shaped device out of silkworm gut. In 1923 Pust described a similar device but attached it to a stem [4]. The next major innovation occurred in Germany in 1930. Ernst Grafenberg started manufacturing rings made out of silkworm gut and silver wire [5]. Four years later, Tenrei Ota of Japan began to use gold and gold-plated silver intrauterine devices. Interest in the use of these types of intrauterine devices then spread to other countries. However, stories soon began to circulate about the development of intrauterine infection and, as a result, IUDs fell into disrepute and their use virtually ceased.

Following this era, very little research was carried out in this field for a considerable period of time. Then, in the late 1950s, with the recognition of the urgent worldwide need for effective means of fertility regulation, interest once again developed in intrauterine contraception. This renewed interest came about also as the result of two favourable articles which appeared in the medical literature in 1959. The first was written by Oppenheimer, and discussed the effectiveness of the Grafenberg and Ota rings; the second, by Ishihama, commented on the clinical usefulness of the Ota ring [6,7].

The first devices to be invented in this era were fashioned out of biologically inert plastics. This new type of IUD had become possible because of advances in plastics technology. Materials had been developed which allowed a device to be given memory during the manufacturing process. After being stretched out into a linear form for insertion into the uterus, it would reassume its original shape.

The first of the plastic non-medicated IUDs were the Margulies spiral and the Lippes loop [8–11]. The spiral had a stem made of plastic which went through the endocervical canal and emerged through the external os. The loop had a thread attached as a tail. These appendages served two purposes: they permitted the doctor and the patient to confirm the continued presence of the device and they could be grasped and traction applied at the time of removal. There were a number of other plastic devices developed about that time: among them were the Saf-T-Coil, Dalkon Shield, Birnberg Bow and Lem [12, 13]. In addition to the plastic IUDs, several metal devices, such as the Majzlin spring, the M device and the stainless steel ring, were developed and evaluated [14–16].

Of all of these devices, only the Lippes loop is still in (diminishing) usage. The rigid tail of the spiral produced discomfort to male sexual partners. Two IUDs, the Bow and the stainless steel ring were closed devices with the potential for producing bowel obstruction should perforation occur [17]. The Dalkon shield was removed from the market when it was shown to be associated with an increased risk of mid-trimester septic abortion [18]. Finally, the Lem and all the metal devices embedded significantly and proved to be quite difficult to remove [13,19,20].

It soon became apparent that in order to evaluate and compare the various IUDs, some central evaluation mechanism must be set up. Therefore, in 1963 the Cooperative Statistical Program was set up by the Population Council under the direction of Dr Christopher Tietze. This programme monitored data accumulated out of 27 000 insertions with 39 000 woman-years of use. In this evaluation, such events as pregnancies, removals for pain, bleeding, infection, and other medical indications, removals for personal reasons such as planned pregnancy, and complications such as perforation and expulsion were identified, and their rates of occurrence calculated [21–24]. In this programme, data were analysed under the life table technique instead of the less accurate Pearl index which had previously been employed [25,26]. Thus, the early anecdotal publications composed of case reports and small studies of a single device were replaced by valid comparative data collected on several IUDs, using a common protocol.

From these studies it became possible to draw several conclusions. It was found that large devices were more effective in preventing pregnancy than small ones; they were not expelled as often, but they produced higher rates of side-effects such as cramping and bleeding and, therefore, had higher rates of medical removal. Smaller devices, on the other hand, had fewer side-effects such as cramping and bleeding; however, they were not as effective and they were more often expelled [24].

As the result of these earlier comparative studies, it was decided to try to develop a small plastic platform which would be T-shaped to conform to the shape of the uterine cavity, which would theoretically decrease the incidence of cramping and bleeding. However, it soon became apparent that pregnancy rates of 18 per 100 woman years would result from the use of such a device. Therefore, copper wire was added to small T- and 7-shaped IUDs. It was thus found to be possible to obtain rates which were approximately equal to the large non-medicated devices, but with lower rates of adverse side-effects [27–30]. Until January 1986 two copper-bearing devices were available in the United States, the Tatum–T, TCu 200 and the Cu–7. Copper devices widely used in other countries include the TCu 200, TCu 220C and TCu 380A, and the 380A Slim-line manufactured by Ortho Canada; the Multiload 250 and 375 by Multilan, Switzerland, the TCu 380 Ag and the Nova T (Leiras Company, Finland). (See below for discussion of the situation in the USA.)

Another type of IUD utilizing a T-shaped platform was subsequently developed, to which was added a reservoir of progesterone [31–34]. This device, the Progestasert, has a decreased total blood loss but induces a moderate amount of intermenstrual spotting. Moreover, all the medicated IUDs have a fixed duration of action ranging from one year for the Progestasert to 3 years for the Cu-7, 4 years for the Tatum-T, TCu 200 and 5 years for the TCu 380A, following which, officially, they should be removed and renewed. However, as more data are obtained the approved life-spans of copper IUDs may be extended [59]. This would be valuable in reducing insertion-related risks (page 149). (See also Table 9.2, page 164.)

Thus the IUD has been used in one form or another for centuries. Its popularity has been intermittent, but it has served as a major component of the world's contraceptive armamentarium since its most recent reintroduction in the late 1950s. An FDA report in 1968 stated that IUDs are generally safe, effective and useful methods of birth control [17]. A second report published 10 years later reiterated this same conclusion [35]. Finally, in the report of a WHO Scientific Group on IUDs, published in 1987, it was concluded: 'In summary, the Scientific Group considered the IUD to be an important method of fertility regulation with high continuation rates and significant advantages in convenience of use. The newer copper-releasing devices are comparable to oral contraception in terms of safety and efficacy, and the use of IUDs in both developed and developing countries should continue to be supported as a reliable and safe method of reversible fertility regulation.' [36]

Mechanism of action

For many years it has been recognized that IUDs are a very effective means of preventing pregnancy. However, their mechanism of action has remained unclear during most of this period of time and is only now beginning to be understood. One reason for the confusion is the fact that there is considerable species variability. IUDs apparently block sperm transport in sheep and fowl and interfere with corpus luteum function and/or implantation in the cow, ewe, pig, rabbit and guinea-pig [17].

A number of theories have been developed over the years, attempting to explain how IUDs work. One of the early explanations, coming out of research on rhesus monkeys, was that the presence of the device induced hyperperistalsis of the fallopian tube [37]. This meant that the ovum traversed the tube and entered the uterine cavity before fertilization could occur. Subsequent studies, however, indicated that this phenomenon occurred only in artifically ovulated animals [38].

A second theory suggested that the intrauterine device produced a hormonal imbalance which somehow interfered with the establishment of a pregnancy. However, no consistent pattern has ever been found to support this concept.

A third proposed mechanism of action was that the foreign body produced endometritis and, therefore, a pregnancy could not be established and maintained. This theory, also, could not be substantiated. Although organisms from the vagina are inevitably introduced into the uterus at the time of insertion, in the majority of cases the fundus rapidly reverts to its previous sterile condition [39]. (But see also [40].)

It is currently believed that IUDs act by producing a number of biochemical changes in the endometrium, due to the stimulation of a sterile inflammatory response. It has been shown that shortly after the insertion of the intrauterine device, white blood cells (WBCs) such as polymorphonuclear leukocytes appear in the endometrium and uterine fluid. The next step is the invasion of foreign-body giant cells, macrophages, plasma cells and mononuclear cells. It is the combined action of these cells which appears to be responsible for the production of the biochemical alterations in the endometrium [41–46].

They appear to prevent pregnancy in one or more ways. The WBCs may phagocytize spermatozoa, oöcytes or blastocysts. The liberation of endocytotoxins from the WBCs may result in the lysis of the sperm, ovum and/or blastocyst and may interfere with implantation by denaturing endometrial enzymes or altering endometrial metabolism of glycogen [43–45].

Another theory suggests that the presence of the IUD causes an increased production of prostaglandins [47–49]. This, in turn, could stimulate uterine and tubal contractions, modifying the tubal transport of sperm, ova and blastocysts, and interfering with implantation. Moreover, the prostaglandins might cause an increased production of immunoglobulins, which could act either to prevent implantation or to disrupt the early implantation site.

Thus, the basic mechanism of action of an IUD is apparently the induction of a localized sterile inflammatory response. In fact, there is evidence to suggest that the effectiveness of any IUD is directly related to the amount of foreign-body reaction that it stimulates. In the case of the non-medicated devices, the tissue response is directly proportional to the surface area and is maximum in the part of the endometrium immediately adjacent to the device [50]. However, cultures taken from these areas of inflammation are almost invariably negative. Moreover, the insertion of a foreign body into one horn of a bicornuate uterus does not protect against pregnancy in the other horn.

Biochemical analyses of endometrium taken from IUD users show a number of changes. RNA:DNA ratios are altered, and acid and alkaline phosphatase, phospholipids, oxygen consumption, glycogen deposition, and total proteins all undergo changes. Other cellular components such as protein, urea, non-protein nitrogen, and lysosomal hydrolases are increased, indicating tissue breakdown [35]. In addition the microvasculature undergoes changes which might interfere with implantation and/or the support of an early pregnancy.

The copper-bearing devices stimulate qualitatively the same types of responses in the endometrium, but they are quantitatively more intense, due to the release of copper ions. These produce a direct toxic effect on ova and sperm, the motility, capacitation and survival of sperm all being adversely affected by copper [51,52]. Copper ions also modify cervical mucus, reducing sperm penetration and their ability to ascend upward into the uterus and tubes.

The progesterone-bearing IUDs also induce a sterile inflammatory reaction but, in addition, produce local hormonal effects [53,54]. The viscosity of cervical mucus is increased, impairing sperm penetration. The endometrium, particularly the areas in direct contact with the device, shows progestational responses such as secretory and decidual changes. Over time, the endometrium becomes somewhat atrophic.[55–57] All these endometrial alterations occur without measurable increases of copper or progesterone in the serum [58].

Beneficial effects

The use of IUDs for fertility regulation offers a number of advantages. They require only a single act of motivation on the part of the user and, unless problems arise, necessitate minimal continuing medical care. While the medicated devices require changing periodically, the non-medicated IUDs may be left in indefinitely.

The cost of IUDs, calculated over time, is usually low. Their continuation rates are high compared to methods that demand daily pill-taking or use with each act of coitus. Discontinuation is easy with methods requiring repetitive performance, but it requires a positive action in the case of the IUD. At the end of 1 year, 75% of women are still using their devices. Continuation rates improve with each succeeding year of use and, at the end of 6 years, almost one-half of those accepting the Lippes loop in one study were still using it. Insertion and removal are most often uneventful and the return of fertility is prompt in most instances [24,35].

IUDs have been and continue to be popular methods of birth control. It has been estimated that 50–60 million women are using them, 40 million of these in China, 3 million in the United States, and the remainder in both developed and lesser developed countries (LDCs). They are particularly useful in LDCs because they are easy to manufacture, ship and store, and because they can be inserted by trained paraprofessional health workers [35].

Effectiveness

The intrauterine device is a highly effective form of contraception (see Table 9.1) [59–65]. Only Depo-Provera and the combined oral contraceptives have efficacy rates, both for method-effectiveness and use-effectiveness, which are higher than those obtained with IUDs. The currently available IUDs have method-effectiveness rates of 96–98 per 100 women users and use-effectiveness rates of 90–96 [24]. The TCu 380 has a method effectiveness of 99+/100 women users (see four-year study by Sivin and Tatum).

It has been found that many factors enter into the effectiveness of any IUD. Amongst these are the basic design of the device, the age and parity of the acceptor, expulsion rates, the technique of insertion and the inserter itself [66]. For example,

Table 9.1 Effectiveness of IUDs over a 2-year period of use

Device	*Pregnancy*	*Pain/bleeding*	*Expulsion*	*Continuation*	*No. of women*	*Reference*
Lippes loop D	3.7	7.9	10.0	54.8	992	[60]
Cu 7	3.6	6.5	7.9	55.5	994	[60]
TCu 200	5.6	18.9	8.3	50.0	1851	[61]
TCu 220C	1.8	17.1	9.8	59.7	1097	[61]
TCu 380A	1.0	23.7	9.5	50.1	1679	[61]
Nova T	1.8	19.1	7.8	51.6	918	[62]
Multiload MLCu 250	2.5	6.1	2.1	74.0	580	[63]
Multiload MLCu 250	1.1	3.8	1.2	89.5	664	[64]
Multiload MLCu 375	0.9	12.3	10.2	65.6	432	[65]

Table based on cumulative event rates per 100 women for discontinuation over 2-year period of use in multiparae. Interval insertions. Largest multicentre studies selected from Table 1 of Treiman and Liskin, *Population Reports* Series B, number 5, March 1988. Population Information Program, the Johns Hopkins University, Baltimore, Maryland 21205, USA [59].

Conclusion from Table 1:

1. The continuation rate with IUDs is far greater than with oral contraceptives. The rates of accidental pregnancies are all quite low.
2. Pain/bleeding seem to increase for a given shape of IUD as the surface area of copper increases.
3. Pregnancy rates do not seem to contribute significantly to the continuation rate.

women who are older and of higher parity have lower expulsion rates. Of major importance is the skill of the individual who performs the insertion [35]. Finally, levels of motivation and socioeconomic factors such as race, religion and cultural attitudes regarding such things as vaginal bleeding greatly affect both the acceptance and continuation rates [35]. For example, it has been found that women are less apt to have their IUDs removed for side-effects such as cramping and bleeding, if they have completed their desired family size.

It is very important that the IUD be placed high in the fundus, since it is only relatively effective, causes more bleeding, and is more readily expelled if left in the lower uterine segment [67]. In general, the push-out technique has higher rates of uterine perforation and poor placement than the inserter-tube withdrawal method in which the IUD is positioned at the top of the fundus, following which the inserter tube is removed [67,68].

Multiple studies have shown that effectiveness and continuation rates vary greatly according to the type of care given to the IUD patient. This is true as regards the competence of the individual doing the insertion; it is also true of the quality of initial counselling and follow-up care. In fact, the differences found in comparative trials are more often reflective of these sorts of considerations than of the nature and configuration of the devices being studied [69].

Adverse effects

Intrauterine devices have always been associated with the development of certain adverse side-effects. The overall morbidity and mortality rates remain low with intrauterine contraception; hospitalizations range from 0.3 to 1.0 per 100 woman-years of use, and deaths range from 1 to 10 per million woman-years of use [35]. In general, IUDs have lower mortality rates but higher morbidity rates than the oral contraceptives [70,71]. However, in younger women and older non-smoking women, the risk of death is lower with both methods than that associated with pregnancy and delivery [72]. Post-IUD infertility has been shown to relate more to multiple sexual partners (and *their* partners), than to the copper-bearing devices especially. The non-medicated IUDs, with the exception of the unique Dalkon shield which has the highest rate of infertility of any known IUD, have a slightly higher incidence of infertility than do the copper-bearing IUDs [73,74].

Problems associated with insertion

At the time of insertion there may be a mild to moderate amount of pain or discomfort as the endocervical canal is dilated and the intrauterine device is inserted through it to the top of the fundal cavity. In a few individuals this discomfort results in a vagal response and may produce syncope. The tendency towards this reaction is increased if the patient is nulliparous, has a long, narrow cervix, is extremely anxious, or if she has a history of vascular instability or seizure disorders [35]. Mild symptoms such as hypotension, pallor, diaphoresis, weakness, and bradycardia or tachycardia may occur, and grand mal seizures have been reported [75]. However, the incidence of severe problems is very low and they can almost always be avoided by giving good psychological support to the patient, along with the administration of mild sedation, local anaesthesia – and intravenous atropine if indicated by bradycardia [75,76].

Perforation

One of the major side-effects of intrauterine contraception is perforation through the uterine wall and into the pelvic or abdominal cavity. The incidence of this complication ranges from 0.0 to 8.7 per 1000 insertions, and is directly proportional to the skill of the individual performing the insertion [75]. One major reason for perforation is the failure to establish the size and orientation of the uterus by careful pelvic examination. This is particularly important where there is sharp ante- or retroflexion of the uterus, and where it is not straightened with traction using a tenaculum prior to the insertion. Other reasons include severe cervical stenosis, congenital uterine anomalies, careless sounding or failure to sound the cavity, and the insertion of a device without sufficient care during the early postpartum period when the uterine musculature may be more easily perforated [75].

The complication occurs most frequently at the time of insertion. It may be suspected because of excessive pain and/or bleeding, and the device may be retrieved. However, the perforation is often silent and is not recognized until somewhat later when it is found that the tail has disappeared, or when a pregnancy is diagnosed [35]. There is some evidence to suggest that delayed perforation may occasionally occur. In this instance the perforation usually begins at the time of insertion and the device is subsequently forced by uterine contractions through the remainder of the uterine wall and into the pelvic cavity [75,77].

Cervical perforations have been reported with the copper T- and 7-shaped IUDs and also with all the IUDs which have a dependent end. In these cases, it appears that uterine contractions progressively force the lower arm of the device downward. It impinges on one of the endocervical rugae and then gradually the tip of the device passes through the cervical wall and appears in the vaginal canal [35,76].

Over a period of time certain devices will become deeply embedded in the endometrium. On occasions this may produce abnormal bleeding but in most instances it is asymptomatic. However, once the device is deeply embedded and covered by endometrium, it loses its effectiveness and a pregnancy may occur [35,75].

If a perforation is suspected, the location of the IUD must be determined. This can be done by probing the uterus or by the use of ultrasound or X-ray [35] with a uterine marker (such as another IUD). If the device is found to be in the pelvic or abdominal cavity, it should in most instances be removed. Copper IUDs must be taken out as soon as feasible because copper ions induce intense tissue reactions, resulting in dense intraperitoneal adhesions; unless a copper device is removed within a few days of the perforation, laparotomy is usually required [76]. Non-medicated IUDs should probably also be removed because they may perforate the bowel or be converted to a closed loop and cause intestinal obstruction. In this instance, however, there is no urgency as far as removal is concerned, and the devices can usually be retrieved by laparoscopy [75,76].

Cervical perforations are usually silent and are only noted at the time of a routine follow-up examination. Since the devices are no longer high in the fundal cavity, they have only limited effectiveness and should be removed. This is easily accomplished by exerting upward pressure on the device through the endocervical canal, followed by its extraction [35,76].

Expulsion

Another major complication found with IUDs is expulsion, since the uterus tends to expel foreign bodies. Rates are higher with smaller devices of various designs. The shape and stiffness of an IUD also have an effect on its expulsion rate. Reported rates for current IUDs range from 0.7 to 19.3 per 100 users [35,75].

Expulsion may occur at any time after insertion, but is most commonly noted at the time of the first postinsertion menses [35,75]. Thereafter the frequency of expulsion decreases; it remains highest during the early months of use and is most apt to occur with a menstrual period. In general, patients who are older, are of higher parity, or who have used a device for longer periods of time have lower expulsion rates [35,75,77].

Expulsion may be complete, the device being expelled by the uterus, following which it passes out of the vagina. An expulsion may also be partial, the device being displaced into the lower uterine segment or the endocervical canal. When this occurs, the protection against pregnancy is reduced and there may be an increased risk of ascending infection. A partial expulsion may be suspected when the transcervical tail is getting longer, the tip of the IUD can be felt in the endocervical canal or there is increased intermenstrual spotting [76].

An expulsion may be detected by the patient, particularly if she has been instructed to feel for the tail of her device after each menstrual period and finds that it is gone [75]. This occurs in about 20% of cases. However, expulsion may pass unnoticed until a pregnancy occurs. One-third of all pregnancies associated with the use of IUDs are the result of an unnoticed expulsion [77].

Women who expel an IUD have a threefold increased risk of expelling the same or another device. However, almost one-half of women who request a reinsertion will retain their second device [24]. Certain of the earlier devices such as the stainless steel Majzlin spring were highly resistant to expulsion. Unfortunately, they were also associated with a greater potential for cramping, bleeding, embedding, and difficult removal [67,78,79].

Cramping and bleeding

These two very common symptoms which occur with IUD usage are responsible for more than one-half of the medical removals [24]. The overall removal rates for currently available devices range from 4 to 14.7 per 100 users [35,75]. It has been found that the frequency and severity of these two side-effects are directly related to the shape and the size of the IUD relative to the dimensions of the uterine cavity. IUDs conforming to the cavity shape have fewer side-effects than those which do not and which distort the walls [75].

It has also been shown that the material of which the device is made has a major effect on the frequency of cramping and particularly on the amount of blood loss. The largest blood loss occurs with the non-medicated devices (70–80 ml), the next with copper (50–60 ml), and the least with the progesterone-bearing devices, the amount with these last actually being lower than the normal menstrual flow of approximately 35 ml [75,76,78].

The majority of the women who experience these two side-effects do so early in the use of their device, and the symptoms tend to disappear with continued use [35]. However, they may continue to be a problem throughout the entire time of usage in certain individuals. When one reviews the literature on cramping and bleeding, and consequent removal, it is found that there is a wide variation in bleeding patterns. Some women experience intermenstrual spotting and/or bleeding, others heavier menses, and still others have both [75].

These complications tend to be more common in nulliparous patients and with the use of larger devices. While the amount of bleeding does not usually constitute a medical problem, if a blood loss of more than 60 ml occurs and is repeated with each menses, there is a fivefold increase in iron-deficiency anaemia [80]. This is of major importance in those areas of the world where women are anaemic, have sub-standard diets, suffer from parasitic infections, and have frequent and numerous pregnancies [77].

There are also variations in removal rates that are primarily reflections of the attitudes of the patients themselves and particularly of the attitudes of their health-care providers. In many instances, when strong support is given to a patient who has cramping and bleeding during the early months of using an intrauterine device, the episode can be passed over and use continued until the symptoms disappear [35,75]. On the other hand, there are areas of the world where abnormal bleeding poses a major problem. In some cultures women who are bleeding are not permitted to cook, to have sexual intercourse, to take care of children, to attend religious services, or to make religious pilgrimages. In these situations intermenstrual bleeding is considerably more serious, and will be a cause for removal more often than in other areas where the cultural prohibitions against bleeding are not so strong [35,69,78].

Because these two side-effects have such a major impact on acceptance and continuation rates, numerous attempts have been made to identify their aetiology(ies) so that appropriate therapy could be instituted. Multiple theories of causation have been formulated. These include a generalized increase in vascularity because of the presence of a foreign body, direct trauma to the endometrial vessels, actual erosion into the endometrium, or biochemical alterations such as an increase in plasminogen activators or fibrin proteolysis [35,75].

A large number of agents have been tried in attempts to reduce the frequency and severity of these complications, and have included antifibrinolytic agents, prostaglandin synthetase inhibitors, vitamins, hormones, coagulants, antihistamines, vasoconstrictors, and prostaglandin antagonists [35,75,81–85]. Thus far, however, no therapy has been found to be consistently successful [75].

Pelvic inflammatory disease

The major problem at the present time with intrauterine contraception is the increased risk of pelvic inflammatory disease (PID). There has been and continues to be considerable debate as to the aetiology, incidence and severity of PID as experienced by IUD users. It is now believed that the overall increase in incidence is approximately twofold [86].

The early concept of these infections was that they were primarily caused by gonorrhoea and were unrelated to the presence of the IUD. This concept is no longer believed to be valid by most experts in the field. Continued research has shown that the IUD itself is associated with a low-level incidence of PID. Moreover, a wide variety of organisms, both aerobic and anaerobic, have been cultured from the endometrial cavities of IUD wearers who have signs and symptoms of pelvic infection.

Of key importance is the number of sexual partners of IUD-users. It has been found that with monogamous women who have sexual partners who are also monogamous, the incidence of pelvic inflammatory disease is very near the background level. The incidence of infection goes up in direct relationship to the number of sexual partners, and the number of sexual partners of the sexual partners.

The diagnosis of PID is based upon symptoms, signs, and laboratory findings. The symptoms are characterized by a vaginal discharge which may be foul smelling and is frequently bloody. The patient complains also of vague lower-abdominal pain which is usually bilateral in distribution. She may attribute this to menstrual cramps or to ordinary gas pains. She may also complain of nausea and/or vomiting. These latter two symptoms are frequently associated with the lower-abdominal pain and they increase in severity as the abdominal pain increases. Tenderness is frequently found in the suprapubic area over the uterus and the patient may also complain of painful intercourse (dyspareunia). She will also usually experience chills and general body aches and pains, somewhat similar to those associated with influenza, and will frequently have a low-grade fever.

In more advance cases of pelvic inflammatory disease there may be a low-grade or spiking fever. Rebound tenderness may be elicited on palpation of the lower and/or upper abdomen. On pelvic examination there may be blood in the vagina and blood may be seen coming through the cervical os. The uterine fundus is generally tender on bimanual examination and may have a softer than normal consistency. Occasionally induration may be detected in the adnexal areas and tubo-ovarian masses may be present.

Frequently, motion of the cervix produces pain and discomfort on the contralateral side, indicating that tension has been placed on the inflamed area. The pain on examination may create enough involuntary resistance and guarding so that the ovaries cannot be detected. It is important to remember that if the adnexa are palpated during this examination, it should be assumed that the fallopian tubes are abnormally large. It is very likely that the patient has a hydro- or pyosalpinx and that the tubes contain infected fluid. On rectal examination the tenderness in the adnexal areas will usually be confirmed. Occasionally a cul-de-sac mass will be detected and may have a characteristic feel which suggests the advisability of drainage.

Laboratory findings will generally include a white blood count which is increased above 10 000 $WBCs/mm^3$. There is frequently a shift to the left in the leukocyte distribution. Although the count is usually increased, it may not be increased in proportion to the severity of the infection. A diffuse extrauterine mass (echogenic to sonography) may suggest fluid within the pelvis and perhaps in the infected area. The sonogram will usually detect the presence of the IUD but may not identify its exact location. An intravenous pyelogram may be helpful. It may demonstrate compression of the bladder and/or uterus by an extrinsic mass. Laparoscopy has been found invaluable, particularly by the Scandinavian workers [86].

After a patient with less severe disease has been on oral antibiotics as an outpatient for between 12 and 24 h, she should be re-evaluated. If she has failed to show significant clinical improvement over this period of time it is mandatory that the IUD be removed, and highly desirable that the patient be hospitalized. In the hospital, active antibiotic treatment can be continued along with general supportive measures.

Both aerobic and anaerobic cultures should be obtained from the IUD when it is removed, looking for the types of organisms as well as for their sensitivity to specific antibiotics. If clinical signs and symptoms do not show fairly prompt evidence of improvement over the 12–24 h after admission, a pelvic examination should again be performed to determine if abscesses are present in the pelvis, and if their location is such that external drainage can be accomplished through the abdomen, vagina, or rectum.

If a cul-de-sac mass is detected which bulges into the vagina, this should be drained by colpotomy and a drain placed within the abscess cavity. If no definite abscess is found but one is nevertheless suggested by abdominal and pelvic examinations and ultrasound, the failure to respond promptly to definitive therapy may mean that exploratory laparotomy is mandatory. If this procedure is carried out, the ovaries should be conserved if at all possible. Drainage and removal of abscess structures should be accomplished whenever feasible, again, with a major effort being made to conserve ovarian function. This conservative approach is especially important since the majority of these patients are still within the childbearing age and have normal ovarian hormonal production.

If, however, surgical castration is the end-result of the definitive surgery, the patient should be given exogeneous oestrogens. In almost all instances this replacement therapy must be continued until the normal age of menopause is reached, and possibly beyond. If ovarian conservation is carried out and the subsequent clinical course is not satisfactory, it may ultimately be necessary to perform another laparotomy to remove infected ovarian tissue. But a second exploration is preferable to initial surgical castration that may not have been absolutely necessary.

Actinomycosis

In most instances, pelvic inflammatory disease associated with an IUD results from a mixed infection. The majority of organisms are found to be anaerobes. In recent years actinomycosis has been publicized as a serious complication of intrauterine contraception. It is certainly true that most proven cases of pelvic actinomycosis are related to the use of an IUD. Actinomycosis is caused by a bacterium which is a strict anaerobe; it is a close relative to a fungus but is a true bacterium. The specific pathogenic species in humans is *Actinomyces israelii*. This organism is a normal inhabitant of the human mouth, nasopharynx and gastrointestinal tract. It has rarely been reported in the vagina except in IUD users. However, there are conflicting reports relevant to this finding [79].

The majority of the surgically documented cases of PID which have been reported in the world literature in association with Actinomyces have also been associated with the presence of other types of anaerobic bacteria. True pelvic inflammatory disease caused primarily by Actinomyces is extremely rare. A recent review of the world literature has disclosed not more than 120 *bona fide* cases of pelvic inflammatory disease where Actinomyces was the predominant organism [H. Tatum, Personal communication to US Centers for Disease Control]. For this reason, great conservatism should be exercised before the diagnosis of PID due to this specific organism is made. The diagnosis requires pathological verification from tissue extirpated at the time of definitive surgery. Experience has shown that when pelvic inflammatory disease is present and is the result of Actinomyces, intensive management is required, using massive doses of penicillin and/or tetracyclines for a matter of several weeks. The mortality from the true pelvic actinomycosis used to be approximately 80%. With appropriate modern antibiotic therapy and definitive surgery, this mortality has dropped to between 10% and 20%. If surgery is necessary, wide excision of all infected structures is mandatory. This usually means a total hysterectomy and bilateral salpingo-oöphorectomy.

However, if Actinomyces-like organisms (ALOs) are found on Pap smears, this should not be construed to mean that there is a pelvic infection with Actinomyces. It merely means that the ALOs are present in the cervix or vagina [88,89]. If there are no symptoms, a study at the Margaret Pyke Centre in London has shown that removal of the IUD – whether or not it is replaced with a new one – leads to disappearance of the finding of ALOs on subsequent careful follow-up with Pap smears [90]. This subject with its clinical implications has been well reviewed by McEwan [91].

Conclusion

It should be clearly understood that neither age, gravidity, nor parity have a significant effect upon the development of pelvic inflammatory disease. The primary factors which increase the risk of ascending pelvic infection are the numbers of sexual partners and the numbers of sexual partners of those sexual partners. With each additional sexual partner, within a relatively short time span, the incidence of pelvic inflammatory disease or ascending infection from the vagina up into the upper genital tract increases. The primary aftermath or clinical result of ascending pelvic infection is that of tubal obstruction and secondary infertility.

The first episode of pelvic inflammatory disease is associated with a statistical incidence of infertility of approximately 10%–20%. With a second episode of PID, this incidence increases from 20% to 40% and with a third episode it increases to somewhere within a range of 50%–70%.

The implications and the psychological impact of infertility is significantly greater when it occurs in a woman who has not borne her desired number of children. Conversely, the implication of reduced fertility is not nearly so important for the woman who has already satisfied her wishes for a family. It is this phenomenon which has led to the philosophy among many clinicians that the nulligravid woman is not a candidate for the use of intrauterine contraception. It has been shown, however, that a truly monogamous couple with no children has no greater risk of developing pelvic inflammatory disease in association with an IUD than does a monogamous couple who have already achieved their desired number of children. Selection of the candidate for an IUD is therefore extremely important and will largely determine the success of this type of contraception. For a women whose sexual life style is either unknown or is admittedly polygamous, the IUD is generally not the contraceptive method of first choice.

Dalkon shield

It seems appropriate at this time to present a comprehensive review of the Dalkon shield inasmuch as publicity about this particular device and the link with pelvic infections has had a major negative effect upon the use of all IUDs throughout the world. The Dalkon shield IUD was developed by Drs Davis and Lesinsky in the late 1960s. After a limited clinical evaluation, it was distributed commercially throughout the United States and the rest of the world by the A. H. Robins Company of Richmond, Virginia. The Dalkon shield had a transcervical tail affixed to the base of the device which extended through the endocervical canal into the vagina. The tail was fixed to the lower portion of the shield by means of a double knot. There was a single knot approximately 2 cm above the end of the dependent tail. The purpose of this single knot was to ascertain the approximate position of the IUD within the uterine cavity.

In June 1974, Dr Donald Christian reported in the *American Journal of Obstetrics and Gynecology* a number of maternal deaths associated with intrauterine devices [18]. A majority of these cases were associated with the use of a Dalkon shield. The clinical entity which Dr Christian described in his report was that of spontaneous mid-trimester sepsis followed by an abortion. In a number of instances there was a rapidly developing systemic infection terminating in maternal death. The clinical sequence of events were the onset of 'flu-like' symptoms followed very quickly by evidence of intrauterine infection and then by a spontaneous septic abortion.

This publication called attention to a clinical syndrome previously exceedingly rare. Because of the widespread negative publicity associated with this serious complication, it became apparent that the aetiology of this problem required clarification in order that the use of IUDs as an important method of family planning be placed in proper perspective. If the spontaneous mid-trimester septic abortion syndrome were generic to all IUDs, then their use as a major contraceptive method would be more limited.

Detailed laboratory studies of the Dalkon shield and other devices, were carried out by Tatum and his associates at the Population Council, looking for potential contributing factors to this clinical entity [92,93]. These studies quickly demonstrated to the scientific community that the Dalkon shield was unique among currently used IUDs in that its transcervical tail consisted of a bundle of many monofilaments enclosed within a sheath. This tail had the physical characteristics of a wick, and could transport fluids and bacteria.

Dalkon shields which were removed electively from women throughout the United States were studied with respect to the presence and type of bacteria found within the sheath of the tail, in the spaces between the fibres. A wide variety of bacteria, both aerobes and anaerobes, were cultured from all areas below the double knot within the sheath of these tails. These bacteria included most if not all of the species known to be associated with ascending pelvic inflammatory disease. By means of electron microscopy, live-appearing bacteria could be demonstrated in all segments of Dalkon shield tails removed from these women.

From these data it was postulated that the mid-trimester spontaneous septic abortions which had been reported in association with the Dalkon shield could be explained by the following sequence of events. Bacteria were growing within the sheath and between the fibres in all segments of the tail. In pregnancy, the IUD along with its dependent tail moved upward into the uterine cavity as the fetus and products of conception increased in size. At about 10 weeks of pregnancy, many of these transcervical appendages had retracted upward through the cervical canal and entered the extraovular space within the pregnant uterus. The bacteria which were within the sheath of the tail were then free to grow out into the extraovular space, and produce intrauterine infections. These ended in fetal demise, and occasionally in maternal death.

In addition to the presence of bacteria within the sheath of these used Dalkon shields, many breaks in the sheath itself were demonstrated by Tatum and others; they occurred from the area immediately below the double knot (which is normally within the endometrial cavity) through various points along the length of the tail. Breaks in the sheath were demonstrated both in unused Dalkon shields as well as in those removed from patients. Clinical observations disclosed that these fractures of the sheath of the Dalkon tail increased in frequency and number in direct proportion to the length of time the IUD was within the uterine cavity. With the fractures in the sheath, the individual fibres within the sheath were exposed to the adjacent environment and were in a position to allow bacteria to exit from the spaces between them and grow out into the surrounding areas.

Because of the clinical findings and adverse publicity surrounding the Dalkon shield in the autumn of 1974, the USFDA pressured the company to discontinue sales and distribution of the device. The use of intrauterine devices was significantly reduced as a result of this adverse publicity, which unfortunately appeared in many lay publications around the world and was interpreted as being characteristic of all IUDs.

During the next decade, a number of publications reported severe pelvic inflammatory disease, associated with IUDs in general. Although the numbers of IUDs in these individual series were so small as to preclude significant statistical analysis relevant to specific types of devices, the majority of them indicated that the Dalkon shield carried a greater risk for the development of pelvic inflammatory disease than the other types of IUDs. One exception to this rule was the Majzlin spring, which also demonstrated an increased risk of PID. Whereas the Dalkon shield multifilament tail was enclosed within a sheath, the tail of the Majzlin spring consisted of multiple woven filaments but no sheath. Multiple bacteria have been shown to be present on the multiple filamented tail.

In 1983 the first large-scale study of the risk factors associated with hospitalized patients using IUDs and pelvic inflammatory disease was published by Lee from the Centers for Disease Control in Atlanta [94]. Within this series there were sufficient numbers of Dalkon-shield users to permit comparisons between different devices and the incidence of PID. The conclusion of this report was that the Dalkon shield carried at least a fivefold increased risk of pelvic inflammatory disease compared with all other IUDs currently in use. These clinical data supported the concepts proposed by the laboratory findings of Tatum and his associates as published in 1975.

Ascending infection also occurs in association with monofilament IUD tails (and indeed when IUDs are not being used at all). Sparks and colleagues studied women undergoing hysterectomy. They found bacteria in the uterine cavities of 12 of 14 women using IUDs with monofilament tails, in all three women using normal Dalkon shields, but in none of five women using tailless Dalkon shields – and also in none of non-users of IUDs [40]. It is thus apparent that any transcervical appendage leading from the vagina into the endometrial cavity may increase the risk of the development of pelvic inflammatory disease. For this reason investigations are being carried out in a number of locations throughout the world [95] in an effort to develop a tail-less IUD. In order for this device to be practical there must be an easy and inexpensive way to detect the location of the IUD, and secondly a method must be found whereby the IUD may be removed with a minimum of manipulation. It is thought that if such an IUD could be developed, along with effective detection and retrieval systems, the small but measureable risk of ascending pelvic infection associated with IUD usage would be significantly reduced.

The Dalkon syndrome

Over the past decade a syndrome has appeared repeatedly among Dalkon-shield users [96]. It is characterized by the using of the Dalkon shield for a varying time, from one up to 10 or more years, without major complications. Often during the initial years of use these patients have few or no signs or symptoms of an ascending pelvic infection. Then, without apparent reason, very severe acute pelvic inflammatory disease develops.

When the devices are removed by traction on the tail, multiple breaks in the sheath are usually present. Multiple filaments can be seen at these points of sheath fractures.

Cultures of purulent material obtained from the tubes and ovaries at surgery as well as from the IUDs are polymicrobial and are primarily anaerobic species.

In most instances this syndrome is of such clinical severity that massive broad-spectrum intravenous antibiotics must be administered. If there is inadequate response to the antibiotics, surgical intervention is essential. In many instances, this includes a total abdominal hysterectomy and bilaterial salpingo-oöphorectomy, with removal of as much diseased tissue as is possible. Following these measures and the continuation of antibiotics there is usually a fairly prompt improvement.

At least two deaths have been reported in long-term non-pregnant users of the Dalkon shield, and every effort should be made to alert the medical community throughout the world of this potential life-threatening problem, and to encourage removal of any Dalkon shield still being used, even though the users are, at the moment, totally asymptomatic.

Pregnancy

Although the intrauterine devices being used today are highly effective, pregnancies with the IUD still *in situ* have occurred with a low order of frequency (0.5%–6%) with all devices studied to date. These pregnancies may be either intrauterine or ectopic. IUDs will protect against intrauterine pregnancy by 99.5%, against tubal pregnancy by 95%, and against overian pregnancy not at all [97]. Pregnancies have been observed at varying times following IUD insertion, but they are most likely to occur during the early months of use. Despite this, there is a continued low-level of risk as long as the device is in place [77].

It was originally believed that if a woman developed an intrauterine pregnancy with an IUD *in situ*, its removal would increase the likelihood of a spontaneous abortion. With continued research, just the opposite has proved to be the case. Over one-half of patients using IUDs will have a spontaneous abortion if the device is not removed [98]. This is three times the risk in women using oral contraceptives, diaphragms, or no method at all. We now know that the spontaneous abortion rate for women wearing IUDs can be approximately halved by removal [98]. Therefore if a woman elects to continue the pregnancy, it is highly desirable to remove any intrauterine device as soon as the diagnosis is made.

There are additional reasons for immediate removal. Firstly it will protect against the development of septic mid-trimester abortion. The potential for this complication was found to be highest with the Dalkon shield, because its multifilament tail acted as a wick, carrying bacteria up into the endometrial cavity. However, there is still a risk with any of the other devices, albeit at a much lower level. Deaths from septic abortion are rare with IUDs other than the Dalkon shield – less than one per 250 000 Lippes loops in one study. In general the risk of death is seven times higher in IUD users, excluding the shield, than in the general population, but five times higher with the Dalkon than with other devices. Secondly, it has been shown that leaving an IUD *in situ* produces a fourfold increase in the incidence of prematurity. Early removal will also reduce this risk [98].

The development of infection in a pregnancy associated with an IUD is potentially a very serious situation. It requires prompt antibiotic therapy and removal of the device, when feasible. If the IUD is a Dalkon shield, preventive measures make the removal of the IUD mandatory, since mortality is so high, and termination of the pregnancy should be recommended (see section on the Dalkon shield).

More conservative management may be possible if the infection is associated with a single- or double-monofilament-tailed IUD. Antibiotic treatment should be initiated promptly and the IUD removed as soon as possible. If membranes rupture as a result of IUD removal, termination of pregnancy is virtually inevitable and should be enhanced by whatever means are appropriate. If the device cannot be removed, or if the tail has retracted up into the uterine cavity, the decision must be made whether to continue antibiotics and the pregnancy, or to terminate the pregnancy. This is a decision which must depend upon the wishes of the patient and upon the severity of the infection and/or the response to the initial antibiotic treatment. In most instances, the recommendation is that the pregnancy be terminated promptly, the IUD removed, and definitive antibiotic therapy administered.

Concern has frequently been expressed about the possibility of damage to a fetus if a woman with an unplanned pregnancy does not have the IUD removed and the pregnancy is allowed to go to term. A number of infants have been born under these conditions, and to date there is no evidence of any damage to the fetus, the IUD always being in an extraovular position [75].

Ectopic pregnancy

Pregnancies may also occur in the fallopian tube, although this is less likely. A number of studies have suggested that tubal pregnancies are increased by the presence of an intrauterine device. However, there are other data showing that IUDs actually protect against ectopic pregnancy for the first 2–3 years, the rate then coming back to the level of non-IUD-users [76].

Evaluating the possible association between IUD usage and the risk of ectopic pregnancy is a particularly difficult task. Many factors enter into the incidence in non-IUD users, such as rates of previous ectopic pregnancy, the prevalence of PID, and prior tubal surgery; all these increase the basic risk. As a result, ectopic rates vary widely in different population groups [75]. This makes it difficult to gather satisfactory control groups which are needed to make valid comparisons between different IUDs. In general the bulk of the evidence to date does not suggest any major increase in risk unless there are additional risk factors present. There appear to be no differences between devices, with the exception of the Progestasert which appears to have a somewhat higher rate.

Return of fertility

Concern has been expressed about the return of fertility following the removal of an IUD. There may be a short delay in establishing a pregnancy, but 70% of women in one study had conceived at the end of one year and 92% in another study had given birth at the end of 2 years [73,99].

However, most of the studies of this particularly issue have been carried out on women who have had an uneventful course during the use of their IUD, and have then had it removed in order to establish a pregnancy. Clearly, studies on this group may have a strong built-in bias. Studies are now under way on fertility rates in individuals who have had their IUDs removed for medical reasons, primarily because of cramping and bleeding, or the diagnosis or suspicion of pelvic inflammatory disease. It appears that in these cases fertility might be somewhat lowered, either temporarily or permanently. The risk of lowered fertility appears to increase with age and with the duration of use of the IUD. While this is probably due to the superimposition of PID, no statistically valid data are yet available to prove this hypothesis.

Case-control studies are largely reassuring with respect to the risk of tubal subfertility in ex-users of copper as compared with inert IUDs [74,100,101]. Moreover, there was no increased risk associated with IUD use among women reporting only one sexual partner [101].

Malignancy

There has been considerable discussion about the possible induction of malignancy with the long-term use of intrauterine devices. This concern has been stimulated by the observation that plastic and metal devices, placed in the subcutaneous tissues of animals, have induced the formation of tumours. However, there is no reason to assume that this observation has any relevance to the human uterus. Studies which have followed women for up to 5 years have shown no evidence of any cellular changes suggesting a transition toward malignancy [75].

Clinical management

Patient selection

At one point it was believed that any woman in the childbearing years who was sexually active, who had a normal reproductive tract, and who wanted to use an intrauterine device was able to do so [76]. After more evaluation was carried out, at the time when only the larger non-medicated devices were available, nulligravid and nulliparous patients were not considered to be candidates. However, with the development of the smaller, medicated IUDs, this form of contraception became a possibility [75].

Now, because of the increasing concern about the possible development of infection, considerable thought has once again been given to this subject. Many clinicians currently feel that women who have not completed their desired family size, women who have had one ectopic pregnancy, and women who have multiple sexual partners may not be good candidates. On the other hand there are patients for whom the IUD holds special advantages. These include women who wish to terminate their childbearing but are unwilling to accept sterilization, those who have medical contraindications to the use of oral contraceptives, and those who are unable to cope with coitally related methods [76].

Contraindications

The *absolute* contraindications for IUDs, as currently listed by the USFDA, are:

1. Intrauterine pregnancy;
2. Suspected pregnancy (intrauterine or ectopic);
3. Genital malignancy, diagnosed or suspected, or a Pap smear, Class 3 or more;
4. Vaginal bleeding of unknown aetiology;
5. Acute vaginitis (until the infection is controlled);
6. Acute pelvic inflammatory disease [35,76];
7. (For Cu IUDs) proven allergy to copper – rare.

A recent addition to this list is known infection with the human immunodeficiency virus (HIV) or any other state of immunosuppression. This is because of a likely increase in the risk of *severe* PID, plus the added transmission danger (from increased uterine bleeding).

The *relative* contraindications for IUDs, as currently listed by USFDA, are:

1. Chronic PID;
2. History of ectopic pregnancy;
3. Untreated cervicitis;
4. Congenital anomalies of the uterus such as cervical stenosis, infantile uterus and bicornuate uterus, unless the size of the cavity is incompatible with the IUD;
5. Uterine fibroids, if causing distortion of the uterine cavity;
6. Anaemia – haemoglobin less than 9 g %;
7. Heart disease – congenital or acquired valvular (insertion under full antibiotic cover, if at all – see Sparks [102]);
8. Leukaemia;
9. (For Cu IUDs) suspected allergy to copper;
10. Wilson's disease (congenital defect in copper excretion) (rare: 1 in 200 000 women) [35,76].

Some authorities would consider numbers 1–3 and 10 as absolute or at least 'near absolute' contraindications. In addition there are a number of other medical conditions which might be considered as relative contraindications:

History of acute PID; postpartum endometritis, or infected abortion in past 3 months; history of sexually transmitted disease; debilitating dysmenorrhoea; repetitive menorrhagia; submucous fibroids; history of partial or complete expulsion of an IUD; sickle-cell disease; vascular coagulopathies; anticoagulant treatment for chronic disease; use of chronic corticosteriod therapy (which may increase susceptibility to ascending infection); age less than 16 years; nulligravidity (if future childbearing is desired); multiple sexual partners or partner(s) with multiple sexual partners [35,76].

While the first two lists reflect the current USFDA guidelines for interval insertions, studies have suggested certain additional uses which are somewhat at variance with these. For example, a large international evaluation showed the incidence of adverse side-effects to be the same or lower when IUD insertion is performed prior to hospital discharge after delivery [103]. Similarly, insertions following incomplete abortion, elective abortion prior to 12 weeks gestation, and use as a postcoital contraceptive have been reported to carry no greater risks than interval insertions [77,103].

Device selection

A woman who has a normal uterus that sounds to a depth of 6.5–8.0 cm can use any of the standard intrauterine devices. A women whose uterus measures more than 5.5 cm but less than 6.5 cm should have one of the smaller IUDs inserted. Conversely, one with a depth greater than 8 cm should be fitted with a larger device [76].

In addition to size, there are several other factors to consider. When the use of a medicated device, e.g. copper, is being considered, it is important to be sure that the patient is not sensitive to the substance released from the IUD. Since the medicated devices must be replaced at periodic intervals, their use may be inappropriate in areas with a minimal health-care infrastructure. Finally, since there is a differential in blood loss with the various devices, this factor must also be taken into account [75].

IUD insertion

For several reasons, insertions have traditionally been carried out near the end of a menstrual period. The cervix is softer and more patulous, which makes the insertion easier and less traumatic. In addition there is minimal chance of pregnancy. Since the woman is already experiencing vaginal bleeding, the post-insertion bleeding is less apparent and therefore, less disturbing to the patient. Finally, there is less menstruum present to provide nutrients for the growth of bacteria [76].

There are many instances, however, in which menstrual insertions are totally impractical. In these situations, the device may be placed at any time, provided that pregnancy has been ruled out [76].

Prior to the insertion of an IUD, a careful assessment of the pelvic organs must be carried out. This includes ruling out lesions of the vulva, vagina, and cervix, and establishing the size and position of the uterus and whether or not there is any evidence of adnexal disease.

A single-toothed tenaculum or less traumatic tissue-holding forceps should always be placed on the anterior lip of the cervix and gentle traction applied in order to straighten out the endocervical canal. Doing so will reduce the number of perforations. Following this, the uterus is sounded to determine the depth of the cavity and to confirm its position. If excessive narrowing of the endocervical canal is found, it may be necessary to dilate it, using a paracervical block.

Originally IUDs were put in under surgically sterile conditions. However, it is now clear that only those parts of the instruments which enter the uterine cavity, and the device itself, need to be sterile. Careful washing of the hands, the use of sterile gloves, and the employment of a 'no touch' technique appear to provide adequate protection [35,76].

The earlier plastic devices were inserted using a push-out technique. The IUD was stretched out and loaded into the introducer immediately prior to insertion. Afterwards, it would return to its original shape in the uterine cavity. With this type of device, the introducer is placed near but not at the top of the fundus, and the device is pushed out slowly with the plunger into the endometrial cavity [75].

A more recent development is the withdrawal technique, used with the copper and hormone-bearing IUDs. In this case, the inserter is introduced to the top of the fundus, withdrawn slightly to free the transverse arms, and then the device is deposited at the top of the fundal cavity. In general, this second technique has been found to be associated with fewer perforations and with better placement [76].

Following the insertion of a tailed device, the threads should be trimmed to about 2–3 cm beyond the external cervical os. These are used for future checking for the presence of the device by the patient and clinicians, and for its removal when indicated. The patient should then be observed for about half an hour for any signs of problems such as syncope and perforation. If she remains asymptomatic, she should be given follow-up instructions and allowed to leave [75].

Follow-up care

Good counselling is an essential part of the care given to an IUD patient. It is important that a woman be told which type of device she has and, if the device has a tail, be taught to feel for the tail monthly to check for any unnoticed expulsion. A return schedule should be described to her. The first post-insertion appointment should be made shortly after the first menstrual period, certainly by 3 months following insertion, since this period carries the greatest risk of expulsion. Thereafter she may be seen at roughly yearly intervals, unless problems develop [35,75].

A woman must also be instructed about what to anticipate in terms of side-effects, particularly those which she should try to ignore and those which should make her seek immediate medical care. She should also make sure that she knows where to obtain that care when required. It is essential that a woman be aware of the fact that there is a slightly increased risk of infection with the use of intrauterine devices. She must be told to report any abnormal vaginal discharge, pelvic pain, and abnormal bleeding. Finally, if she has been given a medicated device, she must know its duration of action and when it must be replaced [76].

Classification of intrauterine contraceptive devices

There are two major classes of intrauterine contraceptives. The first is the non-medicated IUD. The primary examples of these formerly available in the United States are the Lippes loop and the Saf-T-Coil. In the Far East, the Ota ring is another widely used non-medicated device. Although originally fabricated from metal such as gold or silver, this latter ring is now made of plastic. The second major class of device is the medicated IUD. These consist of a self-retaining platform of a relatively non-reactive material such as plastic, upon which is placed an active antifertility agent.

Medicated IUDs

At the present time there are two subclasses of medicated IUDs. The first one to be developed was the Tatum T (made of plastic) on which was wound pure metallic copper wire. The contraceptive effect of the metallic copper was discovered by Dr J. Zipper in Santiago, Chile, as a result of intensive studies of various metals as antifertility agents when placed within the uteri of rabbits and rats. The copper wire wound on the vertical stem of the plastic T constituted the first of the class of medicated IUDs [29].

Since the original copper T, there have been several modifications of the T, with additional copper and with various other shaped platforms upon which have been placed metallic copper wire. The principal copper-bearing IUDs currently available on the world are listed in Table 9.2.

As a result of unwarranted and scientifically unjustified lawsuits against G. D. Searle, the company discontinued making both the Cu 7 and the Tatum T in January 1986. Searle affiliates world-wide were also initially instructed to discontinue sales of these two IUDs. It is imperative to note that the USFDA never removed its approval of any of the copper-bearing IUDs. Fortunately for the women of the USA, in 1988 GynoMed of New Jersey commenced marketing of the T Cu 380 A (ParaGard).

The T Cu 220C was developed by the Population Council in an effort to increase the duration of effective contraception beyond the 3 years recommended for the wire-wound TC 200. This was accomplished by adding copper sleeves to both the transverse arms and the vertical stem. The innovation of using copper sleeves instead of wire permits exposure of the copper to the intrauterine environment on only one surface. This minimizes the possibility of segmental losses of copper.

The third device developed by the Population Council is the TCu 380A. The objective here was to increase contraceptive effectiveness by increasing the surface area of copper on the vertical stem from 200 to 300 mm^2 and to increase the longevity

Table 9.2 Medicated IUDs

Device	*Manufacturer*	*Primary source*	*Minimum duration of action*
Copper-bearing			
T Cu 200	G.D. Searle Ortho Canada	USA Canada	3 years (package insert USFDA). Proven 4 years
Cu 7	G.D. Searle	USA	(Manufacture of both IUDs discontinued in the US Jan 1986 because of unwarranted lawsuits and unavailable product liability insurance)
T Cu 200Ag	Outokumpu Oy	Finland	6 years
T Cu 220C	Ortho Canada Outokumpu Oy	Canada Finland	15–20 years
T Cu 380A	Ortho Canada	Canada	6 years (WHO states 'Indefinite life')
	(& from 1988) GynoMed	New Jersey	4 years
T Cu 380Ag	Outokumpu Oy	Finland	10–15 years
Nova T (Cu Ag 200)	Outokumpu Oy Leiras	Finland Finland	6 years (silver-core copper wire)
Multiload Cu 250	Multilan	Switzerland	4 years
Multiload Cu 375	Multilan	Switzerland	5 years
Progestogen-bearing			
Progestasert (Progesterone)	Alza Corp.	USA	1 year (package insert USFDA)
LNG T (Levonorgestrel)	Leiras	Finland	?6 years (Not yet marketed)

by adding a copper sleeve on each of the transverse arms of the T. Based upon copper loss during *in vivo* use, the estimated life expectancy of both the TCu 220C and the TCu 380A is between 15 and 20 years. An additional reason for copper sleeves on the arms of both IUDs was to increase the biologically active copper high in the fundal cavity. It was anticipated that this modification would counteract some of the diminished antifertility effect which occurs if there is downward displacement of the device.

The clinical data relevant to the addition of this small amount of copper on the transverse arms showed a very significant increase in the contraceptive effectiveness of both devices. The current data indicate that the T Cu 380A has an effective annual rate of about 0.5 pregnancies per year per hundred women over a period of at least 4 full years.

This use-effectiveness rate has been confirmed in four or five separate studies in centres throughout the world. This is proving to be the most effective of the T-shaped copper-bearing IUDs evaluated to date.

Another device in worldwide use and evaluated extensively in clinical trials is the Multiload. The Multiload-Cu250 was designed in 1972 with several unique characteristics. Among these are the flexibility of the side-arms and the simple insertion technique (allowing for high fundal placement and reducing the risk of perforation at insertion). A range of sizes is available, which makes adaptation of the IUD to the size of the uterine cavity possible [105].

The latest version is the Multiload-Cu375, a high dosed copper IUD. It has a very low pregnancy rate of 0.4 after 12 months of use, an effective life span of at least five years, with a cumulative pregnancy rate of 2.9 after 60 months [106].

Progestogen-releasing IUDs

The second subgroup of medicated IUDs carry a reservoir containing a progestogen. The first of these, the Progestasert, was developed with the cooperation of the Population Council, which arranged for the Alza Corporation in California to affix a reservoir of pure natural progesterone on the vertical stem of a T platform.

The second progestogen-bearing IUD is being developed by the Population Council in New York. It consists of a Nova T platform developed as a modification of the Tatum T by Dr Luukainen in Finland, to which is added levonorgestrel in a capsule placed on the vertical stem of the T. Although the levonorgestrel T is not yet available commercially, it is being intensively evaluated, along with variants using different progestogens and carrier platforms, in a number of countries. The levonorgestrel T has a distinct advantage over the Progestasert in that the duration of effectiveness, based upon *in vitro* diffusion rates, is approximately 6 years, whereas the reservoir of progesterone on the Progestasert provides effective contraception for only slightly more than one year.

It is important to note that the progestogen-bearing IUDs, as well as any other progestogen contraceptives which provide a systemic level below that which consistently suppresses ovulation, are all associated with an increased incidence of extrauterine pregnancies among the failures. Indeed the relative risk of 6.7 as compared with two standard copper devices was the reason for the WHO discontinuing further development of their IUD, releasing only 2 μg levonorgestrel per 24 h [107]. (The Population Council device releases 20 μg per day and has a much lower rate of ectopic pregnancies.)

One explanation for the increased likelihood of an accidental pregnancy being tubal rather than intrauterine is that the subovulation-suppressing level of the progestogen modifies tubal transport in such a way that the passage of the fertilised egg is impeded.

Non-medicated IUDs

Among these plastic platform (polyethylene, polypropylene) devices, the Dalkon shield was removed from the market in 1974 because of infections. The Lippes loop and the Saf-T-Coil were subsequently discontinued in 1984/1985, primarily because of inadequate demand for the products. This left no inert devices readily available anywhere in the Western world.

Acceptability

The acceptability of intrauterine devices depends upon the specific requirements of the individual user. Because of the small but real increased risk of PID and possible subsequent infertility, a woman whose primary requirement is to terminate childbearing with a reversible type of contraception would probably find that intrauterine devices would meet her needs.

If child spacing rather than termination of fertility is the primary objective, other methods may be preferable in younger women who wish to retain the potential for future pregnancies. Oral contraceptives or barrier methods may then be the preferred choice.

The level of acceptability also depends upon the level of motivation of the user and her tolerance of side-effects, should they occur. Highly motivated women can accept minor temporary adverse side-effects which would be unacceptable to those less well motivated. In addition there are certain cultural prohibitions against abnormal bleeding which would be of great important to some women but much less so to others.

Future advances in intrauterine contraception

The major recent advance which has been made in the field of intrauterine contraception is the development of the medicated IUD. This has made possible the use of various small vehicles which have potent antifertility action resulting from the additional agents affixed to them. Only copper and progestogens have reached the market-place thus far, but other bioactive agents are of potential benefit. Among those being evaluated, it remains to be seen which will prove themselves useful in future contraceptive practice.

Development of an effective, practical tail-less IUD could further enhance the acceptability and utilization of this important method of fertility control.

Summary and conclusions

The intrauterine device continues to play a major role in fertility regulation worldwide, despite the fact that it does not yet meet all the criteria for the 'ideal' contraceptive. It is '. . . probably the second most commonly used reliable reversible method of preventing pregnancy,' according to a recent comprehensive review by the World Health Organization [36]. IUDs require only a single act of motivation, and when no complications occur, only a minimum of continuing medical care. They do not demand constant attention by the patient, are highly effective, and in most instances produce few or no side-effects after the first few months of use.

Each of the currently available devices has been associated with side-effects such as cramping or bleeding. The more recently developed devices have fewer problems in this respect than some of the older IUDs. While protection against unwanted pregnancy is high, there continues to be a small percentage of unplanned pregnancies, both intra- and extrauterine. Moreover, expulsion and perforation have been noted with all existing devices.

The primary problem and the major concern today is the development of PID. This may result in temporary or permanent infertility. A number of experimental techniques are now being evaluated in attempts to maintain or improve the current efficacy of IUDs and to avoid or reduce the problem of pelvic inflammatory disease.

There is still a great need for a reversible type of long-term contraception for women who have no desire for further childbearing. These individuals constitute a very large group, both in the United States and elsewhere. The IUD has a major role to play in this particular area. Careful selection of patients leads to intrauterine contraception with safety and effectiveness. It therefore remains a technique which has wide applicability and will continue to be an important factor in controlling unplanned and unwanted pregnancies.

References

1. CAUVET, G. *Le Chameau.* Ballière, Paris. (1925)
2. FINCH, B. E. and GREEN, H. *Contraception Through the Ages.* Peter Owen Ltd, London. (1963)
3. RICHTER, R. Ein mittel zur verhutung der konzeption. (*Deutsche Medizinische Wocheuschrift*, **35**, 1525. (1909)
4. PUST, K. Ein brauchbarer Praunenschutz. **49**, 952. (1923)
5. GRAFENBERG, E. The intrauterine method of contraception. *Practice of Contraception* (ed. M. Sanger and H. M. Stone), Williams and Wilkins, Baltimore. (1930)
6. OPPENHEIMER, W. Prevention of pregnancy by the Grafenberg ring method: A re-evaluation after 28 years' experience. *American Journal of Obstetrics and Gynecology*, **78**, 446. (1959)
7. ISHIHAMA, A. Clinical studies on intrauterine rings, especially the present state of contraception in Japan and the experience in the use of intrauterine rings, *Yokohama Medical Bulletin*, **10**, 89. (1959)
8. MARGULIES, L. C. Permanent reversible contraception with an intrauterine plastic spiral. In *Proceedings of the Conference on Intrauterine Contraceptive Devices* (ed. C. Tietze and S Lewit) International Congress Series No. 54. Excerpa Medica, Amsterdam. (1962)
9. LIPPES, J. A study of intra-uterine contraception: development of a plastic loop. In *Proceedings of the Conference on Intrauterine Contraceptive Devices* (eds C. Tietze and S. Lewit), International Congress Series No. 54. Excerpta Medica, Amsterdam. (1962)
10. LIPPES, J. Contraception with intrauterine plastic loops, *American Journal of Obstetrics and Gynecology*, **93**, 1024. (1965)
11. LIPPES, J. Observations after four years of experience with the intrauterine plastic loop at the Buffalo Planned Parenthood Center, *Journal of Sex Research*, **3**, 323. (1967)
12. DAVIS, H. J. The shield IUD. A superior modern contraceptive, *American Journal of Obstetrics and Gynecology*, **106**, 455. (1970)
13. LANE, M. E., SINDHUPAK, S., SOBRERO, A. J. and KOHLI, K. L. Clinical experience with the LEM, an intrauterine contraceptive device. *Fertility and Sterility*, **25**, 563 (1974).
14. HALL, H. H. The stainless steel ring: An effective and safe intrauterine contraceptive device. In *Proceedings of the Conference on Intrauterine Contraceptive Devices* (eds C. Tietze, and S. Lewit), International Congress Series No. 54. Excerpta Medica, Amsterdam. (1962)
15. HALL, H. H., STONE, M. L., SEDLIS, A. and CHABON, I. The intrauterine ring for contraception control, *Fertility and Sterility*, **15**, 618 (1964)
16. SILBERMANN, E., STONE, M. L. and CONNELL, E. B. The 'M', a new IUCD. *American Journal of Obstetrics and Gynecology*, **105**, 279 (1969)
17. United States Food and Drug Administration. *Report on Intrauterine Contraceptive Devices.* Advisory Committee on Obstetrics and Gynecology. Washington, DC, United States Government Printing Office. (1968)
18. CHRISTIAN, C. D. Maternal deaths associated with an intrauterine device. *American Journal of Obstetrics and Gynecology*, **119**, 441 (1974)
19. BORIA, M. C., GORDON, M. and STONE, M. L. Some observations on the use of the 'M' IUCD. *Contraception*, **4**, 193 (1974)
20. TAYLOR, W. N., MARTIN, F. G., PRITCHARD, S. A. and PRITCHARD, J. A. Complications from Majzlin spring IUD. *Obstetrics and Gynecology*, **41**, 404 (1973)
21. TIETZE, C. Intrauterine contraceptive rings: history and statistical appraisal. In *Proceedings of the Conference on Intrauterine Contraceptive Devices* (eds C. Tietze and S. Lewit), International Congress Series No. 54. Excerpta Medica, Amsterdam. (1962)
22. TIETZE, C. Effectiveness and acceptability of intrauterine contraceptive devices, *American Journal of Public Health*, **55**, 1874 (1965)
23. TIETZE, C. and LEWIT, S. Intrauterine contraception: effectiveness and acceptibility. In *Proceedings of the Second International Conference on intrauterine Contraception* (eds S. J. Segal, A. L. Southam and K. D. Shafer) International Congress Series No. 86. Excerpta Medica, Amsterdam. (1964)

24. TIETZE, C. and LEWIT, S. Evaluation of IUD's. Ninth progress report of the Cooperative Statistical Program. *Studies in Family Planning*, **55**, 1 (1970)
25. POTTER, R. G. Application of life table techniques to measurement of contraception effectiveness. *Demography*, **3**, 297 (1966)
26. TIETZE, C. and LEWIT, S. Recommended procedures for the statistical evaluation of intrauterine contraception, *Studies in Family Planning*, **4**, 35 (1973)
27. BERNSTEIN, G. S., ISRAEL, R., SEWARD, P. and MISHELL, D. R. JR. Clinical experience with the Cu 7 intrauterine device, *Contraception*, **6**, 99 (1972)
28. STEWART, W., GIBOR, Y., DEYSACH, L. and NISSEN, C. Clinical studies with the Cu-7: a comparison of results in parous and nulliparous women. In *Clinical Proceedings, South-east Asia at Oceania Congress* (Sydney, 1972) International Planned Parenthood Federation (1973)
29. TATUM, H. J. and ZIPPER, J. A. The 'T' intrauterine contraceptive device and recent advances in hormonal anticonceptional therapy. In *Proceedings of the VI Northeast Obstetrics–Gynecology Congress* (Bahia, Brazil) (1968)
30. MISHELL, D. R., ISRAEL, R. and FIELD, N. A study of the Copper T intrauterine contraceptive device (T Cu 200) in nulliparous women. *American Journal of Obstetrics and Gynecology*, **116**, 1092 (1973)
31. MARTINEZ–MANAUTOU, J., ROSADO, A. and MAQUEO, M. Clinical experience with the intrauterine progesterone-releasing system. In *Proceedings of the Third International Conference on Intrauterine Contraception* (Cairo, Egypt, 1974) (eds F. Hefnawi and S. Segal) North-Holland, Amsterdam (1975)
32. PHARRIS, B. B. Uterine progesterone system. In *Intrauterine Devices – Development, Evaluation and Implementation* (eds R. G. Wheeler, G. W. Duncan and J. J. Speidel), Academic Press, New York (1974)
33. PHARRIS, B. B., ERICKSON, R., BESHAW, J. *et al.* Progestasert: a uterine therapeutic system for long-term contraception. 1. Philosophy and clinical efficacy. *Fertility and Sterility*, **25**, 915 (1974)
34. SCOMMEGNA, A., PANYDA, G. N., CHRIST, M. *et al.* Intrauterine administration of progesterone by a slow releasing device. *Fertility and Sterility*, **21**, 201 (1970)
35. United States Food and Drug Administration. *Second Report on Intrauterine Contraceptive Devices*. Advisory Committee on Obstetrics and Gynecology. Washington, DC, United States Government Printing Office (1978)
36. WORLD HEALTH ORGANIZATION SCIENTIFIC GROUP. *Mechanism of Action, Safety and Efficacy of Intrauterine Devices*. WHO Technical Report Series 753. WHO Geneva (1987)
37. MASTROIANNI, L. and ROSSEAU, C. H. Influence of the intrauterine coil in ovum transport and sperm distribution in the monkey. *American Journal of Obstetrics and Gynecology*, **93**, 416 (1965)
38. KELLY, W. A. and MARSTON, J. H. Contraceptive action of IUD in Rhesus monkeys. *Nature*, **214**, 734 (1967)
39. MISHELL, D. R., BELL, J. H., GOOD, R. G. and MOYER, D. L. The intrauterine device: a bacteriologic study of the endometrial cavity. *American Journal of Obstetrics and Gynecology*, **96**, 119 (1966)
40. SPARKS, R. A., PURRIER, B. G., WATT, P. J. and ELSTEIN, M. Bacteriological colonisation of uterine cavity: role of tailed intrauterine contraceptive device. *British Medical Journal*, **282**, 1189–1191 (1981)
41. GUPTA, P. K., MALKANI, P. K. and BHASIN, K. Cellular response in the uterine cavity after IUD insertion and structural changes of the IUD. *Contraception*, **4**, 375 (1971)
42. MOYER, D. L. and MISHELL, D. R., JR. Reactions of human endometrium to the intrauterine foreign body. 2. Long-term effects on the endometrial histology and cytology. *American Journal of Obstetrics and Gynecology*, **111**, 66 (1971)
43. MOYER, D. L. and SHAW, S. T. IUDs: biological action. In *Human Reproduction* (eds E. S. E. Hafez and T. N. Evans), Harper and Row, Hagerstown (1973)
44. SAGIROGLU, N. Phagocytosis of spermatozoa in the uterine cavity of women using IUD. *International Journal of Fertility*, **16**, 1 (1971)
45. SAGIROGLU, N. and SAGIROGLU, E. Cytology of IUDs. *Acta Cytologica*, **14**, 58 (1970)
46. SEDLIS, A. and REYNIAK, J. V. Endometrial leukocytes in patients using IUCDs. *American Journal of Obstetrics and Gynecology*, **108**, 1209 (1970)
47. CHAUDHURI, G. Intrauterine device: possible role of prostaglandins. *Lancet*, **1**, 480 (1971)
48. CHAUDHURI, G. Release of prostaglandins by the IUCD. *Prostaglandins*, **3**, 773 (1973)
49. THOMPSON, I.E. IUD and PGs: a review of the evidence. *Obstetrics and Gynecology*, **42**, 617 (1973)

50. DAVIS, H. J. and LESINSKI, J. R., JR. Mechanism of action of intrauterine contraceptive in women. *Obstetrics and Gynecology*, **36**, 350 (1970)

51. OSTER, G., SALGO, M. P. The copper intrauterine device and its mode of action. *New England Journal of Medicine*, **293**, 432 (1975)

52. TATUM, H. J. Clinical aspects of intrauterine contraception: circumspection 1976. *Fertility and Sterility*, **28**, 3 (1974)

53. DOYLE, L. L. and CLEWE, T. H. Preliminary studies on the effect of hormone releasing IUDs. *American Journal of Obstetrics and Gynecology*, **101**, 564 (1968)

54. DUNCAN, G. W. and KALKWARF, D. R. Sustained release systems for fertility control. In *Human Reproduction* (eds E. S. E. Hafez and T. N. Evans), Harper and Row, Hagerstown, (1973)

55. PANDYA, G. N. and SCOMMEGNA, A. Intrauterine progesterone releasing devices: clinical trial, In *Advances in Planned Parenthood* (eds A. J. Sobrero and R. M. Harvey). International Congress Series No. 246. Excerpta Medica, Amsterdam (1972)

56. SCOMMEGNA, A., AVILA, T., LUNA, M. *et al.* Fertility control by intrauterine release of progesterone. *Obstetrics and Gynecology*, **43**, 769 (1974)

57. SCOMMEGNA, A., PANDYA, G., CHRIST, M. *et al.* Intrauterine administration of progesterones by a slow releasing device. *Fertility and Sterility*, **21**, 201 (1970)

58. HAGENFELDT, K. Intrauterine contraception with the Copper-T device. *Contraception*, **6**, 37 (1972)

59. TREIMAN, K. and LISKIN, L. IUDs – a new look. *Population Reports, series B*, no. 5 (1988)

60. WORLD HEALTH ORGANIZATION. Special Programme of Research, Development and Research Training in Human Reproduction. Task force on intrauterine devices for fertility regulation. Interval IUD insertion in parous women: a randomized multicenter comparative trial of the Lippes Loop D, TCu220C and the Copper 7. *Contraception*, **26**, 1 (1982)

61. SIVIN, I. and STERN, J. Long-acting, more effective Copper T IUDs: a summary of U.S. experience, 1970–75. *Studies in Family Planning*, **10**, 263 (1979)

62. LUUKKAINEN, T., ALLONEN, H., NIELSEN, N.-C., NYGREN, K.-G., and PYÖRÄLÄ, T. Five years' experience of intrauterine contraception with the Nova-T and the Copper-T-200. *American Journal of Obstetrics and Gynecology*, **147**, 885 (1983)

63. GOH, T. H., HUTAPEA, H., MCCARTHY, T. *et al.* A multicenter randomized comparative investigation of ML Cu250, TCu-220C and Cu7 IUDs. *'Advances in Contraceptive Delivery Systems*, (Monograph 1) p. 126 (1985)

64. THIERY, M., VAN DER PAS, H., DELBEKE, L., and VAN KETS, H. Comparative performance of two copper-wired IUDs (ML Cu 250 and TCu 200): immediate postpartum and interval insertion. *Contraceptive Delivery Systems*, **1**, 27 (1980)

65. SAURE, A., HIRVONEN, E., KIVIJÄRVI, A., and TIMONEN, H. Comparative performance of Fincoid, Nova-T, and ML 375 IUDs. In *Intrauterine contraception: advances and future prospects* (eds. G. I. Zatuchni, A. Goldsmith, J. J. Sciarra and C. K. Osborn), Harper and Row, Philadelphia, p. 104 (1985)

66. MISHELL, D. R. The clinic factor in evaluating intrauterine devices, In *Analysis of Intrauterine Contraception. Proceedings of Third International Conference on Intrauterine Contraception* (Cairo, 1974) (eds E. Hefnawi and S. J. Segal), North Holland, Amsterdam, pp. 27–36

67. ORLANS, F. B. Cu IUDs performance to date. *Population Reports, Series B*, No. **1**, (1973)

68. HUBER, S. C., PIOTROW, P. T., ORLANS, F. B. and KOMMER, G. Intrauterine devices reassessed: a decade of experience. *Population Reports, Series B*, No. **2**, (1975)

69. BERNARD, R. P. Factors governing IUD performance. *American Journal of Public Health*, **61**, 559 (1971)

70. JENNINGS, J. *Report of safety and Efficacy of the Dalkon Shield and other IUDs.* Ad hoc Obstetric–Gynecology Advisory Committee to the US Food and Drug Administration (1974)

71. KAHN, H. S. and TYLER, C. W. JR. Mortality associated with use of IUDs. *Journal of the American Medical Association*, **234**, 57 (1975)

72. ORY, H. W., FORREST, J. D. and LINCOLN, R. Making choices. In *Evaluating the Health Risks and Benefits of Birth Control Methods.* The Alan Guttmacher Institute, New York (1983)

73. VESSEY, M. P., WRIGHT, N. H., MCPHERSON, K. and WIGGINS, P. Fertility after stopping different methods of contraception. *British Medical Journal*, **1** (1608), 265–267 (1978)

74. TATUM, H. J. and CONNELL, E. B. A decade of intrauterine contraception, 1976 to 1986. *Fertility and Sterility*, **46**, 173 (1986)

75. CONNELL, E. B. Intrauterine devices. In *Principles and Practice of Clinical Gynecology* (eds N. G. Kase and A. B. Weingold). **63**, 1033 (1983)
76. CONNELL, E. B. and TATUM, H. J. *Manual of Reproductive Health Care*. Creative Informatics, Durant, USA (1984)
77. PIOTROW, P. J., RINEHART, W. and SCHMIDT, J. C. Intrauterine devices. *Population Reports Series B*, No. **3** (1979)
78. LISKIN, L. and FOX, G. IUDs: An appropriate contraceptive for many women. *Population Reports, Series B*, No. **4** (1982)
79. ADEL, S. K., GHORIEM, M. A. and SOBERO, A. J. Difficult Majzlin spring removals. *Obstetrics and Gynecology*, **38**, 653 (1971)
80. ISRAEL, R., SHAW, S. T. and MARTIN, M. A. Comparative quantitation of menstrual blood loss with the Lippes loop. Dalkon shield, and Copper T intrauterine devices. *Contraception*, **10**, 63 (1974)
81. GUILLEBAUD, J., ANDERSON, A. B. M. and TURNBULL, A. C. Reduction by mefenamic acid of increased menstrual blood loss associated with intrauterine contraception. *British Journal of Obstetrics and Gynaecology*, **85**, 53 (1978)
82. BEDI, P., DEVI, P. K. and CHAUDHURY, R. R. Preliminary report of a trial of a long acting antihistaminic buclizine hydrochloride in patients with bleeding after insertion of IUD. *Indian Journal of Medical Research*, **56**, 884 (1968)
83. HORNE, H. W., JR. and SCOTT, J. M. Adrenosem therapy for bleeding coincident with the use of IUCDs: A double blind study. *Fertility and Sterility*, **21**, 230 (1970)
84. WESTROM, L. and BENGTSSON, L. P. Effect of tranexamic acid in menorrhagia with IUCDs. A double blind study. *Journal of Reproductive Medicine*, **5**, 41–48 (1970)
85. GALLEGOS, A. J., AZNAR, R. and MERINO, G. Intrauterine devices and menstrual blood loss: A comparative study of eight devices during the first six months of use. *Contraception*, **7**, 153 (1978)
86. WESTROM, L. Incidence, prevalence, and trends of acute pelvic inflammatory disease and its consequences in industrialized countries. *American Journal of Obstetrics and Gynecology*, **138**, 880–892 (1980)
87. CURTIS, E. M. and PINE, L. Actinomyces in the vaginas of women with and without intrauterine contraceptive devices. *American Journal of Obstetrics and Gynecology*, **140**, 880–884 (1981)
88. JONES, M. C., BUSCHMANN, B. O., DOWLING, E. A. and POLLOCK H. M. The prevalence of actinomycetes-like organisms found in cervicovaginal smears of 300 IUD wearers. *Acta Cytologica*, **23**, 282–286 (1979)
89. PETITTI, D. B. and MORGENSTERN, L. *Factors Associated with Actinomyces-Like Organisms on Pap Smear in IUD Users*. (Oakland, California, Kaiser–Permanente Medical Care Program) Department of Medical Methods Research and Department of Pathology, p. 16, (Mimeo) (1981)
90 MAO, K. and GUILLEBAUD, J. Influence of removal of intrauterine devices on colonization of the cervix by actinomyces-like organisms. *Contraception*, **30**, 535 (1984)
91. MCEWAN, J. ALOs, Actinomyces, actinomycocis and intrauterine devices: some recent findings reviewed. *British Journal of Family Planning*, **12**, 48 (1986)
92. TATUM, H. J., SCHMIDT, F. H., PHILLIPS, D. *et al.* The Dalkon shield controversy: structural and bacteriological studies of IUD tails. *Journal of the Americal Medical Association*, **23** (7), 711–717 (1975)
93. TATUM, H. J., SCHMIDT, F. H. and PHILLIPS, D. M. Morphological studies of Dalkon shield tails removed from patients. *Contraception*, **11** (4), 465–477 (1975)
94. LEE, N. C. Type of intrauterine device and the risk of pelvic inflammatory disease. *Obstetrics and Gynecology*, **62**, 1 (1983)
95. TATUM, H. J. *et al.* Presented at the annual meeting of the American Fertility Society and Canadian Andrology Society, Toronto, September 1986 and at the International Congress of Obstetricians and Gynaecologists, Singapore, October (1986)
96. TATUM, H. J. and CONNELL, E. B. *Intrauterine Contraception*, Creative Informatics, Durant, USA (1985)
97. LEHFELDT, H., TIETZE, C. and GORSTEIN, F. Ovarian pregnancy and the IUD. *American Journal of Obstetrics and Gynecology*, **108**, 1005 (1970)
98. TATUM, H. J., SCHMIDT, F. H. and JAIN, A. K. Management and outcome of pregnancies associated with the Copper T intrauterine contraceptive device. *American Journal of Obstetrics and Gynecology*, **125** (7), 869–879 (1976)

99. BATAR, I. Fertility after IUD removal. In *Medicated Intrauterine Devices: Physiological and Clinical Aspects*. (eds E. S. E. Hafez and W. A. A. Van Os), Martinus Nijhoff, The Hague, pp. 159–168 (1980)

100. DALING, J. R., WEISS, N. S. *et al.* Primary tubal infertility in relation to the use of an intrauterine device. *New England Journal of Medicine*, **312**, 937–941 (1985)

101. CRAMER, D. W., SCHIFF, I. *et al.* Tubal infertility and the intrauterine device. *New England Journal of Medicine*, **312**, 941–947 (1985)

102. SPARKS, R. A. Endocarditis and the IUD. *British Journal of Family Planning*, **11**, 16 (1985)

103. BANHARNSUPAWAT, L. and ROSENFIELD, A. G. Immediate postpartum IUD insertion. *Obstetrics and Gynecology*, **38**, 276–285.

104. TATUM, H. J. Intrauterine contraception. *American Journal of Obstetrics and Gynecology*, **112**, 1001–1023 (1972)

105. VAN OS, W. A., THIERY, M., VAN DER PAS, H. et al. Comparison of four different models of the Multiload copper IUD. *Contraceptive Delivery Systems*, **2**, 275 (1981)

106. THIERY, M. and VAN DER PAS, H. The MLCu375 intrauterine contraceptive device. *Advances in Contraception*, **1**, 37 (1985)

107. WORLD HEALTH ORGANIZATION. Task force on intrauterine devices. Microdose intrauterine levonorgestrel for contraception. *Contraception*, **35**, 363–379 (1987)

Chapter 10

Male and female barrier contraceptive methods

Walli Bounds

Male and female barrier methods are techniques of fertility regulation which, as the name implies, form a barrier to prevent the sperm from reaching the ovum. There are three groups: Condoms, diaphragms and caps, and spermicides.

Condoms

The condom, also known as sheath, protective, rubber, and French letter, is one of the oldest and most widely used forms of contraception. It is a valuable method both as an interim measure and for long-term use. Its history dates back to Roman times, when animal bladders were used to prevent the spread of sexually transmitted diseases. The earliest published description of the condom is that of the Italian anatomist Gabrielle Fallopio who, in 1564, recommended a linen sheath moistened with lotion to be used as protection against venereal infection. It was, however, not until the eighteenth century that condoms began to be used as a means of preventing pregnancy. Condoms made from animal intestines, known as 'skin condoms' are still available, but they are difficult to test, relatively expensive and not widely used [1]. The vast majority of present-day condoms are made of vulcanized latex rubber and come in a great variety of shapes, sizes, textures and colours, as listed in Table 10.1. Thanks to marked improvements in rubber technology, manufacturing techniques and quality control over the past fifty years, the products available nowadays are generally of a very high standard and provide an effective means of contraception.

Table 10.1 Types of condoms

Plain-ended
Teat-ended
Straight-sided
Shaped
Lubricated
Unlubricated
Spermicidally-lubricated
Smooth
Textured (ribbed)
Natural colour
Coloured

Mechanism of action and method of use

A condom physically prevents the transmission of semen into the vagina. For maximum protection, the following rules must be observed:

1. Use a condom every time.
2. Open the foil pack carefully to avoid damaging the condom.
3. Before genital contact, unroll the condom over the erect penis, holding the teat (or plain end) together to expel air.
4. After intercourse, withdraw the penis before it becomes soft, holding the condom firmly against the man's body and taking care not to spill any semen.
5. For maximum effectiveness ask your partner to use a spermicide at the same time.
6. Use only good-quality condoms. (In the UK this means only those brands which carry the British Standards Institution Kitemark.)
7. Use each condom only once.
8. Do not use Vaseline or other oil-based lubricants on your condom. If necessary, use a grease-free jelly (K–Y Jelly) or, better still, spermicidal cream or jelly.

Effectiveness

Because of vast improvements in condom manufacture and stringent quality control, product defects that could lead to failure are rare. There are no reliable data on how often a condom breaks during actual use, but it has been suggested that about one in every 1000 good-quality condoms may burst [2]. Estimated theoretical failure rates range from 0.4 to 2.0 pregnancies per 100 couple-years. However, because successful use depends largely on the motivation of the couple and the care with which the condom is employed, failure rates reported in the medical literature vary widely from a low of 0.4 per 100 woman-years [3] to a high of 31.9 per 100 woman-years [4]. In four UK studies, use-effectiveness pregnancy rates ranged from 3.1 to 4.8 per 100 woman-years [3,5–7], as illustrated in Figure 10.1.

The principal factors affecting efficacy are inconsistent and/or incorrect use. Failures are more frequent with young, inexperienced users and with couples who wish to delay rather than prevent pregnancy. The lowest failure rates are in older couples using the method consistently. For example, in the Oxford/Family Planning Association study in Great Britain, women aged 35 and older, with husbands who had used condoms for more than four years, had a pregnancy rate of only 0.7 per 100 couple-years of use. In comparison, women age 25–34 years, whose husbands had used condoms for more than four years, experienced failure at a rate of 3.6 per 100 couple-years [8]. The influence of pregnancy intention on condom efficacy shows in the results of a 1975 survey of about 5000 British women. Condom users with one or two children experienced a failure rate of 5 per 100 women in one year, whereas those who had not been pregnant before experienced accidental pregnancies at a rate of 14 per 100 women [9]. Similar patterns have been found in other countries.

Use of a spermicide in addition to the condom may increase contraceptive protection. However, since the pregnancy rate among *consistent* condom users is already very low, it would be difficult to measure the degree of protection afforded by the addition of a spermicide. While some couples may prefer to combine the two methods, others may find the use of a spermicide too inconvenient. However, to insist

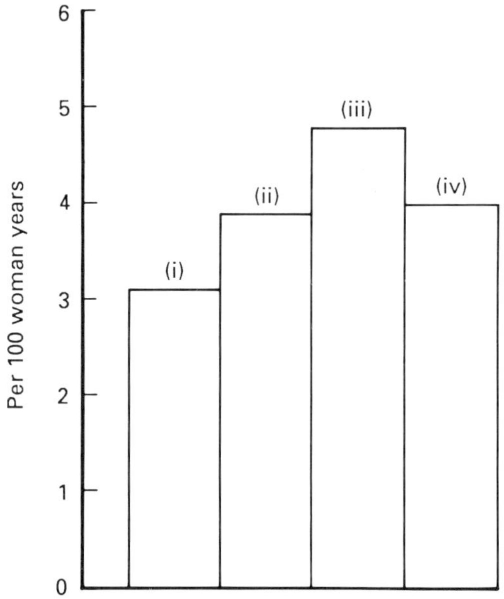

Figure 10.1. Condom use-effectiveness failure rates in the UK (Pearl formula). (i) Peel (1969) [6]; (ii) Peel (1972) [7]; (iii) John (1973) [3]; (iv) Glass *et al.* (1974) [5].

on this requirement may actually inhibit regular use of the condom and thus lead to unwanted pregnancy.

For couples who do not wish to use extra spermicides, a spermicidally lubricated condom may be more appropriate. Already available in many countries, this type of condom was introduced to the UK in 1978, where it is now the market leader. The question of whether a spermicidally lubricated condom affords the same degree of protection as a condom used in combination with a separate spermicide is virtually impossible to answer because of the vast number of patients that would be required for a comparative study. An uncontrolled trial, involving 397 highly motivated couples in the older age group who had completed their families, gave an overall failure rate of only 0.83 per 100 woman-years. The authors, however, admitted that these results should not be considered applicable to the general population of condom users [10].

Acceptability and use

An estimated 40 million couples use the condom worldwide, but with striking geographical differences, as can be seen in Figure 10.2. Japan alone accounts for more than one-quarter of condom users in the world, with 50% of married couples relying on this method. In fact 75% of contracepting couples in Japan use the condom. Factors contributing to this exceptional situation are the availability of ultrathin, virtually flawless condoms, attractive packaging, imaginative marketing, and restricted availability of alternative methods. By contrast, condom use is unusually low in Africa, the Middle East, and Latin America, which together account for only 4% of worldwide use. In the UK there has been a gradual decline in condom acceptance over

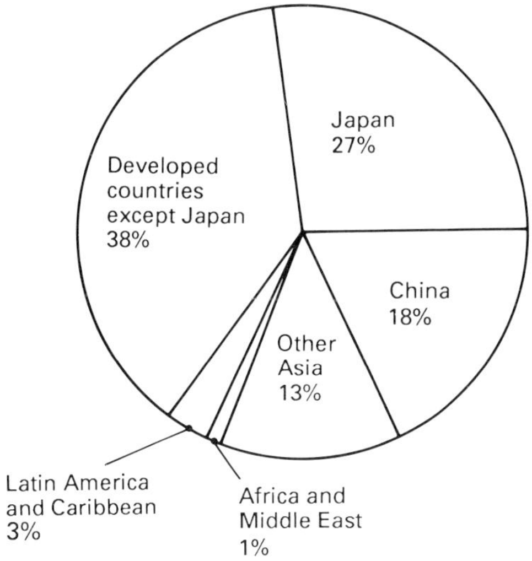

Figure 10.2. Percentage of condom-users; geographical distribution (1981). (From Sherris *et al.* (1982) [1].)

the past decade, with a corresponding increase in sterilization. Recent estimates suggest that only 13% of UK women aged 18–44 years rely on the condom [11], but current concerns over AIDS (acquired immunodeficiency syndrome) have already led to renewed interest in the method and may result in its more widespread use. See section 'The condom and AIDS' in this chapter.

In the past, condoms have been largely ignored by the medical profession and consumers because of their poor image, misconceptions about efficacy and perceived disadvantages in terms of inconvenience and reduced sensitivity. For centuries condoms have been associated with prostitution and viewed as immoral, an image which persists today in some societies. Even in the UK, where family planning has achieved a considerable degree of respectability over the past 50 years, the advertising of contraceptives, including the condom, is still heavily restricted although improvements are on the horizon.

More education and promotional campaigns similar to those undertaken in Japan and Sweden are needed to achieve the favourable image the method deserves. Advertising material similar to 'Proud Pete' (see Figure 10.3) could serve as a humorous and acceptable introduction to the method. Special efforts are required to create a more positive attitude in teenagers, who often begin sexual relations without any contraceptive protection. Since the method does not require medical supervision, is discreet and relatively inexpensive, it is especially suitable for this group. Moreover, its non-contraceptive benefit of protection against some sexually transmitted diseases is of particular value to the young. If adolescents could be encouraged to regard condom use as a sign of responsible adult behaviour, a great number of teenage tragedies could be averted.

In the UK condoms are obtained mainly through retail outlets, by mail order, and vending machines, but family planning clinics play an important role in promoting the method and they should offer supplies freely to male and female clients. That this is not always the case has been clearly demonstrated by Howard [12] in a survey of selected UK family planning clinics. It seems that a more positive approach is needed,

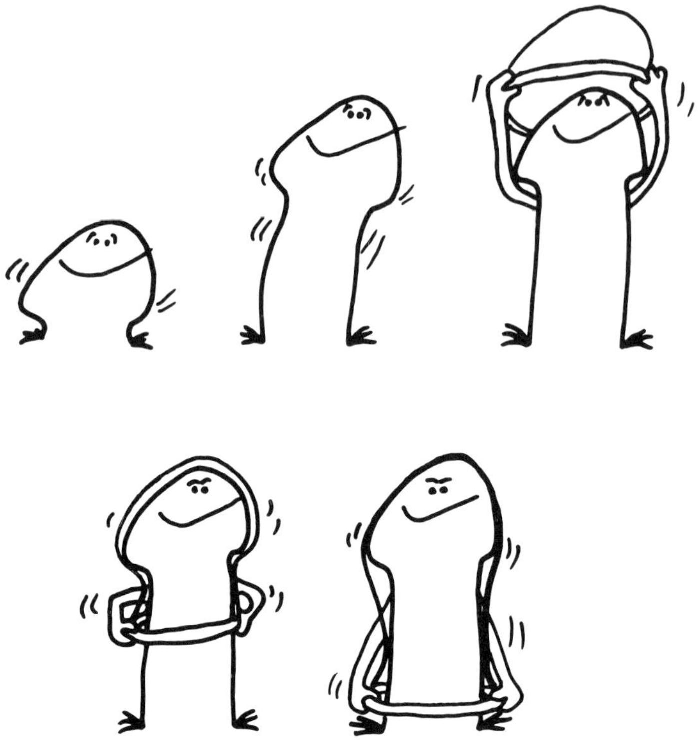

Figure 10.3. 'Proud Pete'. (By courtesy of the Swedish Association for Sex Education (RFSU).

not only by the public at large, but also by those who provide contraceptive care and advice.

Advantages and disadvantages

These are listed in Table 10.2. Ease of obtainability is probably the main advantage, especially for those who are unable or unwilling to make use of formal family planning services. Since no medical supervision is required, couples can pursue their sex lives in complete privacy. Apart from being an excellent long-term method, the condom is particularly suitable for those who require short-term contraception, e.g. while waiting to start oral contraceptives or for intrauterine-device insertion. Likewise, couples who have intercourse only infrequently may find the condom an ideal choice. Freedom from health risks and side-effects is a benefit which is becoming more relevant as our knowledge about the medical hazards associated with the Pill and the IUD widens.

Another increasingly important feature is the condom's protective effect against some *sexually transmitted diseases* (STDs) and their sequelae, although the degree of protection depends on consistent and correct use. For example, in a study of men attending a London STD clinic, Barlow found that those who had used a condom consistently had a significantly lower probability of acquiring *gonorrhoea* ($P<0.001$)

Table 10.2 Advantages and disadvantages of the condom

Advantages	*Disadvantages*
1. Easily obtainable	1. Requires high degree of motivation
2. Free from medical risks	2. Interrupts love-making
3. Highly effective if used consistently and correctly	3. Decreases sensitivity
4. No medical supervision required	4. Perceived to be messy
5. Protection against some sexually transmitted diseases	5. Coitus-related
6. Possible protection against cervical carcinoma	
7. Relatively inexpensive	
8. Offers visible evidence of use	
9. Involves the male in sharing contraceptive responsibility	
10. Useful in cases of premature ejaculation.	

Table 10.3 Relative risk of severe cervical dysplasia with barrier methods as against oral contraceptives [17]

Duration of use (years)	*Barrier methods*	*Oral contraceptives*
None	1.0	1.0
Less than 5	0.9	1.7
5–9	0.4	3.6
More than 10	0.2	4.0

and a significantly higher chance than no sexually transmitted disease would be diagnosed ($P < 0.0005$) compared to the rest of the clinic population [13]. Likewise, in a retrospective study of 246 Australian soldiers who had served in Vietnam, none of 55 consistent condom users acquired an STD, whereas of the 191 who did not use condoms, 35% did. Occasional use or washing after intercourse appeared to make little difference [14].

It is not yet known to what degree the use of condoms also protects against *genital herpes*. *In vitro* studies involving condoms containing herpes virus suspended in nutrient broth showed the condom to be an effective barrier to transmission of the virus [15]. However, since the herpes lesions often cover a wide area, involving buttock, vulva, and thighs, the use of condoms in these circumstances may not be as beneficial as presumed [M. W. Adler, Personal communication].

There is also evidence that the condom may guard against *pelvic inflammatory disease (PID)*. Analysing data from the Women's Health Study in the USA on hospitalization for initial episodes of PID, Kelaghan found that partners of condom users had a relative risk of 0.6 of developing PID compared to women using no contraception. The same protective effect was found for all barrier method users [16].

Recent studies suggest that the condom may have a protective and even possibly a therapeutic effect on *cervical-cell abnormalities* by limiting transmission of agents believed to be responsible for cervical carcinoma. In a UK case-control study, the relative risk of developing severe cervical dysplasia decreased with duration of condom or diaphragm use, while it increased with duration of oral contraceptive (OC) use. After 10 years of use, the relative risk for women using barrier methods was 0.2 compared to 4.0 for OC users (Table 10.3). This trend was also apparent when the data for condom and diaphragm users were analysed separately, and when adjustments were made for the number of sexual partners [17]. In another study, involving 139 women with cervical-cell abnormalities who received no treatment apart from their partners adopting the use of the condom, 136 showed complete reversal of the disease [18]. More research involving a comparison group and more detailed analyses of the various degrees of cellular abnormalities is needed to confirm these findings, however. If evidence for these non-contraceptive benefits is strengthened, the condom could undoubtedly play an important role in the prevention and treatment of these diseases.

The condom and AIDS

Indubitably, the most profound impact on the condom's role in disease prevention has been the emergence of AIDS (acquired immunodeficiency syndrome). This fatal, new disease, for which there is at present no cure, has become a major public-health problem worldwide. Prompt and effective national and global strategies to halt the spread of AIDS are urgently required, involving public education about the nature of the disease and ways of reducing its transmission. AIDS is caused by infection with the human immunodeficiency virus (HIV), which is transmitted mainly through homosexual and heterosexual intercourse. Apart from sexual abstinence or a stable mutually faithful relationship with an uninfected partner, using condoms regularly and correctly seems the best protection against sexually transmitted HIV infection. Several *in-vitro* studies have shown that condoms block the transmission of HIV and other viruses [19, 19a, 19b, 19c; L. Liskin, Personal communication].

Epidemiological evidence of a protective effect of the condom *in actual use* is encouraging, but as yet is not conclusive. A study in the US followed 24 uninfected sexual partners of people diagnosed with AIDS over a 3-year period. Among the ten couples who regularly used condoms, only one partner became infected, whereas among the 14 who did not use condoms, 12 became infected [20]. Similar encouraging results have been reported from other countries [21,22]. Large epidemiological studies among homosexual men using condoms are now under way in the USA. For maximum protection it is obviously essential that the rules for correct condom use described above are followed, and family planning providers play an important role in reinforcing this teaching. Morever, condoms should be offered freely to anyone in need of protection, *including* those whose contraceptive requirements are covered by other methods e.g. the Pill or IUD.

Manufacture and quality control

The manufacture of condoms, a highly automated process, involves dipping condom-shaped metal or glass moulds into cooled latex solution, from where they pass to a drying oven. After a second immersion in latex solution, the moulds pass into another oven for drying and vulcanization. Finally the condoms are removed from the moulds by water jets or brushes and are then subjected to quality control testing. The vast majority of condom-producing countries have national standards for condom quality, although the precise specifications vary from country to country. The standards generally require:

1. Visual inspection for packaging defects
2. Measurement of length, width, thickness and/or mass
3. A test for holes
4. A test of strength

Nearly all manufacturers screen condoms electronically for pinholes. In addition, most national standards require testing for holes by means of water and air-inflation tests. A typical sheath produced by the leading UK manufacturer would hold approximately 40 litres of air before bursting. But because of differences in national testing requirements it has hitherto not been possible for consumers and family planning providers to compare the quality of condoms produced in different parts of the world. To overcome this problem, the International Standards Organization (ISO) has created an international standard for condom testing [23] which, it is hoped, will be accepted by most if not all countries.

Future advances

Entirely new developments in the condom field seem unlikely. Studies designed to determine if a water-soluble condom could be produced, using biocompatible films and plasticisers, have been undertaken [24], but this approach appears to have been abandoned. The kind of changes one can expect in the near future are possibly improvements in packaging design, the manufacture of more ultrathin condoms, and the introduction of a greater variety of spermicidally lubricated condoms. Moreover, in view of the condom's increasing importance in the prevention of transmission of AIDS, it is likely that stronger condoms and more stringent quality control specifications will be introduced. These aspects have recently been addressed by the British Standards Institution, which has now published new quality control and consumer information criteria.

Diaphragms and caps

Diaphragms and caps are small, dome-shaped rubber devices which, when placed in the vagina, form a physical barrier over the cervix and serve as a carrier for spermicides. See Figure 10.4. Details of specific devices are listed in Table 10.4.

History

Although ancient cultures lacked a clear understanding of the mechanisms involved in fertilization and implantation, they were aware that pregnancy could be avoided by preventing semen from entering the uterus. Thus, over many centuries, various substances have been employed to form occlusive barriers. Hungarian women used melted beeswax, while the Chinese and Japanese covered their cervices with oiled silky

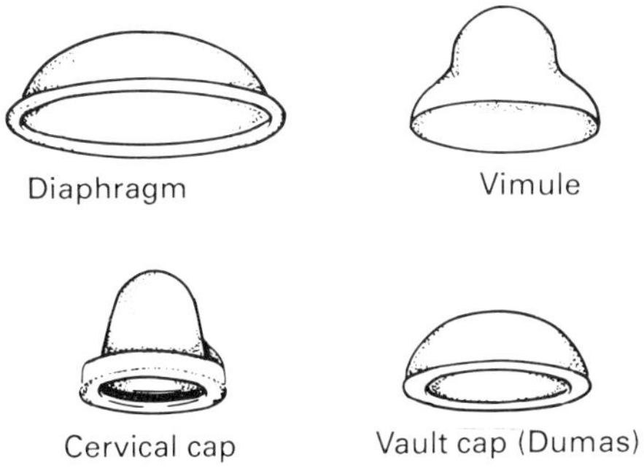

Figure 10.4. Diaphragms and caps.

Table 10.4 Diaphragms and caps available in the UK

Product and manufacturer	*Description*	*Size*	*On DoH drug tariff*
Diaphragms			
Durex LRC Products Ltd	Flat-spring diaphragm	55–95 mm (rising in 5-mm steps)	Yes
Durex Arcing-spring LRC Products Ltd	Arcing-spring diaphragm	60–95 mm (rising in 5-mm steps)	No
Ortho Ortho–Cilag Pharmaceutical Ltd	Coil-spring diaphragm	55–100 mm (rising in 5-mm steps)	Yes
Ortho-White Ortho–Cilag Pharmaceutical Ltd	Flat-spring diaphragm	55–95 mm (rising in 5-mm steps)	Yes
All Flex Ortho–Cilag Pharmaceutical Ltd	Arcing-spring diaphragm	65–95 mm (rising in 5-mm steps)	No
Caps			
Dumas Lamberts (Dalston) Ltd	Vault cap	55–75 mm (rising in 5-mm steps)	Yes
Prentif Cavity Rim Lamberts (Dalston) Ltd	Cervical cap	22–31 mm (rising in 3-mm steps)	Yes
Vimule Cap Lamberts (Dalston) Ltd	Vimule cap	45–51 mm (3 sizes)	Yes

paper. Contraceptive tampons made of 'lint' and soaked in honey and certain drugs were used by the Egyptians as early as 1550 BC, and in the Talmud of AD 230 reference is made to 'mokh', a spongy absorbent substance made of cotton or wool, which Hebrew women were advised to insert [25]. Intravaginal sponges came into use in European society in the seventeenth and eighteenth centuries, and are said to have been a popular method in France, where they were moistened with a mixture of water and brandy prior to insertion. Over the past decade this form of barrier method has attracted renewed interest among researchers, and one type of synthetic sponge has recently become generally available in America and Great Britain.

Present-day diaphragms and caps were developed in the nineteenth century. The cervical cap was first described in 1838 by the German gynaecologist Friedrich Adolphe Wilde. He recommended that the cap should be custom-fitted for each woman by making a wax impression of her cervix, and that it should be worn throughout the menstrual cycle, except during menses [26]. This type of cap was introduced in England in the latter part of the nineteenth century, prior to the diaphragm, where it was widely distributed by the birth control clinics run by Marie Stopes. The first description of the diaphragm in 1882 is credited to the German physician Dr C. Hasse who, in order to protect his reputation, used the pseudonym Wilhelm P. Mensinga. This device rapidly gained popularity in Germany and especially in Holland, hence its name 'Dutch Cap'. Use of the diaphragm spread to England, where it became the most frequently prescribed method in family planning clinics until the arrival of oral contraceptives in the early 1960s.

Historically, diaphragms and caps have normally been used in conjunction with a spermicide in order to provide maximum effectiveness [27,28]. No trials were done, which is not surprising. Bearing in mind the hostile political and public climate of opinion towards birth control at the turn of the century, it was imperative that women who had the courage to attend family planning clinics were offered the most reliable contraception available. However, this teaching about spermicides has recently been called into question, and some physicians now no longer recommend spermicides as adjuncts to mechancal barrier devices [29–31]. See section on 'Future Advances'.

Mechanism of action

Diaphragms and caps form a physical barrier against sperm and they serve also to retain spermicides against the cervix.

Types and sizes of diaphragm

There are three types of diaphragms, all of which are currently available in the UK. See Figure 10.5.

The flat-spring diaphragm

This consists of a rubber dome with a flat metal spring encased in the rim. It is currently the most frequently fitted type in the UK. Although appropriate for most women, its sturdy rim makes it also suitable for women with less firm vaginal muscle tone. It is available in sizes ranging from 55 mm to 95 mm.

The coil spring diaphragm

This diaphragm is less firm because of its wire spiral spring, and as it exerts less pressure, it is more comfortable for some women than the flat-spring version. It is available in sizes ranging from 55 mm to 100 mm.

The arcing-spring diaphragm

This consists of a rubber dome with a firm, double metal spring which when

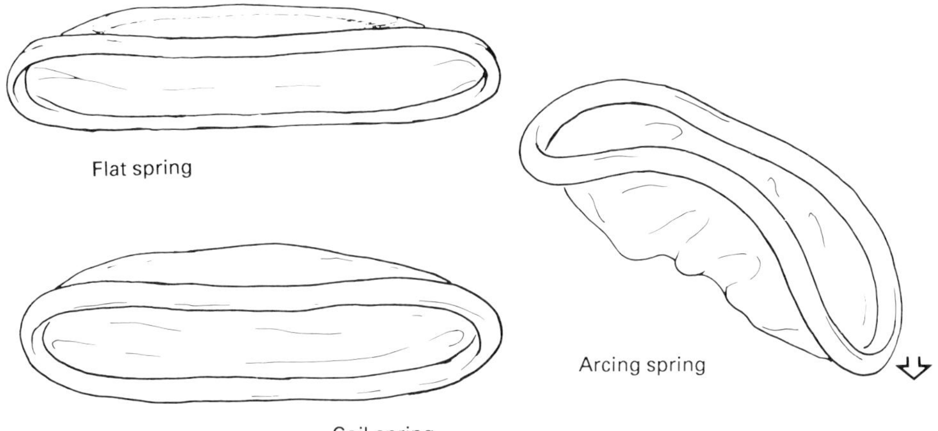

Figure 10.5. Flat-spring, coil-spring, and arcing-spring diaphragms. Note the *downward* direction of the leading rim of the arcing-spring diaphragm, which facilitates easy insertion over the cervix.

compressed forms an arc and allows the diaphragm to be easily directed posteriorly; this makes it particularly suitable for the woman who too readily inserts her diaphragm into the anterior fornix, without, or especially with, a retroverted uterus. It is the most widely used type of diaphragm in America, and is now also available in the UK. The 'All-Flex' model may be compressed at any point of the rim, while the 'Durex Arcing-spring' model must be compressed at the location marked 'press'.

Contraindications for using a diaphragm

Uterovaginal prolapse
Cystocele
Rectocele
Septate vagina or similar congenital abnormalities
Deficient perineal muscle (after tearing at childbirth)
Poor vaginal muscle tone
Absence of retropubic ledge
Toxic shock syndrome (TSS)
Allergy to rubber
A past history of recurrent cystitis or vaginal ulceration should be regarded as a relative contraindication.

Clinical practice and procedures

Two of the most crucial elements in successful diaphragm/cap use are correct fitting and thorough teaching. These procedures need not necessarily be carried out by a doctor. Most nurses can easily acquire the required skills, and since the teaching involves touching the patients' genitalia, many women feel less embarrassed in the presence of a nurse. What is important is that whoever undertakes the fitting/teaching should do so in an unhurried manner, and he/she should be sensitive to the woman's feelings about her sexuality and to her attitude towards vaginal self-examination. (Women who, because of their cultural upbringing or other reasons, have a strong dislike of touching their genitals are unlikely to use the diaphragm successfully.) Privacy is, of course, essential. A three-dimensional plastic pelvic model is a most useful aid to educating the woman about her pelvic anatomy and teaching diaphragm/cap insertion.

How to fit the diaphragm

To be effective, the correct type and size of diaphragm needs to be fitted.

1. The woman should have emptied her bladder.
2. Inspect the vagina and cervix with a speculum.
3. With the woman in the dorsal position, carry out a gentle bimanual examination, noting the length of the vagina, degree of vaginal muscle tone, presence or absence of a retropubic ledge, size and direction of the cervix, and position of the uterus.
4. With the index and middle fingers deep in the vagina, measure the distance between the posterior fornix and the symphysis pubis. Mark the point at which the symphysis pubis touches the index finger with the thumb of the same hand and withdraw your fingers.

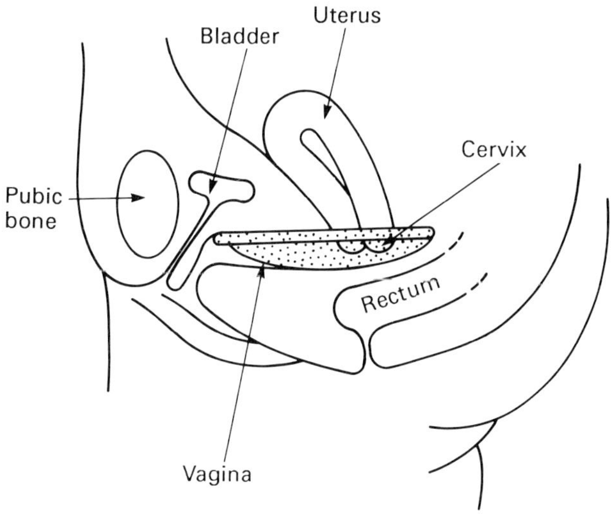

Figure 10.6. Properly fitted, the diaphragm fits snugly between the posterior fornix and the symphysis pubis. (Courtesy of the Williams and Wilkins Co., Baltimore, USA.)

5. Select the correct size by placing the rim of the diaphragm on the tip of the middle finger and the opposite rim in front of the thumb.
6. With the index finger placed inside the rim, compress the diaphragm between thumb and the remaining fingers and insert it with a downward movement deep into the vagina, tucking the anterior rim behind the symphysis pubis.
7. Now check that the cervix is covered by the soft dome of the diaphragm.
8. Ask the woman to cough and bear down to ensure that the device does not become dislodged.
9. To avoid possible discomfort during the insertion and teaching procedures, a small amount of lubricating jelly may be placed on the diaphragm.

Selecting the right size is important, as too large a diaphragm will cause discomfort to the woman and/or her partner. Moreover, if it does not tuck in behind the pubic bone there is a risk that the penis may enter on the 'cervical side'. Too small a diaphragm may become dislodged during intercourse or be accidentally inserted into the anterior fornix, leaving the cervix exposed. A correctly fitted diaphragm is illustrated in Figure 10.6.

How to teach diaphragm insertion and use

Thorough teaching in how to insert the diaphragm correctly and confidently is essential for successful use. One of the main aspects often overlooked by the trainer is that of teaching the woman the correct position to adopt to enable her fingers to reach the cervix. This important omission may be responsible for some of the so called 'cap failures' because the women were unable to check that the device was correctly positioned. Unless instructed to the contrary, many women will automatically adopt a half-standing/half-squatting position when inserting the diaphragm. This should be strongly discouraged, as it will usually not permit the fingers to reach the cervix.

1. Teach the woman to locate her cervix. She can do this while squatting right down or standing with one foot raised on a chair. (A right handed woman should raise her left leg and *vice-versa*).
2. By using both index and middle fingers, the majority of women can learn to identify the cervix.
3. She should then insert the diaphragm as described above and check that it is correctly positioned (i.e. she should feel the cervix covered by the soft rubber dome). The fact that a diaphragm fits snugly behind the symphysis pubis and feels comfortable is no guarantee of correct insertion. This must be explained to the prospective user.
4. To remove the diaphragm, the woman should hook her index finger behind the anterior rim and pull gently downward and out. If the device fits very tightly behind the symphysis pubis, grasping the rim between the index and middle fingers allows it to be removed more readily. This latter manoeuvre is unfortunately often ignored by the teacher, which can result in a woman abandoning the method altogether because of difficulty in removing the device in the more usual manner.
5. The woman should be asked to practise the insertion and removal techniques for a week while still using another method of contraception.
6. At the next visit the doctor or nurse will check that the woman is confident in correct diaphragm insertion, and that the device does not cause any discomfort. Often a larger size needs to be fitted at this visit, as the woman is more relaxed.
7. Before using the diaphragm, the woman should apply two strips, each measuring one inch (two centimetres), of spermicidal cream or jelly on each side of the dome and smear it minimally over each surface. This is standard UK teaching. (In some countries, e.g. the USA, the spermicide is applied only on the cervical side of the diaphragm, while in Australia the addition of spermicide is optional.)
8. The diaphragm may be inserted several hours before intercourse. But if the interval is more than 3 h, more spermicide should be added before love-making begins. This can be done by using an applicator or by simply inserting a pessary.
9. If intercourse is repeated, extra spermicide needs to be added before each new act, with the diaphragm left in position.
10. If intercourse takes place fairly regularly, it is best to insert the diaphragm routinely every night before going to bed, so as not to interrupt love-making.
11. After coitus, the diaphragm must remain in position for a minimum of 6 h, but may be worn longer, if desired. It should, however, be removed once a day for cleansing.
12. The woman should be taught to wash and dry the diaphragm carefully after use and to inspect it regularly for holes.
13. The size of the diaphragm should be re-checked after childbirth, miscarriage, or termination, after a gain or loss of weight of more than 3 kg and after any pelvic surgery.

The question of whether a diaphragm should be inserted 'dome up' or 'dome down' is one which often worries and confuses diaphragm users to such a degree that they ignore the more important aspect of checking that the cervix is covered. In the majority of women it makes little difference which way up a diaphragm is inserted. In the rare situations where a distinctly better fit is achieved one way rather than another, the woman should be advised accordingly. Finally, remind the woman that for maximum protection she must observe the following rules:

1. Use a diaphragm for *every* act of intercourse, including towards the end of, and just after menstruation.
2. Always be sure that the cervix is covered.
3. Use the prescribed amount of spermicide.

Whether or not a diaphragm is used successfully depends on a variety of factors, among which the skill, confidence, and supportive approach of the teacher are of prime importance.

Cervical, vault (Dumas) and Vimule caps

These types of caps form a valuable though much neglected part of our contraceptive armamentarium. They are a little more difficult to fit and teach than the diaphragm, which may account for their relatively infrequent use. They are particularly indicated for women who, because of their anatomical make-up or other reasons (e.g. cystitis), cannot use a diaphragm. Unlike the diaphragm, they are held in place over the cervix by suction.

The cervical cap

This is a thimble-shaped rubber cap with a hollow rim, which is available in four sizes: 22 mm, 25 mm, 28 mm and 31 mm diameter. A prerequisite for this type of cap is that the cervix is long, parallel-sided, not pointing backwards, free from cervical laceration, erosion and nabothian cysts, and accessible to the woman's fingers. A size that fits snugly around the base of the cervix should be selected. Plastic caps, suitable for women who are allergic to rubber, are unfortunately no longer available in the UK.

The Dumas

The Dumas is a shallow bowl-shaped cap made of thick rubber, suitable for the woman with a short, wide cervix. It comes in five sizes and, like the cervical cap, requires a healthy cervix.

The Vimule

This cap bears characteristics of the cervical and Dumas caps in that it has a high, narrow dome and a wide, flat side, which adheres to the vaginal vault. Available in four sizes, it is more appropriate for the irregular or cone-shaped cervix.

As is the case with the diaphragm, these caps need to be used in conjunction with a spermicide. The woman should fill the cap about one-third full with spermicidal cream or jelly before insertion. Too much spermicide may interfere with suction. After insertion, she must check for correct placement by gently pressing against the side of the dome to feel the fullness of the cervix within it and by running her fingers around the rim of the cap to ensure that the cervix is covered. An extra measure of spermicidal cream/jelly or a pessary should be added prior to intercourse and whenever love-making is repeated. To remove the cap, the woman should slide her finger under the rim to release the suction and then guide the cap out. In the UK it is accepted practice to wear the cap for no longer than 24 h to avoid the risk of malodour formation, trauma, and infection. Longer wear, for up to 7 days, appears to be common among some American cap users. [32,33] However, the United States

Food and Drug Administration (USFDA) directions, issued with the granting of marketing approval of the Prentif cavity rim cervical cap in the USA (May 1988), specify that the cap may be left in place for up to 48 h only.

Effectiveness

As has been shown with other types of barrier methods, the documented effectiveness of the diaphragm and caps varies widely, depending on the characteristics and motivation of the population studied and on the type of study undertaken. Retrospective studies based on national samples, such as the 1970 United States National Fertility Study [34], the 1973 National Survey of Family Growth [35], and the 1975 survey Family Planning Services: Changes and Effects [36] carried out by M. Bone on behalf of the UK Department of Health and Social Security, showed failure rates ranging from 13 to 23 pregnancies per 100 women during the first year of use. It should be noted that, in the first and third of these studies, the failure rates represent 'extended use-effectiveness', i.e. if a pregnancy occurred after the use of the diaphragm was abandoned and not replaced by another method, the pregnancy was considered a diaphragm failure. These studies give only a very general picture of contraceptive success in a given population during the period of time under investigation.

A more reliable indicator of a method's contraceptive potential are results derived from prospective clinical trials. Two such studies, published within the past 15 years, have shown exceptionally good results. In the Oxford/Family Planning Association study in the UK, Vessey recorded a use-effectiveness failure rate for the diaphragm of 2.4 per 100 woman-years (Pearl index), based on 5909 woman-years of observation [37]. This study comprised 4052 women from 17 family planning clinics in England and Scotland. To be eligible for recruitment, a woman had to be married, at least 25 years old, with at least five months experience of the method. These factors may have contributed to the remarkably low pregnancy rate, since failures are more likely to occur among young users and during the initial months following adoption of the method. In a more recent analysis of this ongoing study, the failure rate had dropped to 1.9 per 100 woman-years, based on 25 146 woman-years of observation [38].

Equally low failure rates have also been observed in a prospective clinical trial conducted at the Margaret Sanger Research Bureau in New York City in 1971–1972 [39]. The study group of 2168 new diaphragm acceptors differed from the population in the Vessey study in that they were all new to the method; 70% were unmarried; and more than 60% were less than 25 years old. The observed accidental pregnancy rate during the first 12 months of use was 1.9–2.2 (Life table), ranging from a low of 1.9 per 100 users younger than 18 years to a high of 3.0 among those 30–34 years old. In discussion of these exceptionally favourable results, the investigators stated:

'In our opinion, the objectivity with which methods were offered and the thoroughness with which they were described allowed the full exercise of patient self-selection and played a role in successful diaphragm use which was at least as important as the social characteristics of the client. This view is supported by the findings of the British study that there was no clear association between social class and the rate of accidental pregnancy.'

Although the study participants cannot be considered representative of all women, these two trials demonstrate the high level of efficacy achievable with good teaching and selection. In general, however, overall pregnancy rates of around 10–15% during the first year of use are more common [40–42], with the majority of failures being due to inconsistent and/or incorrect use.

Published data on the cervical cap suggest that its reliability is similar to that of the diaphragm. In reviewing the records of 143 women attending a private practice who had used the cap for periods ranging from one month to more than 20 years, Tietze calculated a failure rate of 7.6 per 100 woman-years. This was based on a total of 4415 woman-months of experience, 92% of which was contributed by the 72 women who had used the cap for longer than a year [43]. In a more recent study, Koch reported on the experience of 363 patients fitted with a Prentif Cavity-Rim cervical cap in his private practice between 1977 and 1979 [44]. The pregnancy rate observed in this group was 8.4 per 100 women at 12 months of use (Life table). The largest cervical cap study published to date, which reported on 3433 women, documented a pregnancy rate of 11.3% in the first year of use, with risks of 8.3 and 3.8% for user and method failures respectively [44a].

Acceptability and use

Before the arrival of the Pill and the IUD, diaphragms were widely used in Europe and the USA, since they were the most effective means of fertility regulation available to women. At the peak of its popularity in the 1950s, about one-third of American couples practising contraception were using the diaphragm. But as oral contraceptives and IUDs became widely available in the 1960s, use of barrier methods rapidly declined. Thus, by 1976 only 3% of surveyed American women were using a diaphragm. Similar shifts have also been noted in the UK where, according to 1979 estimates, about 3% of women in their fertile years used this form of contraception, compared to 28% relying on the Pill.

However, in recent years there has been renewed interest in barrier methods, particularly the diaphragm, in the USA and the UK. Among Californian women receiving contraceptive services in state-funded clinics, diaphragm use increased from 7.1% in 1976 to 12.8% in 1979 [45]. Likewise, in a UK family planning clinic serving 11 000 first clinic visits per year, the proportion of diaphragm acceptors rose from 5% in 1975 to 8% in 1978 [46]. Clinic statistics from the Margaret Pyke Centre for Study and Training in Family Planning, UK, show the proportion of diaphragm acceptors to have risen from 14% in 1984 to 18% in 1986 [47]. Increased awareness about general health and fear over real and perceived risks associated with the medical methods probably account for this trend.

Diaphragms and caps have always been more methods for the educated woman in the higher socioeconomic group; they are particularly favoured by doctors, nurses, and other health-care professionals [48,49]. Conversely, use of vaginal contraceptives in general and of the diaphragm in particular is minuscule in developing countries, as shown by the World Fertility Survey and other recent surveys. This is not surprising, considering the high degree of user motivation required for successful use, the need for trained personnel for the fitting and teaching of the method, and the lack of cleaning and storage facilities among the poor.

Advantages and disadvantages

The diaphragm's main advantage is undoubtedly its freedom from serious health hazards. Moreover, there is evidence that the method confers protection against pelvic inflammatory disease (PID). This is one of the most important non-contraceptive benefits, bearing in mind the dramatic rise in the incidence of this disease in the past two decades. In analysing data from the Women's Health Study in the USA, Kelaghan and co-workers found that the risk of hospitalization for PID in women currently using barrier methods relative to women using all other methods, and to women using no method, was 0.6 for both comparisons [50]. Based on these findings, the researchers estimated that, in the USA barrier method users experience 20 000 fewer episodes of PID annually and 5000 fewer hospitalizations for PID per year than they would have if they had used no method. Other advantages include high effectiveness when properly used, is used only when required, is under the control of the user, and possible protection against cervical carcinoma [51–53].

The drawbacks of the diaphragm are that it requires a high degree of user motivation and trained personnel to fit and teach; it is less effective than the Pill, the IUD or sterilization; it requires the woman to handle her genitalia; in rare instances it can be felt by the woman or her partner; and it is perceived to be messy because of the spermicide. Furthermore, diaphragm users have been shown to be at a higher risk of acquiring urinary-tract infections and possibly haemorrhoids [54]. If these occur, changing to one of the caps described above (cervical cap, Dumas or Vimule) may be more satisfactory.

Potentially major health hazards are extremely rare, and the question of whether use of the diaphragm increases the risk of developing toxic shock syndrome (TSS) requires further study. To date, the number of cases of TSS among diaphragm users is very small and does not suggest an increased risk. A small minority of women develop vaginal irritation due to the latex rubber or to the spermicide. Switching to a different spermicide often resolves this problem. Rare observations of vaginal or cervical ulceration and laceration, usually associated with wearing the device for longer than 24 h, have been reported. To minimize this small risk, it seems prudent to remove the diaphragm or cap at least once a day.

Future advances

Renewed interest in vaginal contraception has led to the development of new barrier techniques which it is hoped will prove more acceptable than the currently available methods. Below is a description of a number of such innovations.

Today (Collatex) contraceptive sponge

Sponges soaked in or smeared with substances thought to have spermicidal properties have been used for many centuries, but the concept of a spermicide-impregnated sponge appears to be a relatively recent one. Describing possible methods for fertility regulation in *The Wife's Handbook* in 1888, the UK physician H. A. Allbutt suggested that:

'A kind of artificial sponge or tampon containing in its centre a friable capsule filled with slightly acidulated quinine solution would, I believe, make a very good and cheap preventitive. All that the woman would have to do before intercourse would be to take one of the tampons and squeeze it, which would break the capsule, setting free the solution, which would then permeate the whole sponge. She would then insert it into the vagina as far as possible. It would be better to have a string attached so as to be able to withdraw it easily. If these tampons were made in large numbers they would have a ready sale [27].

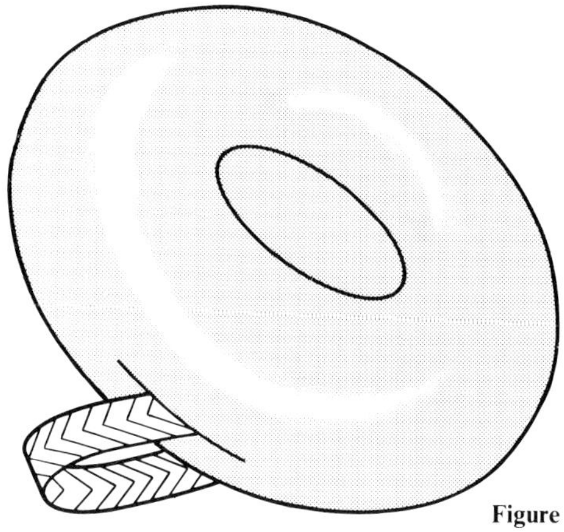

Figure 10.7. Today (Collatex) vaginal contraceptive sponge.

It is of interest that nearly one hundred years elapsed before Allbutt's concept became a reality in the form of the Today (Collatex) vaginal contraceptive sponge. Developed in the mid-1970s by Vorhauer Laboratories, USA, the Today is a small, circular, disposable sponge made of polyurethane foam and impregnated with the widely used spermicide nonoxynol-9. It has a polyester loop to facilitate easy removal. (Figure 10.7). To use the sponge, the woman simply moistens it prior to insertion (to start off the release of spermicide) and inserts it high into the vagina, covering the cervix. As with a diaphragm, the sponge must be kept in position for a minimum of 6 h after intercourse. One of its attractive features is that it can be inserted up to 24 h in advance of anticipated coitus, and that intercourse can be repeated as often as desired without the need to add more spermicide before each new act. Permitted maximum wearing time is 30 h. The sponge should not be used during menstruation. Its advantages are:

1. It can be purchased without prescription from retail outlets.
2. It can be inserted long before intercourse and thus does not diminish sexual spontaneity.
3. No waiting time is required between insertion and intercourse.
4. It is easy to use and not messy.
5. No special fitting (as with a diaphragm) is required.
6. It offers continuous protection, regardless of how often intercourse is repeated.

Multicentre clinical trials, involving various sponge designs and comparisons with other vaginal barrier methods, conducted under the auspices of Family Health International (formerly International Fertility Research Program), gave varying results. In randomized studies, comparing the sponge with Neo Sampoon foaming tablets, pregnancy rates of 9.2 and 11.2 per 100 women at one year of use respectively were observed [42]. A trial in the US, involving 733 sponge users and 721 diaphragm users, yielded failure rates of 17.0 for the sponge and 12.5 for the diaphragm (one year cumulative Life table rates) [41]. The highest pregnancy rates were documented in a UK study, which randomly compared 127 sponge users with 124 diaphragm acceptors, with a rate of 24.5 for the sponge and 10.9 for the diaphragm at 12 months of use [40]. It is worth noting that, as in the US trial, a higher proportion of failures in the sponge group in the UK study was due to method failure – 68% – compared to

40% in the diaphragm group. Moreover, parous women seem to be at a greater risk of pregnancy than nulliparae. Overall, the sponge appears to be as effective as other spermicidal products, but probably less effective than a diaphragm plus spermicide.

In an attempt to increase the reliability of this method, sponges impregnated with different types of spermicides are now being evaluated. One study involves a sperm enzyme (acrosin) inhibitor [55] while another measures the efficacy of the new spermicide RS-37367 [56]. On the question of acceptability, there were striking differences between the populations studied. In Bangladesh, Taiwan, and Yugoslavia sponge users tended to discontinue the method because of difficulty with insertion and removal, discomfort, and partner's objection, whereas in the UK the few complaints voiced centred mainly on vaginal irritation, sponges being displaced from the cervix or expelled during urination/defaecation, and sponges tearing on removal. Despite these problems, the majority of UK users found the method highly acceptable.

The question of whether sponge users are at an increased risk of developing toxic shock syndrome (TSS) is still unresolved, although recent evidence from the USA suggests that the risk is very small. At the time of writing, only 19 cases of TSS in sponge users have been reported in the USA, in relation to over 70 million sponges sold. [57]

Contracap

This is a custom-fitted cervical cap developed by Professors Goepp and Freese in the USA in the mid-1970s. In principle, it is similar to the original cervical cap described by Wilde in 1838, in that the cap is fitted individually for each woman to achieve an absolutely precise fit. The Contracap is designed to be worn continuously for up to 12 months and has a built-in one-way valve to permit the passage of cervical secretions and menstrual flow. One of its most attractive features is that, because of the very precise fit, the cap is meant to be used without spermicides. Since the messiness associated with spermicide use is probably the most off-putting factor with current female barrier devices, this is an important advantage. Preliminary studies of the efficacy of the Contracap have given mixed results, but a clinical trial undertaken at the Margaret Pyke Centre, UK showed an unacceptably high failure rate [58]. Among 29 women who used the Contracap as their sole contraceptive, nine accidental pregnancies occurred during 72 months of use. Further clinical trials in China of a modified version of the cap also revealed a high failure rate. As a result, the manufacturer is likely to abandon further development of this device.

Disposable spermicide-coated diaphragms

Research designed to produce easier-to-use and thus more acceptable types of diaphragms is under way in the USA, although data on clinical experience are not yet available.

Non-spermicide fit-free diaphragm (NSFFD) method – Honeycap

The value of using a spermicide in combination with a diaphragm has been questioned in recent years [31]. It is argued that the requirement for addition of spermicides lowers the acceptability of the diaphragm and leads to inconsistent use and hence to high failure rates. Stim, a New York gynaecologist, proposed that all women be fitted with a small (60 mm) arcing-spring diaphragm; that they should wear the device continuously day and night and only remove it once a day for washing; and that the use of spermicides be omitted. He called this the non-spermicide fit-free diaphragm method. Stim reported a failure rate of only 1 per 100 woman-years among more than 1000 women who had used the diaphragm in this fashion [59a]. However, these exceptionally good results have not been duplicated. In a study at the Marie Stopes clinic in London, involving approximately 100 users of the NSFFD method, a pregnancy rate of 25 per 100 women at one year was observed [C. Smith, Personal communication]. Obviously, more research is required to demonstrate the effectiveness of this technique in relation to other vaginal barrier methods.

A randomized comparative study of women using a diaphragm with and without spermicide and women using spermicide only is in progress at the Margaret Pyke Centre in London. Until the results of this and similar studies become available, it is prudent to recommend that women use the diaphragm in the conventional manner if avoidance of pregnancy is important.

A more recent modification of the NSFFD method is the Honeycap, which involves presoaking the diaphragm in honey for one week before it is issued to the patient. Claims that the presence of honey on the diaphragm will reduce the risk of vaginal infections during prolonged (up to one week) continuous use still require confirmation by appropriate laboratory studies.

Vaginal rings

Another recent innovation are silastic rings designed to release hormones, and clinical trials are now in progress in several countries. The aim is to deliver contraceptive steroids in a simpler fashion and thus increase user acceptance. The rings, placed in the upper vagina, are meant to be worn continuously for varying periods of time, e.g. 3 weeks, during which a controlled release of the active ingredient(s) should take place. To date, much of the published documentation relates to hormone-releasing rings, although rings containing nonoxynol-9 have also been considered.

Sperm electrocution

A novel approach by Dr Steven Kaali in the USA is the development of a tiny electrical battery device, placed in the cervical canal, where it creates a weak electrical field in the cervical mucus. Trials in baboons showed the device to be effective in immobilizing sperm before they reached the uterus. Clinical studies in humans involving a modified device which is placed in the upper vagina rather than in the cervix are planned to start in the near future [S. Kaali, personal communication].

Female condom

One of several inventions of this type is expected to be marketed in 1991 as 'Femidom'. This model was hitherto referred to as 'Femshield'. Made of pliable polyurethane, it is a plastic pouch inserted as a lining to the whole vaginal surface. Intercourse takes place within it, aided by a lubricant. At its rim an integral lower (vulvar) ring prevents the condom from being dislodged into the vagina, and an upper loose ring may be used by the woman as an aid to insertion. (Figure 10.8). This device would appear promising, but at the time of writing too few data are available to assess its possible success in the market place. A pilot study of its user acceptability undertaken at the Margaret Pyke Centre, UK, suggests that, with appropriate modifications to

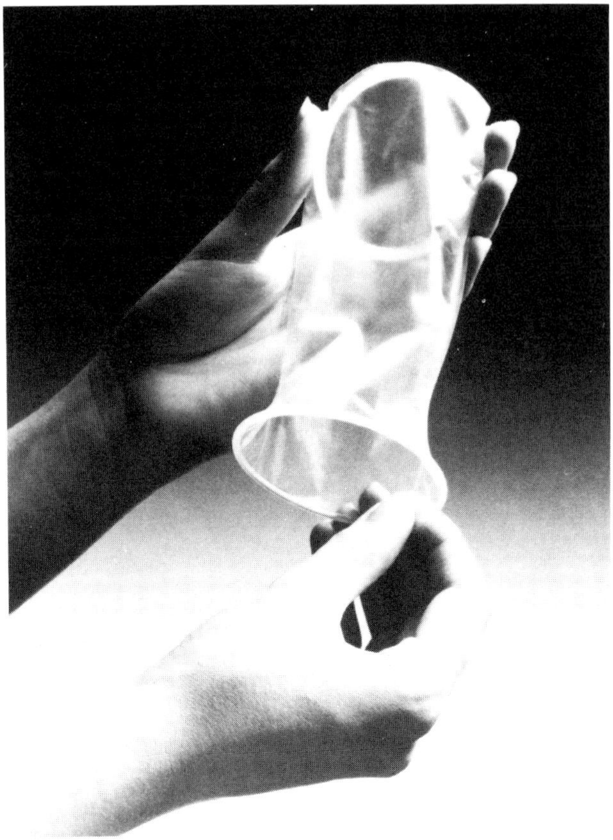

Figure 10.8 'Femidom' female condom.

its present physical design, the Femidom could play a useful role in the prevention of unwanted pregnancy and sexually transmitted diseases [59b].

A device similar to the 'Femidom', but made of latex rather than polyurethane, has been developed in the USA and is expected to become generally available there in early 1989 [59c].

Sterilization of practice diaphragms and caps

Concern over possible transmission of sexually transmitted organisms, notably the human immunodeficiency virus (HIV), human papilloma virus (HPV), and hepatitis B, by means of practice caps from one patient to another, has led to a review of sterilizing procedures in clinics and general practices. The current recommendations adopted by the Clinical and Scientific Advisory Committee of the National Association of Family Planning Doctors (UK) are:

1. Autoclaving is the most satisfactory if it is possible.
2. Milton (1000 ppm chlorine) – soaking for 30 min.

3. Domestos (10 000 ppm chlorine) – soaking for 30 min if there is heavy blood contamination.

   Both 2 and 3 should be followed by thorough washing [60].

Women suffering from vaginal candidiasis (thrush) should sterilize their diaphragms/caps in Milton prior to resuming use, in order to avoid reinfection [J. M. Holton, Personal communication].

Spermicides

Spermicides are chemical agents which immobilize and destroy sperm. They are one of the oldest and simplest forms of fertility control and, although not as effective as the Pill and the IUD they make a useful contribution to family planning because of attributes not found in other methods. Substances presumed to have spermicidal properties have been used by numerous cultures over many centuries. For example, a mixture of honey, natron and crocodile dung was used by the Egyptians in the nineteenth century BC, and during the middle ages people tried to prevent pregnancy by using rock salt and alum. In the more recent past, vinegar, carbolic soap, and quinine solution were recommended. The first commercial spermicide was developed in 1885 by W. H. Rendell, an English pharmacist, who prepared a suppository of soluble cocoa butter and quinine sulphate. A major technological advance occurred in the 1950s with the development of surface-active agents (surfactants), which are now the principal active ingredients in spermicidal products worldwide.

Mode of action

Spermicidal action causes a breakdown of the sperm membrane, involving interaction with the lipoprotein cell membrane, osmotic imbalance, and subsequent leakage of cell components. This leads to irreversible loss of motility. In addition, disruption of acrosome production reduces and even abolishes sperm fertilizing capacity [61–63]. Spermicidal products have two main components: an active spermicide and a relatively inert base material. The base materials differ mainly in their physical characteristics, some being water soluble, others water insoluble. The active ingredients fall into three main groups: Surface-active agents (surfactants), of which the most widely used is nonoxynol-9; bactericides; and acids. Some formulations contain a combination of several active constituents.

Types available and method of use

Spermicides are available in the form of creams, jellies, pessaries (suppositories), aerosol foams, foaming tablets/pessaries, and films. Details of spermicides currently marketed in the UK are listed in Table 10.5. To be effective, the products need to disperse quickly and evenly in the vagina and to release the actual spermicide rapidly. Specific instructions vary with the product but, generally speaking, creams and jellies are applied directly to the diaphragm/cap or inserted high into the vagina by means of an applicator. Pessaries should be inserted about 10–15 min before coitus to allow

Table 10.5 Spermicides available in the UK

Name	*Manufacturer*	*Active ingredients*
Foams		
Delfen Foam	Ortho–Cilag Pharmaceutical Ltd	Nonoxynol-9 12.5%
Creams		
Delfen Cream	Ortho–Cilag Pharmaceutical Ltd	Nonoxynol-9 5%
Duracreme	LRC Products Ltd	Nonoxynol-11 2%
Orthocreme	Ortho–Cilag Pharmaceutical Ltd	Nonoxynol-9 2%
Jellies		
Duragel	LRC Products Ltd	Nonoxynol-11 2%
Ortho Gynol Gel	Ortho–Cilag Pharmaceutical Ltd	Di-isobutylphenoxypolyethoxyethanol 1%
Gynol II	Ortho–Cilag Pharmaceutical Ltd	Nonoxynol-9 2%
Staycept jelly	Syntex Pharmaceuticals Ltd	Octoxynol 1%
Pessaries		
Double Check	FP Sales Ltd	Nonoxynol-9 6%
Orthoforms	Ortho–Cilag Pharmaceutical Ltd	Nonoxynol-9 5%
Staycept	Syntex Pharmaceuticals Ltd	Nonoxynol-9 6%
Film		
C-Film	Arun Products Ltd	Nonoxynol-9 67 mg

* Do not use with diaphragm or caps

sufficient time for them to melt and disperse. Likewise, foaming tablets need to be inserted about 10 min in advance to allow sufficient foam to build up to release the active ingredient. Aerosol foam is supplied in a pressurized container and needs to be released into an applicator, from which the foam is discharged high into the vagina. Soluble film is folded once and inserted by hand 3–5 min prior to coitus. If intercourse is repeated, a further dose of spermicide needs to be applied before each new act.

Tests of the ability of spermicides with different base materials to disperse evenly in the vagina have shown marked differences, with foams and creams giving better coverage than jellies and pessaries [64]. How far these differences affect use-effectiveness is difficult to measure, since in practice many failures appear to be associated with inconsistent and/or incorrect use. In the UK, spermicides are generally recommended as an adjunct to other methods, e.g. diaphragm/cap, the condom, or IUD rather than as a sole contraceptive, although exceptions are made when a patient considers spermicides to be the only acceptable option. However, when a high degree of protection is essential, they should not be relied upon on their own.

Effectiveness

Reported efficacy rates vary widely, with failures ranging from less than one to over 30 pregnancies per 100 woman-years [65]. The best rates are usually obtained in clinic-based studies involving carefully selected, highly motivated women who use the method consistently and correctly. The wide range of failure rates reported for similar or even identical products suggests that the differences are more likely due to the characteristics of the users and to study design rather than the inherent spermicidal potential of the contraceptive. For example, in a study of foam among 2932 well-motivated women attending six family planning clinics in the USA, who received proper instructions and follow-up, Bernstein documented a pregnancy rate of only 3.98 per 100 woman-years [66]. In contrast, in the 1970 United States National Fertility Survey, which measured extended use-effectiveness, Ryder observed a failure rate of 31% during the first year of use in women using a foam [67]. The above examples clearly demonstrate that it is misleading simply to state a specific failure rate for spermicides in general, or for a particular product. When counselling patients it is more appropriate to cite a *range* of failure rates, based on more recent studies, pointing out that careful and consistent users can expect a risk of pregnancy of about 5%, whereas among those who take chances or use the method incorrectly the risk increases to around 15%.

The way in which a product's spermicidal potential is assessed has been questioned in recent years. While in the past great emphasis was placed on *in vitro* and postcoital tests, some researchers now regard these tests as an unreliable predictor of a product's efficacy in actual use. Zaneveld and co-workers have suggested that animal studies would be more appropriate. In two separate studies of Delfen cream in monkeys, they had demonstrated that, although the product had consistently immobilized all sperm in the postcoital tests, half the animals had become pregnant within an average of 3.7 breeding cycles. As a result of these tests the researchers recommended that primate breeding experiments be performed before a spermicide is evaluated in women for its contraceptive effect [68].

Acceptability and use

Both in developed and developing countries spermicides are used by only a small fraction of contraceptive acceptors. Surveys carried out between 1970 and 1982 showed that the percentage of currently married women of reproductive age using vaginal contraceptive methods ranged from below 0.5% in African, Asian and Middle Eastern countries to 8.0% in Europe and the USA [65]. In developing countries spermicides appear to be used more often as the principal method, while in the developed world, spermicide-only and spermicide with diaphragm use seem to be equal. A United Kingdom survey undertaken in 1970 showed that 4% of the women interviewed used each method [69]. The reasons for the relatively low acceptance of spermicides are many and include:

1. Little or no knowledge about the method among health care providers and potential users, especially in developing countries.
2. Spermicides are perceived to be ineffective and unacceptable.
3. The products need to be used near the time of intercourse.
4. They need to be used at every coitus.
5. Their use requires that the woman touches her genitalia.
6. Some products require a waiting time between insertion and coitus.
7. Some spermicides tend to increase vaginal lubrication noticably and leave a liquid residue. Hence they are perceived to be messy.
8. Foaming tablets/pessaries generate heat on dissolving, which some women and/or

their partners find unacceptable. (Conversely, in Ghana men liked foaming tablets because they found the sensation of heat stimulating and increasing sexual pleasure. In the Philippines advertisements cite the heat production as an added bonus, with T-shirts carrying the slogan 'Neo Sampoon – for that warm sensation'.)

On the whole, there appears to have been little change in spermicide usage on a global basis over the past two decades, with small geographical exceptions. Social marketing programmes have been used in selected developing countries to increase knowledge, availability and usage of spermicides, in particular Neo Sampoon, (a foaming tablet containing menfegol). But despite these efforts, spermicide acceptance has been significantly lower than oral contraceptives, condoms, or the IUD [65]. It appears that when spermicides are selected, it is often not because of their intrinsic attributes, but because of fear over real and perceived hazards associated with the Pill and the IUD. Users then view this form of contraception as a last resort.

The traditional view that use of vaginal contraceptives is entirely dependent on characteristics of the product and the motivation of the user is now being questioned. Recent experience suggests that the acceptance of a method, including spermicides, can be greatly influenced by the attitude of family planning providers. Often doctors and nurses are biased against vaginal barrier methods and underrate their usefulness. Inevitably this negative attitude is transferred to the potential user. For example, a survey among family planning personnel in two American cities showed that respondents tended to quote *theoretical* effectiveness rates for the Pill and the IUD, whereas they rated vaginal barrier methods according to *use*-effectiveness or even lower [70]. In contrast, the women's self-help movement in the United States and the UK has a very positive approach towards barrier contraceptives and encourages their use. Since health care professionals obviously play a crucial role in the choice of method, it is important that they are educated about the merits and disadvantages of *all* methods.

Advantages and disadvantages

These are listed in Table 10.6. Ease of obtainability, freedom from major health hazards, and no need of medical supervision are probably the main positive attributes of vaginal spermicides. These factors are of particular importance in countries with only limited health-care facilities. Moreover, they are a useful contraceptive option for women, particularly teenagers, who are unwilling or unable to use existing family planning services and who would otherwise use none, or only ineffective, methods.

Table 10.6 Advantages and disadvantages of spermicides

Advantages	*Disadvantages*
1. Easy availability	1. Perceived to be messy
2. Freedom from major health risks	2. Not highly effective in general use
3. No medical intervention/supervision required	3. Are coitus dependent, and thus inconvenient to use
4. Need only be used when required	4. Can cause local irritation
5. Provide some protection against some sexually transmitted diseases	
6. Allows the female to be in control of contraception	
7. Are a valuable adjunct to other methods	

Women who have intercourse infrequently may find spermicides particularly appropriate.

In vitro and *in vivo* studies suggest that spermicides provide protection against some sexually transmitted diseases, and hence they may also afford protection against pelvic inflammatory disease (PID). Laboratory tests have demonstrated that surface active agents such as nonoxynol-9 are highly effective against *Neisseria gonorrhoea*, *Trichomonas vaginalis*, *Candida albicans* and *Herpes* virus [71,72]. Moreover, some carrier materials, e.g. foam, may in themselves be lethal to specific microorganisms. The small number of *in vivo* studies published to date have shown promising results, but more research is needed to confirm the laboratory findings in clinical practice. An American case-control study which examined medical records of 241 women found that spermicide users had a gonorrhoea rate about one-quarter that of Pill users or women who had been sterilized [73], and a double-blind study using two spermicidal products and a placebo in 78 women exposed to the risk of gonorrhoea found a statistically significant reduction in the incidence of the disease among the spermicide groups [74]. More recently, a comparative clinical trial of the effect of the contraceptive sponge (containing nonoxynol-9) among high-risk women in Bangkok, Thailand, demonstrated that sponge users had a lower risk of acquiring chlamydial and gonorrhoeal infections than non-users, although users had a higher incidence of candidiasis [75].

Of paramount current interest is the question of whether spermicides also protect against AIDS. Limited evidence from *in vitro* studies looks promising, but further research is required to confirm the early results. Nonoxynol-9, the most widely used spermicide worldwide, has been shown to inactivate the human immunodeficiency virus (HIV) in laboratory tests [76, 76a], as has benzalkonium chloride, the active ingredient of several spermicidal products sold in Europe and Canada [77]. In addition, studies are under way to determine if a combination of interferon and nonoxynol-9 inactivates HIV. *In vitro* studies have shown that the two products together inactivate the herpes simplex virus more effectively than either component alone. Preliminary *in vitro* studies suggest that this is also true for HIV. If further laboratory studies prove successful, the developers plan to produce a condom containing an interferon-nonoxynol-9 gel. Thus, spermicides could play an increasingly important role in preventing the spread of AIDS, particularly for women whose partners are reluctant to use a condom. However, as is the case with condoms, the success of such prophylactic measures will depend largely on the regularity and care with which the spermicides are employed.

Disadvantages

On the side of disadvantages, messiness and only moderate effectiveness in actual use seem to be the main complaints against the method. The former may be minimized by delivering the active spermicide in new base materials, as is already the case with the Today contraceptive sponge. (See section on Diaphragms and Caps.) Local irritation does occur in a small number of spermicide users, but changing to a product with a different carrier and/or a different active ingredient usually resolves the problem. True allergic reactions are rare. It is also worth bearing in mind that local reactions may be due to a concurrent vaginal infection (e.g. candidiasis) rather than to the spermicide.

In recent years, questions concerning the possibility of *systemic effects* have been raised. It is well known that the vagina is capable of absorbing a wide range of substances, including nonoxynol-9 [78]. Animal studies have given mixed results, but to date no evidence of systemic effects in humans has been reported. The conclusion of a recent World Health Organization review of the effects of contraception on women's health during the postpartum period and during lactation was that: 'There has not been any suggestion, for lactating or for non-lactating postpartum women, of an adverse health effect resulting from the use of spermicidal creams or suppositories, [79]. Nor is there any evidence that spermicide use could adversely affect the milk of a lactating woman, and in turn the health of her breast-fed child.

Another area of spermicide safety was questioned when a US study carried out by Jick and co-workers suggested a connection between spermicide use and *fetal abnormalities*. Of the 763 infants born to women presumed to have used spermicides, 2.2% exhibited congenital disorders, compared to 1.0% of the 3902 infants born to non-users [80]. The validity of this study has been queried because, (a) it is not known whether the women actually used spermicides around the time of conception, (b) there was no well-defined pattern of fetal abnormalities, as would be expected if a causal relationship existed, and (c) the rate of 1.0% in the control group is well below the US national norm. Other studies suggested a link between spermicide use and Down's syndrome and an increased risk of spontaneous abortion. In contrast to the few studies questioning the safety of spermicides, there are numerous others that have found no association between spermicide use and congenital defects [81–85], nor between spermicide use and spontaneous abortion [86]. Obviously more research is needed to clarify these issues, but the more convincing evidence to date suggests there is no risk [87].

Future advances

Research is under way for new and better spermicides and for better carrier materials. New delivery systems as well as entirely new types of spermicidal agents are being tested. These include enzyme inhibitors which operate by immobilizing sperm or preventing them from penetrating the ovum, and drugs normally used for non-contraceptive indications. In 1973 several drugs including propranolol, chlorpromazine, and phenoxybenzamine were reported to inhibit the motility of spermatozoa *in vitro*. One of these, propranolol, is now being tested more extensively in humans. In a study by Zipper *et al.*, involving vaginal insertion of 80 mg propranolol tablets by 198 Chilean women, a pregnancy rate of only 3.9 per 100 woman-years was documented, and no major adverse effects were encountered [88]. More recently, postcoital tests comparing various doses of D-propranolol (which has only very weak beta-blocking activity) with nonoxynol-9 at the Margaret Pyke Centre in London demonstrated complete immobilization of spermatozoa by 80 mg D-propranolol but not with nonoxynol-9 [Y. Tayob, Personal communication].

Gossypol, a derivative of cotton seed oil, which has been tested in China as a systemic contraceptive for men, is also being studied as a potential spermicide. Postcoital tests in 15 Finnish women who had used a gossypol gel showed complete sperm immobilization in 11 women and partial immobilization in the remaining four [89].

Research is also under way to evaluate the antiseptic *chlorhexidine* as a possible new spermicide. Unlike nonoxynol-9, chlorhexidine does not possess surfactant properties but does have a spermicidal effect. Moreover, in a recent in-vitro study, Sharman and co-workers observed that chlorhexidine penetrates into the cervical mucus, whereas nonoxynol-9 does not [90]. This important finding could explain some of the failures associated with the use of current spermicide products. A pilot study in human volunteers is now in progress at the University of Manchester, UK [E. Chantler, Personal Communication].

If some of the research described above comes to fruition, spermicides could in future play a more important role in the control of human fertility.

References

1. SHERRIS, J. D., LEWISON, D. and FOX, G. Update on condoms products, protection, promotion. *Population Reports* Series H. No. **6** (1982)
2. KESTELMAN, P. Standards and quality control in contraception. Presented at the International Family Planning Association seminar for pharmacists. Dublin, January (1980)
3. JOHN, A. P. K. Contraception in a practice community. *Journal of the Royal College of General Practitioners*, **23**, 665 (1973)
4. TIETZE, C., PAI, D. N., TAYLOR, C. E. and GAMBLE, C. J. A family planning service in rural Puerto Rico. *American Journal of Obstetrics and Gynecology*, **81**, 174 (1961)
5. GLASS, R., VESSEY, M. and WIGGINS, P. Use-effectiveness of the condom in a selected family planning clinic population in the United Kingdom. *Contraception*, **10**, 591 (1974)
6. PEEL, J. A male-orientated fertility control experiment. *The Practitioner*, **202**, 677 (1969)
7. PEEL, J. The Hull family survey. II. Family Planning in the first 5 years of marriage. *Journal of Biosocial Science*, **4**, 333 (1972)
8. VESSEY, M., LAWLESS, M. and YEATES, D. Efficacy of different contraceptive methods. *Lancet*, **1**, 841 (1982)
9. BONE, M. In: *The Family Planning Services: Changes and Effects*. Her Majesty's Stationery Office, London (1978)
10. POTTS, M. and MCDEVITT, J. A use-effectiveness trial of spermicidally lubricated condoms. *Contraception*, **11**, 701 (1975)
11. WELLINGS, K. Trends in contraceptive method usage since 1970. *British Journal of Family Planning*, **12**, 15 (1986)
12. HOWARD, G. and WHITTAKER, J. Difficulties in obtaining condoms on the NHS. *British Journal of Family Planning*, **7**, 12 (1981)
13. BARLOW, D. The condom and gonorrhoea. *Lancet*, **2**, 811 (1977)
14. HART, G. Factors influencing venereal infection in a war environment. *British Journal of Venereal Diseases*, **50**, 68 (1974)
15. CONANT, M., SPICER, D. W. and SMITH, C. Herpes simplex virus transmission: condom studies. *Sexually Transmitted Diseases*, **11**, 94 (1984)
16. KELAGHAN, J., RUBIN, G. L., ORY, H. W. and LAYDE, P. M. Barrier-method contraceptives and pelvic inflammatory disease. *Journal of the American Medical Association*, **248**, 184 (1982)
17. HARRIS, R. W. C., BRINTON, L. A., COWDELL, R. H. *et al.* Characteristics of women with dysplasia or carcinoma in situ of the cervix uteri. *British Journal of Cancer*, **42**, 359 (1980)
18. RICHARDSON, A. C. and LYON, J. B. The effect of condom use on squamous cell cervical intraepithelial neoplasia. *American Journal of Obstetrics and Gynecology*, **140**, 909 (1981)
19. CONANT, M., HARDY, D., SERNATINGER, J. *et al.* Condoms prevent transmission of AIDS-associated retrovirus. *Journal of the American Medical Association*, **255**, 1706 (1986)

19a CONANT, M., HARDY, D., SERNATINGER, J. *et al.* Condoms prevent transmission of AIDS-associated retrovirus. *Journal of the American Medical Association*, **255**, 1706 (1986)

19b VAN DE PERRE, P., JACOBS, D., and SPRECHER-GOLDBERGER, S. The latex condom, an efficient barrier against sexual transmission of AIDS-related viruses. *AIDS*, **1**, 49 (1987)

19c RIETMEIJER, C. A. M., KREBS, J. W., FEORINO, P. M. *et al.* Condoms as physical and chemical barriers against human immunodeficiency virus. *Journal of the American Medical Association*, **259**, 1851 (1988)

20. FISCHL, M., DICKINSON, G. M., SCOTT, G. B. *et al.* Evaluation of heterosexual partners, children and household contacts of adults with AIDS. *Journal of the American Medical Association*, **257**, 640 (1987)
21. SMITH, G. L. and SMITH, K. F. Lack of HIV infection and condom use in licensed prostitutes. *Lancet*, **2**, 1392 (1986)

22. MANN, J. M., QUINN, T., FRANCIS, H. *et al.* Sexual practices associated with LAV/HTLV-III seropositivity among female prostitutes in Kinshasa, Zaire. (Abstract) Presented at the International Conference on AIDS, Paris, June (1986)
23. MELLSTAM, S. International standardisation of mechanical contraceptives. *IPPF Medical Bulletin*, **17**, 2 (1983)
24. BELSKY, R. Water-soluble condom and vaginal contraceptive film insert. In: *Vaginal Contraception: New Developments* (eds Zatuchni G. I., Sobrero, A. J., Speidel, J. J. and Sciarra, J. J.) Harper and Row, Hagerstown (1979)
25. KEOWN, K. K. JR. Historical perspectives on intravaginal contraceptive sponges. *Contraception*, **16**, 1 (1977)
26. HIMES, N. E. *Medical History of Contraception*, Williams and Wilkins, Baltimore, p. 319 (1936)
27. ALLBUTT, H. A. *The Wife's Handbook*, Forder, London, p. 49 (1888)
28. PEEL, J. and POTTS, M. *Textbook of Contraceptive Practice*. Cambridge University Press (1970)
29. STIM, E. The non-spermicide fit-free diaphragm: A new contraceptive method. *Advances in Planned Parenthood*, **15**, 88 (1980)
30. AUSTRALIAN FEDERATION OF FAMILY PLANNING ASSOCIATIONS (AFFPA Medical Task Force). Guidelines on contraception. *British Journal of Sexual Medicine*, **10**, 33 (1983)
31. CRAIG, S. and HEPBURN, S. The effectiveness of barrier methods of contraception with and without spermicide. *Contraception*, **26**, 347 (1982)
32. KOCH, J. P. The Prentif contraceptive cervical cap: A contemporary study of its clinical safety and effectiveness. *Contraception*, **25**, 135 (1982)
33. LEHFELDT, H. Cervical cap. In: *Manual of Family Planning and Contraceptive Practice* (ed Calderone, M. S.) Williams and Wilkins, Baltimore p. 368 (1970)
34. RYDER, N. B. Contraceptive failure in the United States. *Family Planning Perspectives*, **5**, 133 (1973)
35. VAUGHAN, B., TRUSSEL, J., MENKEN, J. and JONES, E. F. Contraceptive failure among married women in the United States, 1970–1973. *Family Planning Perspectives*, **9**, 251 (1977)
36. BONE, M. *The Family Planning Services: Changes and Effects*, Her Majesty's Stationery Office, London (1978)
37. VESSEY, M. and WIGGINS, P. Use-effectiveness of the diaphragm in a selected family planning clinic population in the United Kingdom. *Contraception*, **9**, 15 (1974)
38. VESSEY, M., LAWLESS, M. and YEATES, D. Efficacy of different contraceptive methods. *Lancet*, **1**, p. 841 (1982)
39. LANE, M. E., ARCEO, R. and SOBRERO, A. J. Successful use of the diaphragm and jelly by a young population: Report of a clinical study. *Family Planning Perspectives*, **8**, 81 (1976)
40. BOUNDS, W. and GUILLEBAUD, J. Randomised comparison of the use-effectiveness and patient acceptability of the Collatex (Today™) contraceptive sponge and the diaphragm. *British Journal of Family Planning*, **10**, 69 (1984)
41. EDELMAN, D. A., MCINTYRE, S. L. and HARPER, J. A comparative trial of the Today contraceptive sponge and diaphragm. *American Journal of Obstetrics and Gynecology*, **150**, 869 (1984)
42. SHERRIS, J. D., MOORE, S. H. and FOX, G. New developments in vaginal contraception. *Population Reports*, Series H, No. 7 (1984)
43. TIETZE, C., CHURCH, F., LEHFELDT, H. and LIEBMANN, H. G. The effectiveness of the cervical cap as a contraceptive method. *American Journal of Obstetrics and Gynecology*, **66**, 904 (1953)
44. KOCH, J. P. The Prentif contraceptive cervical cap: A contemporary study of its clinical safety and effectiveness. *Contraception*, **25**, 135 (1982)
44a RICHWALD, G. A., GREENLAND, S., GERBER, M. M. *et al.* Effectiveness of the cavity-rim cervical cap: results of a large clinical study. *Obstetrics and Gynecology*, **74**, 143 (1989)
45. AVED, B. M. Trends in contraceptive methods of use by California family planning clinic clients aged 10–55, 1976–1979. *American Journal of Public Health*, **71**, 1162 (1981)
46. NUTTALL, I. D., BURSLEM, R. W., ELSTEIN, M. *et al.* Current trends in contraception. *British Medical Journal*, **2**, 641 (1979)
47. Clinic statistics. Margaret Pyke Centre for Study and Training in Family Planning, UK. Data on file.
48. JACKSON, M., BERGER, G. S. and KEITH, L. G. (eds.) *Vaginal Contraception*. G. K. Hall Medical Publishers, Boston (1981)

49. BACHMANN, G. Medical students like diaphragm, but use inconsistently. *Contraceptive Technology Update*, **4**, 3 (1983)

50. KELAGHAN, J., RUBIN, G. L., ORY, H. W. and LAYDE, P. M. Barrier method contraceptives and pelvic inflammatory disease. *Journal of the American Medical Association*, **248**, 184 (1982)

51. HARRIS, R. W. C., BRINTON, L. A., COWDELL, R. H. *et al.* Characteristics of women with dysplasia or carcinoma in situ of the cervix uteri. *British Journal of Cancer*, **42**, 359 (1980)

52. MELAMED, M. R., KOSS, L. G., FLEHINGER, B. J. *et al.* Prevalence rates of uterine cervical carcinoma in situ for women using the diaphragm or contraceptive oral steroids. *British Medical Journal*, **3**, 195 (1969)

53. WRIGHT, N. H., VESSEY, M. P., KENWARD, B. *et al.* Neoplasia and dysplasia of the cervix uteri and contraception: A possible protective effect of the diaphragm. *British Journal of Cancer*, **38**, 273 (1978)

54. VESSEY, M., DOLL, R., PETO, R. *et al.* A long-term follow-up study of women using different methods of contraception – An interim report. *Journal of Biosocial Science*, **8**, 373 (1976)

55. QUIGG, J. M., KAMINSKI, J. M., WALLER, D. and ZANEVELD, L. J. D. Development of a vaginal sponge delivery system for an aryl 4-guanidinobenzoate with and without nonoxynol-9. *Advances in Contraception*, **2**, 288 (1986)

56. REMINGTON, K. M., JENSEN, R. H., ESSIG, M. G. *et al.* The Today (R) contraceptive sponge as a delivery system for a new vaginal contraceptive compound. *Advances in Contraception*, **2**, 289 (1986)

57. Toxic shock syndrome not only linked to tampon or sponge use. Women's Health Update. *Contraceptive Technology Update*, **8**, 3S (1987)

58. BOUNDS, W., KUBBA, A., TAYOB, Y. *et al.* Clinical trial of a spermicide-free custom-fitted, valved cervical cap (Contracap™). *The British Journal of Family Planning*, **11**, 125 (1986)

59a. STIM, E. M. The non-spermicide fit-free diaphragm: A new contraceptive method. *Advances in Planned Parenthood*, **15**, 88 (1980)

59b. BOUNDS, W., GUILLEBAUD, J., STEWART, L. and STEELE, S. A female condom (Femshield ™): A pilot study of its user acceptability. *British Journal of Family Planning*, **14**, 83 (1988)

59c. Editorial. *Contraceptive Technology Update*, **9**, 98 (1988)

60. JEFFRIES, D. J. What are the safest sterilization procedures for practice 'caps' in clinics and general practice? *British Journal of Family Planning*, **12**, 64 (1986)

61. SOBRERO, A. J. Spermicidal agents: Effectiveness, use and testing. In: *Vaginal Contraception: New Development* (eds. Zatuchni, G. I., Sobrero, A. J., Speidel, J. J. and Sciarra, J. J.) Harper & Row, Hagerstown, p. 48 (1979)

62. WILBORN, W. H., HAHN, D. W. and MCGUIRE, J. J. Scanning electron microscopy of human spermatozoa after incubation with the spermicide nonoxynol-9. *Fertility and Sterility*, **39**, 717 (1983)

63. SCHILL, W. B. and WOLFF, H. H. Ultrastructure of human spermatozoa in the presence of the spermicide nonoxynol-9 and a vaginal contraceptive containing nonoxynol-9. *Andrologia*, **13**, 42 (1981)

64. JOHNSON, V. E. and MASTERS, W. H. Intravaginal contraceptive study. Phase 1: anatomy. *Western Journal of Surgery, Obstetrics and Gynecology*, **70**, 202 (1962)

65. SHERRIS, J. D., MOORE, S. H. and FOX, G. New developments in vaginal contraception. *Population Reports*, Series H, No. 7 (1984)

66. BERNSTEIN, G. S. Clinical effectiveness of an aerosol contraceptive foam. *Contraception*, **3**, 37 (1971)

67. RYDER, N. B. Contraceptive failure in the United States. *Family Planning Perspectives*, **5**, 133 (1973)

68. ZANEVELD, L. J. D., BHATTACHARYYA, A. K., KIM, D. S. *et al.* Primate model for the evaluation of vaginal contraceptives. *American Journal of Obstetrics and Gynecology*, **129**, 368 (1977)

69. BONE, M. *Family Planning Services in England and Wales. Her Majesty's Stationery Office,* London, p. 167 (1973)

70. TRUSSELL, T. J., FADEN, R. and HATCHER, R. A. Efficacy information in contraceptive counselling: those little white lies. *American Journal of Public Health*, **66**, 761 (1976)

71. BOLCH, O. H. and WARREN, J. C. *In vitro* effects of Emko on *Neisseria gonorrhoea* and *Trichomonas vaginalis*. *American Journal of Obstetrics and Gynecology*, **115**, 1145 (1973)

72. SINGH, B. and CUTLER, J. C. Vaginal contraceptives for prophylaxis against sexually transmitted diseases. In: *Vaginal Contraception: New Developments* (eds. Zatuchni, G. I., Sobrero, A. J., Speidel, J. J. and Sciarra, J. J.) Harper and Row, Hagerstown, p. 175 (1979)

73. JICK, H., HANNAN, M. T., STERGACHIS, A. *et al.* Vaginal spermicides and gonorrhoea. *Journal of the American Medical Association*, **248**, 1619 (1982)

74. RENDON, A. L., COVARRUBIAS, J., MCCARNEY, K. E. *et al.* A controlled comparative study of phenylmer-

curic acetate, nonoxynol-9 and placebo vaginal suppositories as prophylactic agents against gonorrhoea. *Current Therapeutic Research*, **27**, 780 (1980)

75. ROSENBERG, M. J., ROJANAPITHAYAKORN, W., FELDBLUM, P. J. and HIGGINS, J. E. Effect of the contraceptive sponge on chlamydial infection, gonorrhea and candidiasis. *Journal of the American Medical Association*, **257**, 2308 (1987)
76. HICKS, D. R., MARTIN, L. S., GETCHELL, J. P. *et al.* Inactivation of HTLV III/LAV-infected cultures of normal human lymphocytes by nonoxynol-9 in vitro. *Lancet*, **2**, 1422 (1985)

76a. MALKOVSKY, M., NEWELL, A. and DALGLEISH, A. G. Inactivation of HIV by nonoxynol-9. *Lancet*, **1**, 645 (1988)

77. CHERMANN, J. C., BARRE-SINOUSSI, F., HENIN, Y. and MARECHAL, V. HIV inactivation by a spermicide containing benzalkonium chloride. *AIDS-Forschung (AIFO)*, **2**, 85, February (1987)
78. BENZIGER, D. P. and EDELSON, J. Absorption from the vagina. *Drug Metabolism Reviews*, **14**, 137 (1983)
79. WHO Task Force on oral contraceptives. Contraception during the postpartum period and during lactation: The effect on women's health. *International Journal of Gynaecology and Obstetrics*, **25** [Supplement] 13 (1987)
80. JICK, H., WALKER, A. M., ROTHMAN, K. J. *et al.* Vaginal spermicides and congenital disorders. *Journal of the American Medical Association*, **245**, 1329 (1981)
81. CORDERO, J. F. and LAYDE, P. M. Vaginal spermicides, chromosomal abnormalities and limb reduction defects. *International Family Planning Perspectives*, **9**, 15 (1983)
82. MILLS, J. L., HARLEY, E. E., REED, G. F. and BERENDES, H. W. Are spermicides teratogenic? *Journal of the American Medical Association*, **248**, 2148 (1982)
83. POLEDNAK, A. P., JANERICH, D. T. and GLEBATIS, D. M. Birth weight and birth defects in relation to maternal spermicide use. *Teratology*, **26**, 27 (1982)
84. SHAPIRO, S., SLONE, D., HEINONEN, O. P. *et al.* Birth defects and vaginal spermicides. *Journal of the American Medical Association*, **247**, 2381 (1982)
85. LINN, S., SCHOENBAUM, S. C., MONSON, R. R. *et al.* Lack of association between contraceptive usage and congenital malformations in offspring. *American Journal of Obstetrics and Gynecology*, **147**, 923 (1983)
86. HUGGINS, G., VESSEY, M., FLAVEL, R. *et al.* Vaginal spermicides and outcome of pregnancy: Findings in a large cohort study. *Contraception*, **25**, 219 (1982)
87. BRACKEN, M. B. Spermicidal contraceptives and poor reproductive outcomes: the epidemiologic evidence against an association. *American Journal of Obstetrics and Gynecology*, **151**, 552 (1985)
88. ZIPPER, J., WHEELER, R. G., POTTS, D. M. and RIVERA, M. Propranolol as a novel, effective spermicide: preliminary findings. *British Medical Journal*, **287**, 1245 (1983)
89. RATSULA, K., HAUKKAMAA, M., WICHMANN, K. and LUUKKAINEN, T. Vaginal contraception with gossipol. A clinical study. *Contraception*, **27**, 571 (1983)
90. SHARMAN, D., CHANTLER, E., DUKES, M. et al. Comparison of the action of nonoxynol-9 and chlorhexidine on sperm. *Fertility and Sterility*, **45**, 259 (1986)

Chapter 11

Natural family planning

Anna M. Flynn and John Bonnar

Natural methods of family planning (NFP) have been defined by the World Health Organization (WHO) as methods for planning or avoiding pregnancies by observation of the natural signs and symptoms of the fertile and infertile phases of the menstrual cycle. Developments in family planning over the past decade in western societies have shown that increasing numbers of couples are taking up natural methods to plan their families [1,2]. Motivations for using natural methods are various; many couples believe their sexual life is manipulated by technology and welcome NFP as a liberating influence, allowing them to take autonomous control of their fertility; for others the educative approach of fertility awareness and shared responsibility by both partners for family planning is the attraction; concern about the complications of some contraceptive techniques make yet others choose NFP as an alternative; finally, contrary to what the media suggest, a small percentage choose natural methods for religious and/or cultural reasons in our western society.

In contrast to artificial contraception, natural methods are mainly educative and depend on sufficient numbers of competent teachers or advisors being available for the clients. Although their number is gradually increasing in England and Wales, the preparation of NFP teachers is a slow process and limits the number of clients who can be offered NFP. The recent creation of a National Association of NFP Teachers should help to develop and diffuse natural methods throughout the country as an efficient alternative method of family planning for those requesting and motivated to use these methods. Further expansion may be expected when simple home-based tests to detect female fertility, now in the research stage, become available.

Historical background

The problem of fertility control has taxed people's imaginations for centuries. In primitive societies fertility was regulated by taboos, customs and traditions, and this still holds to a greater or lesser degree among certain well-organized communities in different parts of the world. Although it was always recognized that the female exhibited only cyclical fertility in contrast to the ever-fertile male partner, until recently, fertility awareness was still inaccurate and sometimes anecdotal. Scientific and technological developments in the second half of this century have had beneficial repercussions in the field of reproductive medicine and natural birth control. The work of Ogino [3] and Knaus [4] which was carried out independently in Japan and in Austria, showed that in any individual menstrual cycle, ovulation precedes menstruation by approximately 12–16 days. From these studies, both developed formulae to determine the fertile and infertile days in the menstrual cycle. The birth-control method based on these days of fertility and infertility was popularly described as the rhythm method and even today, despite much more precise indicators of fertility, for many people the rhythm method and natural family planning are synonymous.

Definition

The World Health Organization has defined natural family planning as 'methods for planning or avoiding pregnancies by observation of the natural signs and symptoms of the fertile and infertile phases of the menstrual cycle. It is implicit in the definition of natural family planning, when used to avoid contraception, that drugs, devices and surgical procedures are not used, there is abstinence from sexual intercourse during the fertile phase of the menstrual cycle, and the act of intercourse, when it occurs, is complete [5]. Variations from the above are commonly practised, however, e.g. the use of barriers or coitus interruptus during the fertile phase.

Fertility awareness

The World Health Organization's definition of natural family planning indicates that there are two separate components involved. The first of these is fertility awareness; the second is the application of this knowledge to help in planning one's family or what we term the methodologies.

Fertility awareness implies some knowledge of the clinical manifestations of the physiological processes involved in conception and reproduction, and can be summarized as follows: The male is potentially fertile from puberty to old age and this fertility is neither rhythmic nor periodic. The fertilizing capacity of the spermatozoon is not yet completely elucidated.

Published work suggests that although the mean fertilizing life of the sperm appears to be quite short (2–3 days), under optimal conditions in the female reproductive tract a fertilizing capacity of up to 7 days may, in exceptional circumstances, be possible [6].

In contrast to the male, the female exhibits a natural monthly fertility cycle in which the fertilizable span of the female gamete (ovum) has been established as not longer than 10–24 h [7]. Natural methods, therefore, aim at identifying as precisely as possible the female fertile period, and this process is described as fertility awareness. Once the fertile period is identified, a pregnancy may be achieved or avoided by planned sexual intercourse.

Several methods are available to detect this fertile time with reasonable accuracy. Serial follicular measurements by ultrasonic techniques and cyclical studies of steroid hormones in the blood, urine, and saliva are some of the more sophisticated technological approaches used to determine the beginning and end of these potentially fertile days. Advances in monoclonal antibody techniques have facilitated the development of simple urine tests to enable luteinizing hormone (LH) and pregnanediol glucuronide (PDG) to be monitored at home by the couple. However, these are still in the research stage, and NFP Programmes utilize the signs and symptoms which these hormones produce on target organs in the body which women can observe objectively. These are known as the *clinical indicators* of the fertile period,

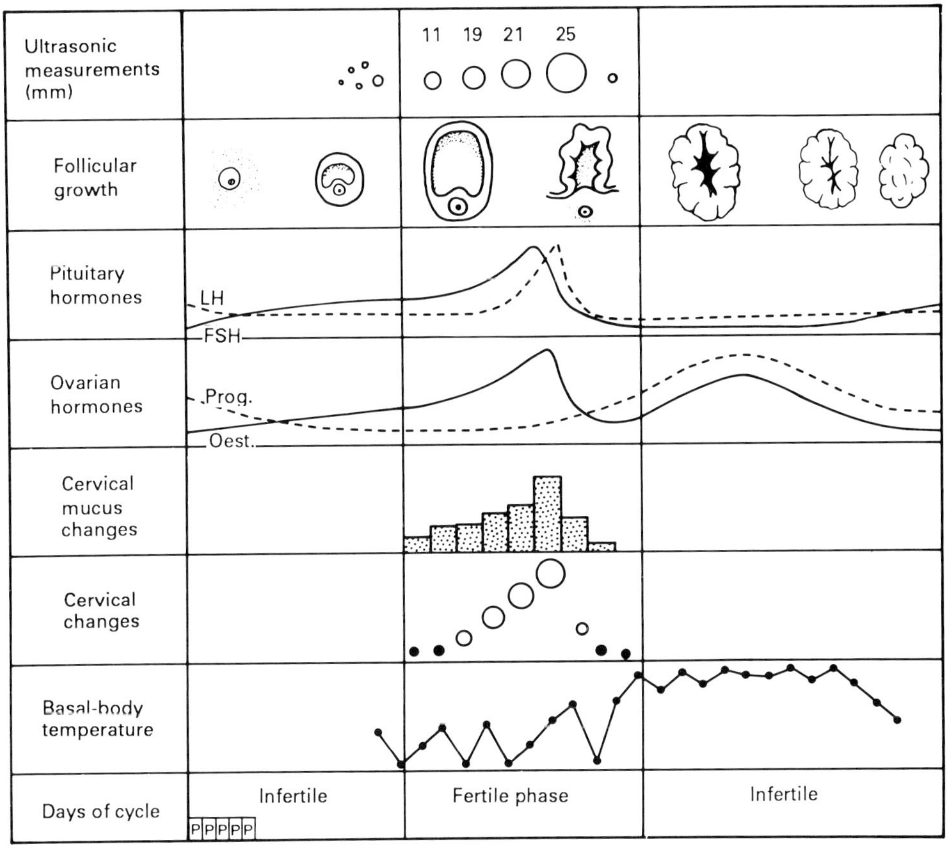

Figure 11.1 Relationship during cycle between serial ultrasonic measurements, hormonal control, and clinical indicators of fertility.

and an important part of the art of natural family planning lies in the woman and/or her sexual partner being able to identify and interpret these for themselves.

Figure 11.1 is a composite picture of the hormonal sequences that occur during each fertile cycle. At the end of menstruation the low levels of oestrogen and progesterone stimulate the production of increased amounts of follicle-stimulating hormone (FSH) and luteinizing hormone (LH) and the growth of an egg follicle in the ovary. The follicle, as it grows, causes the secretion of ever increasing quantities of oestrogen into the blood stream, reaching peak levels just prior to ovulation. These increasing amounts of oestrogen cause the production of increased quantities of mucus in the cervical crypts and certain changes in the cervix itself.

After ovulation the corpus luteum produces increasing quantities of progesterone, but in the absence of conception the corpus luteum begins to disintegrate 8–10 days after ovulation. The levels of oestrogen and progesterone fall, and menstruation occurs [8]. This high concentration of progesterone after ovulation stops the secretion of oestrogenic mucus and reverses the changes in the cervix initiated by the oestrogen. It also causes an increase in basal body temperature (BBT), producing a bi-phasic temperature chart.

The fertility cycle

Allowing for gamete survival, one can now describe fertile and infertile phases in the cycle (Figure 11.1).

Phase 1 covers the time from menstruation until the earliest time that any sperm could survive and cause a pregnancy. (It is assumed that the beginning of follicular growth coincides with an increase in oestrogen and mucus, producing conditions favourable to sperm survival, either in the cervical crypts or in the fallopian tube, until ovulation occurs.) This is often referred to as the first infertile phase and it varies in length depending on the rapidity of the follicular response to the pituitary hormones.

Phase 2 or the fertile phase, extends from the end of Phase 1 as just defined until that time after ovulation has occurred when the ovum is no longer fertilizable [7]. The preovulatory fertile days in this phase result from the potential capacity of the spermatozoa to live in genital-tract mucus (page 24). The post-ovulatory fertile days result from the fact that, although the ovum has a fertilizable lifespan of 12–24 h [9,10] only, the moment of ovulation cannot be exactly estimated [11]; therefore the potential fertile days have to be extended for 48 h after the estimated ovulation. The fertile phase refers therefore to the combined fertility of both sexual partners.

Phase 3 extends from the end of *Phase 2* until the onset of menstruation which marks the end of that cycle. This is the absolute infertile phase having a mean duration of 14 days with a range of 10–16 days [12,13]. Once ovulation has occurred, the luteal hormonal levels rise rapidly to prevent the possibility of a second ovulation later in the cycle. Thus, provided that ovulation is accurately determined, conception is impossible in this phase.

Methods of determining these phases in the cycle

1. *Biophysical methods* such as serial ultrasonic monitoring of follicular growth, changes in vaginal, ovarian and digital blood flow, and electrical impedance are so far not appropriate for NFP users.
2. *Biochemical methods* which detect the changing concentrations of the sex steroids in blood, urine and saliva are still for the most part limited to laboratories, but home kits have been developed and are available. (See New Techniques for NFP.)
3. *The biological or clinical indicators* – see below.

The clinical indicators

In the ovulatory cycle the ovarian hormones, oestrogen and progesterone, have their most marked effects on:

1. The cervix
2. The body in general (basal body temperature and others)
3. The psyche and emotional centres.

Mucus as an indicator of fertility

Just after menstruation the levels of oestrogen and progesterone in the woman's blood stream are very low, so little if any mucus is produced and, if present, it is thick and tacky. Held between thumb and forefinger and stretched, this infertile-type mucus breaks quickly (Figure 11.2a). The woman feels a positive sensation of dryness

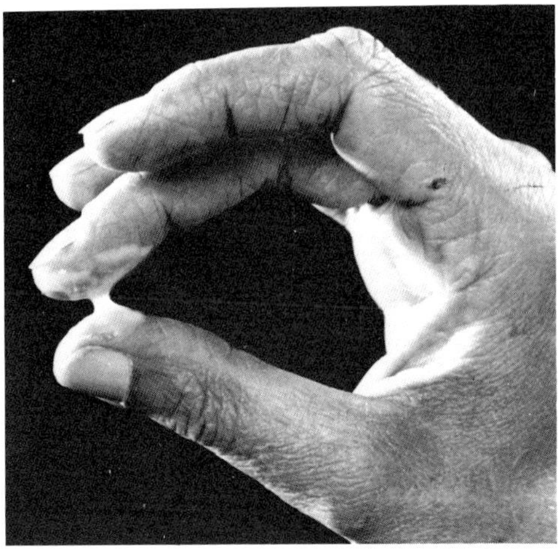

(a)

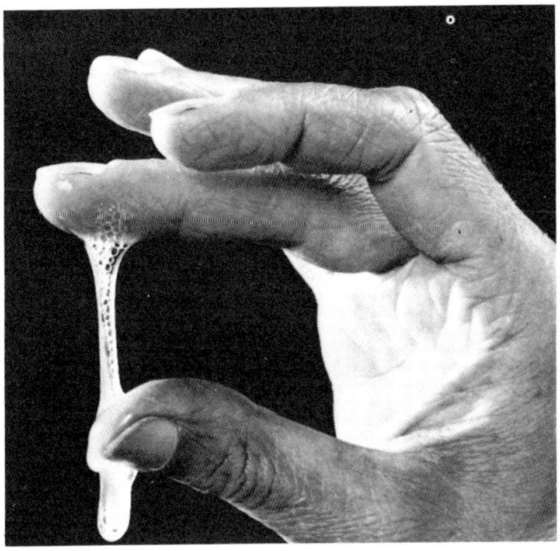

(b)

Figure 11.2 (a). Infertile-type mucus. (b) Fertile-type mucus (From Hibbard B. M. *Principles of Obstetrics*, Butterworths, p. 25 (1988) by permission)

in the vulva, indicating the absence of mucus. This absence of mucus denotes infertility, and on a mucus chart these days are coloured green. When follicular growth occurs rapidly during or just after menstruation, mucus appears immediately and this first infertile phase is absent or greatly reduced in days.

The fertile phase

As the follicles begin to ripen, the increasing amounts of oestrogen stimulate the cervical crypts to step up mucus production, which is perceived by the woman as a feeling of dampness or increasing quantities of mucus at the vulva. As oestrogen from the growing follicle increases, the mucus becomes more abundant and increasingly thinner, stretchier, clearer and more watery, being 98% water when close to ovulation. Because of the high content of mineral salts, it is often discharged in threads and has an elastic quality, allowing it to be stretched for several centimetres before the strand breaks (Figure 11.2b). Some women have likened this type of mucus to raw egg white, although occasionally it may be cloudy, yellowish or pinkish.

The peak mucus symptom

The peak mucus day, which corresponds closely with the peak secretion of oestrogen in the blood, is the last day of the fertile type mucus, and is identified retrospectively. Physiologically therefore we can conclude that the peak mucus day precedes ovulation by not more than three days [14]. If we allow 24 h for ovum fertilization, then the evening of the fourth day after the peak indicates the end of the fertile phase. There is an abrupt change from the fertile-type characteristics to the infertile-type mucus which makes the peak mucus day very easy to recognize.

The second infertile phase

After ovulation, the sudden drop in oestrogen and the rise in progesterone cause a rapid change in the amount and characteristics of the mucus. The quantity of mucus drops sharply or disappears completely, and if present it resembles the infertile type described in the first infertile phase. Having allowed 3 days for ovulation and one day for ovum fertilizability, the second infertile phase begins on the fourth day past the peak symptom.

How does one detect these changes over the cycle?

Mucus can be identified at the vulva both by sensation and by observation of the mucus. This sensation may be one of dryness indicating infertility, one of wetness indicating maximum fertility, or a feeling of being neither wet nor dry. This is referred to as a sensation of moistness or dampness, which always indicates potential fertility when it occurs before ovulation.

Mucus when present is observed at the vulva, usually on toilet paper at the time of micturition. By stetching the toilet paper between the fingers, one can note the colour, fluidity, glossiness, transparency and stretchiness, and fertile and infertile types can be differentiated. The mucus is observed over the entire day and charted last thing at night. The most fertile characteristics of the mucus over the entire day are charted, and mucus charts have open boxes for each day of the cycle. In these boxes the client either fills in a colour (green for dry, yellow for mucus, red for bleeding or spotting) or writes in a description of the mucus seen (Figure 11.3).

Cyclical changes in the cervix

The increasing amounts of oestrogen produced by the developing follicle also cause changes in the cervix during the cycle. These were first described by Keefe [15]. During the first infertile phase the cervix is situated low in the pelvic cavity, close to the vulva. It is quite firm and dry to touch and the external os is closed. With the development of the follicle and increasing production of oestrogen indicating the beginning of the fertile phase, the cervix begins to move upwards in the pelvis, away from the vulva, and becomes more difficult to reach. It also feels softer and wet from the mucus present on the surface, and opens slightly, but only enough to admit a fingertip. At the

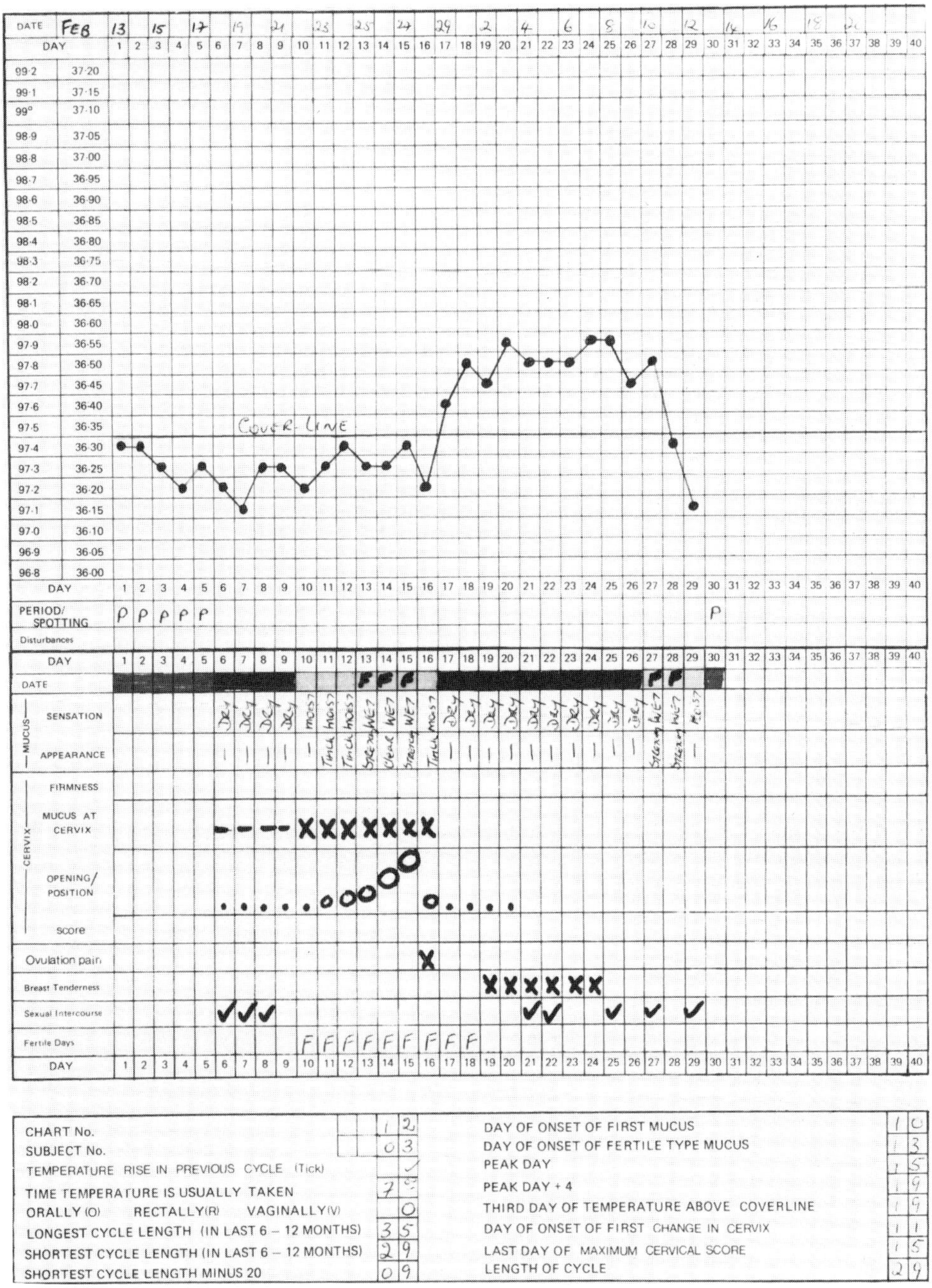

Figure 11.3 Multiple-index chart.

time of the peak oestrogen, these changes are at their maximum. As the oestrogen levels drop sharply around ovulation, the cervix changes abruptly back to its condition during the first infertile phase, becoming dry, closed, firm and once more close to the vulva.

These changes can be seen by observing the cervix with the aid of a vaginal speculum or they can be ascertained by autopalpation (or palpation by one's sexual partner) using two fingers in the vagina to feel the cervix. Daily palpation is recommended to detect these cyclical changes.

Changes in the basal body temperature

The increased quantities of progesterone produced by the corpus luteum after ovulation cause a rise or shift in the basal body temperture (BBT). To detect this shift, a woman measures her temperature after a period of sleep and before beginning any actions, usually in the morning before rising. In order to detect the small shift, which is normally between 0.2 and 0.6°C, a special expanded-scale mercury thermometer (fertility thermometer) is used. The temperatures may be taken orally (5 min), rectally (3 min) or vaginally (3 min) and are plotted daily on a special chart designed to enhance the small change from the lower to the higher level and to facilitate the later interpretation of the graph (Figure. 11.4). At the end of the cycle the temperature usually drops, reflecting the decrease in progesterone prior to menstruation. Should conception occur during the cycle, the temperature remains at a high level.

Certain variables, such as a disturbed night, illness, or variation in the hour when the temperature is taken can alter the temperature.

The major clinical indicators of fertility

Changes in the uterine cervix, in the cervical mucus, and in the BBT are always present when the cycle is a fertile one. Since they are important and consistent, they are called the major indicators of fertility.

The minor clinical indicators of fertility

There are, however, certain other indicators, which are specific to individual women or only occur in some ovulatory cycles, which we describe as minor indicators. When present, these minor indicators are very helpful in confirming and helping to interpret the major signals. Among the minor indicators are ovulation pain, mid-cycle bleeding, breast symptoms, acne and skin changes, variations in mood, and increased excitability.

Fertility awareness is not only important in the context of family planning, but is also a general educative process applicable to all stages of a woman's reproductive life. At puberty, when adolescents are undergoing rapid and profound physical, psychological and emotional changes consequent on the increased concentrations of sex hormones, an awareness of the developmental processes underlying these changes can help them adjust less traumatically to the situation. Fertility awareness can also help to increase understanding between partners in a sexual relationship. An awareness of their different but complementary fertility and sexuality often helps to enhance the quality of a couple's relationship.

The methodologies

These refer to the selection and combination of the fertility indicators to detect as precisely as possible the fertile and infertile phases in the cycle.

Some couples, if they have chosen fertility awareness for reasons other than religious ones, may wish to use barrier methods during the fertile phase rather than abstinence from sexual intercourse as a means of avoiding a pregnancy. It is important, however, that they realize that barrier methods must be used with obsessional care during the highly fertile phase if a pregnancy is to be avoided. In addition if a spermicide is used with the barrier, it will interfere with the accuracy of mucus observations and can cause problems with the identification of the fertile phase, especially during the learning period. Condoms which have the spermicide within the rubber barrier are available and should preferable be used. Once the woman knows her mucus pattern she usually has no great difficulty in distinguishing mucus from spermicidal cream or jelly.

The choice of indicator or indicators used to detect the beginning and/or end of the fertile phase determines the method of natural family planning used. Historically and traditionally, four methods are described:

1. The calendar method (also described as calendar rhythm, Ogino–Knaus, or the rhythm method).
2. The temperature method (BBT).
3. The mucus symptom or ovulation method. (This is often referred to as the Billings method.)
4. The symptothermal methods, of which there are several varieties, all of which suppose the use of the BBT.

The calendar or calculation method

Historically this is the earliest of the natural methods, and stemming from the work of Ogino is sometimes described as the rhythm method. By allowing at least 5 days for sperm survival and 24–48 h for ovum survival, a formula is used to detect the beginning and the end of the fertile phase. Thus the potential fertile phase is calculated by:

1. Defining the shortest and longest menstrual cycle over the previous 6 or 12 cycles.
2. Subtracting 20 from the length of the shortest cycle, when one derives the first day of the fertile phase.
3. Subtracting 11 from the longest cycle, when one derives the last day of the fertile phase.

The problem with the calendar method is the biological variation in menstrual cycles, and consequently, long periods of abstinence are involved. It is not surprising therefore that the calendar method as a single index of fertility fell into disrepute, and today is only used as one of the indicators in the multiple-index methods.

The BBT method of NFP

The temperature can only detect the end of the fertile phase, which is recognized by a sustained elevation of the temperature for 3 days after the shift. To make it easier to detect the shift, the use of a 'coverline' drawn 0.05°C over the low phase temperatures, of which there should be a minimum of six and excluding the first four days and any disturbances, is recommended (Figure 11.4).

Couples who wish to avoid a pregnancy by the use of the BBT method alone must restrict sexual intercourse to the second infertile phase, i.e. from the morning of the third sustained high temperature after the shift until the end of the cycle. Because of the length of abstinence required, the method as a single indicator may not be very acceptable, but is very effective. In practice it is usually combined nowadays with another indicator such as the calendar calculations or the mucus symptom in a multiple-index combination. It has the advantage of being an objective indicator of the end of the fertile time, which can be seen and discussed by NFP teachers, sexual partners, and the medical profession.

How to use the mucus indicator as a method of natural family planning

Cervical mucus methods are single-index methods by which women assess the changes in the quality of the cervical mucus as a means of detecting the fertile phase in the cycle in order to achieve or avoid a pregnancy. There are several different sets of guidelines on the use of the mucus indicator, one of the earliest and best known being that of Drs E. and J. Billings [16]. The cervical-mucus method proposed here is based on the guidelines set out in the Family Fertility Education Learning Package of WHO/British Life Assurance Trust (BLAT) [5], and differs slightly from the Billings method, although they are similar in most respects.

Rules for using the mucus method of family planning

The mucus method allows the identification of all phases – fertile and infertile – in the cycle. For this reason it can be used both as a method of avoiding a pregnancy or a method for achieving conception if this is desired.

To avoid a pregnancy, the first 5 days of a true menstrual bleed and alternate dry days before ovulation are considered to be infertile days. Alternate days are used because the presence of seminal fluid may mask the observation of the mucus and makes the day potentially fertile.

The fertile phase

The first fertile day in the cycle is the first day on which either the sensation of moistness or mucus occurs. The last fertile day is the fourth day after the peak symptom. The postovulatory infertile phase extends from the evening of the fourth day after the peak symptom until the end of the cycle and is a highly effective phase.

Rule for the use of changes in the cervix in natural birth control

Any change in the cervix opening (softening or shift upwards in the pelvis) before ovulation has occurred indicates the start of the fertile phase. Three days after the cervical findings have returned to the prefertile state one can detect the end of the fertile phase. To date, changes in the cervix have not been used consistently and singly as a method of NFP. Recently an increasing number of women and their partners find this indicator a more objective and clear-cut one than the mucus indicator, and its use is becoming more popular. A few women who have used it as a single indicator of the fertile phase have found it both satisfactory and efficient. In special physiological situations such as the premenopausal years, returning fertility after childbirth, and discontinuing hormonal contraception, the changes in the cervix appear to be a more reliable indicator of impending ovulation than cervical mucus [17]. This, however, requires confirmation in a prospective formal trial.

The single-index and multiple-index approach

Each woman has a unique hormonal production during the cycle. In addition, the effect of these hormones on specific target organs in her body are also individual to her, and as a consequence so are her predominant clinical signs and symptoms of fertility. To expect an individual woman to fit into one or other of the methods just outlined may be too rigid and confining, and not necessarily in her best interests. A better approach allows each woman to discover which are the best indicators for her, given her specific requirements. In this way the methods can be tailored to her as a unique individual.

Viewed in this way, one can classify all natural methods as follows:

Single-index methods

Where only one indicator is used to define the fertile phase (BBT, cervix, mucus).

Multiple-index methods

Where several indicators are combined to detect the fertile phase. This differs from the symptothermal method in that the temperature is not necessarily one of the indicators used. From an initial combination of several indicators, women can freely change to other combinations or to a single-index if that is sufficient for the moment. The important point is that each one can choose freely whatever is the most effective combination for the couple.

Depending on the combination of indicators used, there are several varieties of multiple-index methods. For our clients wishing to avoid a pregnancy, we recommend the double-check method in which the following indicators of fertility are observed:

To detect the beginning of the fertile phase

1. Calendar calculations – the shortest cycle minus 20, where at least six cycle-lengths have been recorded and the woman has noted a temperature shift and a high-temperature phase in her previous cycle (to ensure that it is a menstrual and not an ovulatory bleed); or
2. The first mucus symptom, whether detected by sensation or appearance. Whichever of these indicators comes *first*, marks the beginning of the fertile phase.
3. Changes in the cervix can be used as a check on the other indicators, though this is not essential.

To detect the end of the fertile phase and the beginning of the postovulatory infertile phase

1. The temperature shift – the infertile phase begins on the morning of the third consecutive high temperature after the temperature shift.
2. The peak mucus symptom – the infertile time begins on the evening of the fourth day after the peak mucus symptom.

Whichever of these indicators comes *last* marks the beginning of the infertile phase.

3. Again, changes in the cervix can be used, if desired, to confirm the information supplied by the other indicators (Figure 11.3).

The effectiveness of NFP

Table 11.1 summarizes some of the prospective studies made to determine the efficiency of NFP methods [18–23]. A study of this Table shows that in common with artificial contraception, the number of biological (signal) or 'method failures' are substantially lower than the 'user failures', whichever natural method is used. However, it can also be seen that all varieties of the symptothermal method appear to have a substantial lower failure rate than the cervical mucus methods, and finally that where sexual intercourse is restricted to the postovulatory infertile phase, the chances of an unplanned pregnancy are greatly reduced. In one study, no unplanned pregnancies occurred in the postovulatory phase [22, 23].

Further analysis of these surveys highlight three important factors which seem to contribute to the successful or unsuccessful use of natural methods, namely: the motivation of the users to avoid a pregnancy, the quality and type of teaching they receive, and the physiological characteristics of the women practising the methods.

Motivation is important for all methods of family planning, but of the highest importance for the successful use of coitally related contraceptive techniques such as the barrier methods and natural family planning. Furthermore, in the case of natural methods, it is the motivation of the couple (and not just one or other partner) and their joint ability to cope with abstinence during the fertile time which achieves success or failure with the method. Table 11.1 illustrates that the motivated couple using natural methods to limit their family do so with much greater success than couples who use natural methods to space or delay the next pregnancy [19].

Efficient teaching

NFP is mainly an educational delivery service, and competent teaching is essential to the successful use of natural methods, the efficiency of any natural method being directly proportional to the user's ability to identify the fertile time during the cycle. NFP programmes use different pedagogical approaches such as couple-to-couple and group lectures, and the clinic situation with a doctor or nurse dealing with the individual woman or couple. Whatever approach is used, it is the teacher's basic scientific knowledge and her ability to communicate which are important, not only in imparting knowledge, but also in providing a high motivating influence. Evidence suggests also that teaching the male partner with the woman is important for the successful use of natural family planning [24]. Kambic *et al.* [Personal communication] also found that the partners were more likely to practise periodic abstinence than couples where wives only were trained.

Reflecting the recent emphasis on efficient teaching in natural family planning services, the WHO in collaboration with BLAT have published a skeleton learning package designed to set out the minimum programme content for training NFP teachers [5]. Further emphasis on the importance of efficiency in teaching for the success of an NFP method is shown by the introduction of a new category to classify

Table 11.1 Effectiveness of natural family planning methods based on prospective studies

Authors	*Year*	*NFP method followed*	*Subjects*	*Months of exposure*	*Failure rate (Pearl formula; pregnancies per 100 woman-years)*				
					Method related	*Teaching related*	*Combined method-user failure*	*Rate for those spacing*	*Rate for those limiting*
Marshall [18]	1968	BBT postovulation	321	4 739	1.2	–	6.6		
Marshall [18]	1968	BBT-calendar	255	3 545	5.0	–	19.3		
Rice *et al.* [19]	1981	Symptothermal (pre- and postovulation)	1 022	21 736	0.93	–	7.47	14.56	4.13
World Health Organization [20]	1981	Ovulation method (pre- and postovulation)	869	10 215	2.2	0.3	22.3		
Perez *et al.* [21]	1983	Ovulation method (pre- and postovulation)	660	5 140	2.8	–	13.3	(16.8 Inexperienced instructors 4.7 experienced instructors)	
Barbato *et al.* [22]	1987	Sympto-thermal (double-check)	460	8 140	0.44	1.47	2.2	–	–
Frank-Hermann [23]	1988	Sympto-thermal (double-check)	203	2 630	0.7	–	1.8	–	–

unplanned pregnancies which occur when a couple have not learned the method properly, now termed teaching-related pregnancies [20, 25].

Perez [21] in a 2-year prospective study of the efficiency of the ovulation method at Santiago in Chile, was able to show that where the instructors of the method were inexperienced (first-year instructors) the total pregnancy rate (method + user-failure) was 16.8 per 100 woman-years of use, in contrast to a total pregnancy rate of 4.7 per 100 woman-years of use when the instructors had already one year's experience in teaching the method (second-year instructors).

The physiological characteristics of the woman can be a factor in the success of a natural method. The question has been asked 'Can most women learn to observe their cervical mucus patterns.' There are conflicting reports in the literatures on the number of women who can observe and identify their cervical mucus at the vulva [26–28]. However, the WHO prospective multicentre trial which made a cross-cultural assessment of cervical mucus observations in five centres, some urban and some rural, reported that 93% of the participants showed an interpretable mucus pattern, i.e. the woman was judged to be identifying her symptoms correctly, in the first cycle following instruction [20].

In a further analysis of this study Bonnar [29] found that the pregnancy rate was highest in those women who required teaching for more than three cycles; those learning the method within three cycles had 1.3% pregnancies per cycle while those who required extended teaching beyond three cycles had 7.02% pregnancies per cycle, results which seem to confirm experiences with individual clients attending our clinics.

Even in those women who quickly master their mucus patterns, one must accept that for some the difficulty of accurately identifying the fertile time in the cycle by mucus observations may be a contributory factor in an unplanned pregnancy. The probability of conception outside the fertile phase in the cycle has been shown to be very low [6,30]. The difficulty for the couple wishing to avoid a pregnancy may be the presence of mucus many days before the peak day.

Retrospectively these days can be seen to be those with a very low probability of conception, but this cannot be predicted at the time and some couples may have several unnecessary days of abstinence; yet others may be warned too late. For NFP clients, this is the grey area in the cycle, requiring further research to improve predictability. At present some couples find changes in the cervix to be a more reliable indicator; yet others choose the use of a barrier during these days. For the future, simple tests based on increasing levels of urinary oestradiol or the changing ratio of oestrone to pregnanediol (dual analyte) may help to improve reliability at this time in the cycle [31].

Continuation and discontinuation rates for NFP

No study of efficacy is complete without some reference to the numbers who abandon the method after one or more years of use. In the WHO multicentre study [20], 85% of women entered the effectiveness phase, which suggests a low discontinua- tion rate. Other studies in the US have found similar or better continuation rates [32]. In a retrospective survey among Australian couples using NFP, four important factors appear to influence the continuation/discontinuation of the client, i.e. the NFP method learned, the place where it is learned, the experience (good or bad) of the client when exposed to the method, and the capability of the couple to modify their sexual behaviour to the NFP challenge [33].

Advantages and disadvantages

Natural methods do not interfere with normal physiology and have no physical side-effects for users. They also help to introduce an awareness of fertility which some couples find psychologically beneficial to helping them develop a more responsible attitude to family planning, together with increased dialogue and sharing of responsibility within the relationship. These methods are culturally and morally acceptable to many persons who find other methods distasteful. The fact that natural methods can be used to achieve or avoid a pregnancy allows couples to be in autonomous control of their fertility. Further, the knowledge about peak fertility time may be an advantage in helping sub-fertile couples to achieve a pregnancy. When ovulation occurs only sporadically in the female, or the number and quality of sperm in the ejaculate is below the normal, planned sexual intercourse or insemination at a time of high fertility offers the optimal conditions for conception (Table 11.2) [32–36].

Finally, the fact that the couple, once they become autonomous users of a natural method, do not require any further expenditure on medication or medical follow-up over a period of years, guarantees long-term cost-effective benefits. In countries which have restricted resources of money and/or medical or nursing manpower, this can be a very important advantage.

Disadvantages

On the debit side, it must be recognized that the use of natural methods requires accurate detection of the fertile phase and a certain modification of sexual behaviour by both partners if it is to be successful. Many situations can be envisaged in which such *cooperation* may be lacking, and even highly motivated cooperative couples may experience difficulty in observing the required abstinence. This is apparent from the high user-failure rate in comparison with the biological (signal) failure rate. The *psychological problems* related to periodic abstinence are not, as yet, fully investigated. Preliminary studies, however, seem to suggest that where couples really wish to use a natural method, periodic abstinence is not considered detrimental, and the majority of such users believe the method helpful to the marriage relationship.

A further potential hazard which must be kept in mind is the possibility of *chromosomal abnormalities* leading to spontaneous abortions, or abnormal infants due to conceptions resulting from fecundation by ageing gametes. Animal studies clearly document such an association and some fears have been expressed that this may also be true for humans. Jongbloet [37] in a retrospective study of 35 couples using the 'rhythm' method suggests the association. However, Oechsli [38] and later Bracken [39] in prospective studies found no statistically significant difference in the

Table 11.2 Effectiveness of fertility awareness to achieve pregnancy

Authors	*Date*	*Number of women*	*Method*	*Months of exposure*	*% Achieving pregnancy*
Klaus and Fagan [32]	1981	27	CM* or STM†	122	74
Dolack [34]	1978	42	CM	Within one year	33
Bernard [35]	1980	187	CM	Within one year	46
Weissman *et al.* [36]	1972	18	CM	–	39
Johnston *et al.* [33]	1978	33	CM	270	57
Johnston *et al.* [33]	1978	27	STM	380	48

*CM = Cervical mucus method; †STM = Symptothermal method

incidence of birth defects between users of a natural method and a control group. This was also the finding in the WHO multicentre study [20] where neither spontaneous abortions nor babies with congenital malformations in those women who got pregnant during the study (whether a method- or user-failure) showed any increased incidence over those in the general population.

In an epidemiological review on adverse pregnancy outcomes and aged gametes associated with natural methods of family planning, Gray [40] found that although studies suggest a possible increased risk of birth defects associated with NFP use, the evidence is far from conclusive. Since the implication for NFP depends on the frequency of method failures in the user populations, it is not likely to constitute a major hazard. However, he suggests a method for further research on the subject.

Breast-feeding and infertility

Full or ecological breast-feeding tends to prolong the physiological infertility of pregnancy and thus can be considered an efficient natural contraceptive [41]. Certain variables, however, influence the duration of this natural infertility, notably the frequency and duration of suckling and the introduction of artificial feeding [42]. The result is that the return of fertility is very often a prolonged process during which spurious attempts at follicular growth and ovulation occur over weeks or months before the actual ovulatory event occurs [43].

Gross reported on the pattern of returning fertility in 54 breast-feeding mothers [44]. She found the probability of a normal ovulation before the first menses and before 30 weeks after delivery in ecological (on-demand) breast-feeding women to be 2%, which confirms the incidence found by Chilean workers [45]. In the weaning stage, however, 29.6% of the group showed evidence of ovulation (hormonal 9%, clinical indicators 20%) with a normal luteal phase ($\geqslant$11 days). In general however, women had cycles with shorter than normal luteal phase lengths (7 days), and in some women this pattern persisted over several cycles. Gross found that the presence of a continuous mucus pattern of vaginal discharge over several weeks creates problems for NFP users in that very often it is not possible to distinguish an ovulatory from an anovulatory cycle. The appearance of mucus can, however, indicate when artificial contraception should begin if the couple intend to use such methods. For those who wish to continue with natural methods, the addition of changes in the uterine cervix to the mucus observations is helpful, and we have found that marked changes in the patients' cervix (opening, consistency, position) occur only in the days immediately preceding the first ovulation [17]. In a multicentre prospective study in breast-feeding women in Australia, Canada and the UK financed and co-ordinated by Family Health International (FHI), Durham, NC, USA, urinary hormone concentrations of E_1-3-G and Pd-3a-G were determined from 42 days to the second ovulatory cycle post-partum. The women also did daily BBT, mucus and cervix graphs over the same period. Results are now being analysed to determine the reliability of the different clinical indicators (BBT, muchs, cervix) either alone or in combination to indicate the onset of returning fertility during breast-feeding and weaning. Guidelines will then be written to help women use this period of natural infertility without having to have recourse to unnecessary contraception during this time.

Research and the development of new techniques in NFP

Rapid development in medical technology over the past decade has resulted in the production of simple tests and devices for the prediction and detection of ovulation and the fertile days in the cycle.

Digital thermometers

A digital thermometer gives a digital read-out of a temperature to two decimal points without the need to 'read' the temperature as with the ordinary mercury thermometers. It requires no preliminary shaking down and registers the temperature after 45 to 60 seconds. Most digital thermometers emit a beeping sound at the end of this time to advise that registration is complete. There are several brands on the market, all clinically tested, reliable and battery-operated.

Electronic thermometers

The electronic thermometer is battery-operated and a temperature probe is used to measure the BBT which can be displayed on a small screen. The most widely used and clinically researched electronic thermometer is the Bioself 110 fertility indicator. This device, by means of a microchip uses the calendar calculations to detect the onset and the BBT shift to determine the end of the fertile days in the cycle. The device is 'set' at the beginning of the cycle and it indicates by signal lights the fertile, highly fertile and infertile days in the cycle. The temperature graph can be obtained at the end of the cycle by plugging the thermometer probe into a printer. Studies with ultrasound and hormonal determinations have proved the technical reliability of the device [46,47]. The contraceptive efficiency of the device was determined in 100 women who used the device to avoid a pregnancy in a 2-year study in the UK. There was only one unplanned pregnancy directly related to the malfunctioning of the device (unpublished data). The results of this study are being prepared for publication and the device will be available in the UK early in 1991.

Home-based tests and dipsticks

Serum concentrations of E_2, LH and Pd (and their metabolites in urine) have been used for several decades to determine respectively, the onset of fertility, the highly fertile days and the postovulatory infertile phase of the cycle. Such tests are not practical for NFP users. However, developments in monoclonal antibody technology have resulted in the production of rapid and simple urine tests designed for home use by non-medical, non-technical persons.

LH test kits

Home kits to detect changes in LH concentrations in urine are now used daily by non-medical individuals. There are several kits on the market but the most popular and the most recent is the Clearplan One Step which only requires a woman to hold a dipstick in the stream of early morning urine to obtain results within 5 minutes.

LH tests are designed to indicate high fertility in the cycle for women who wish to conceive; they do not indicate the beginning of the fertile phase sufficiently early to accommodate for sperm survival in couples wishing to avoid a pregnancy. Consequently, they have only a limited use in NFP programmes.

RAMP progesturine (PDG assay)

This simple urine self-test measures the urinary metabolite of progesterone pregnanediol glucuronide (PDG). The assay is not done by dipstick but by a rapid absorbent matrix pad (RAMP) to which is added a monoclonal antibody specific for PDG. Depending on the amount of PDG present in the urine, the binding sites will be totally bound (high concentrations of PDG in the urine) or only a few will be found (low concentrations of PDG). When the enzyme-treated PDG solution is added, one can assess how much PDG is taken up by adding water to the pad and noting the colour change. When a high quantity of the enzyme PDG is taken up an intense blue colour denotes low concentrations of PDG in the urine; conversely, when the binding sites are saturated by PDG from the urine there is no colour change on the pad.

Although this test only indicates the end of the fertile phase, we found in a small clinical trial in Birmingham that it was 100% reliable on days 4–8 past the peak mucus day, and 90% on day 3 past the peak day. Where the temperature shift is uncertain, this test could be used to confirm that ovulation has occurred and the postovulatory phase of the cycle has begun. It is a very simple and relatively rapid test to perform, but in its present package of 50 tests it is not suitable for individual home use. The 50-test kit is available from Medimar Laboratories, Sarum House, 17 The Queensway, Chalfont St Peter, Bucks SL9 8NB, UK.

Ovulation predictors

Home-based tests for urinary oestradiol concentrations to predict fertility and ovulation have proved much more difficult to develop than LH or Pregnanediol glucuronide and no single test has yet come on the market. Brown in Melbourne University has developed a kit to measure total urinary oestrogen [48]. It is not available for clinical trials outside Australia and personally, having seen the test performed, I believe it is not simple enough for a lay person to use at home at least in the UK! However, there is intensive interest by laboratories in this development and we can expect new productions over the next 3–5 years.

Measurement of changes in body fluids

The most important body fluid used to detect fertility in the cycle is that of cervicovaginal fluid (CVF). It is a well-established fact that CVF, which is a combination of cervical mucus and vaginal transudate, changes in volume over the menstrual cycle. Only recently, however, has it become possible to aspirate and reliably measure these volume changes, thanks to the development of a calibrated disposable plastic aspirator, the Rovumeter.

Preliminary studies show that the CVF volume changes correlate with cycle variations of oestrogen, progesterone, and LH, and can be used to predict ovulation and determine the fertile phase [49]. The Rovumeter is easy to use, objective, and generally acceptable to clients. It is as reliable as the LH dipstick to signal the highly fertile days in the cycle and is comparatively cheap. Further studies are under way in a multicentre WHO-sponsored project to refine the rules for CVF volume changes in order to establish the fertile phase limits with greater precision and accuracy.

Measurement of changes in electrical resistance

The electrical resistance of skin, saliva, and vagina changes over the menstrual cycle, and these electrical changes can be measured and used to delineate the fertile and infertile phases of the cycle. The Cue Fertility Monitor is a battery-operated instrument which measures the changes in electrical resistance of saliva and in the vagina. It is produced by Zetek, Aurora, Colorado and so far has only had limited use in the US and West Germany.

Conclusion

Attempts to develop some form of natural family planning are evident from the beginning of history. The results were not very successful, however, and with the introduction of the more efficient methods of artifical contraception at the beginning of this century, natural methods fell into disuse.

Recently, though, developments in reproductive research have led to an increased interest in the cyclical fertility of women, leading to more accurate and scientific approaches and renewed interest in natural family planning. This interest is reinforced by present-day ecological trends and a general concern about the complications of drugs and devices, including those used in the field of contraception. One must realize however, that natural methods in their present form are still very crude indicators of the fertile time and to be efficient, require a modification of sexual behaviour. The development of more accurate and simpler methods to detect the potentially fertile days may refine the methodology, leading to easier charting and a reduction in their number. At present, the capriciousness of sperm survival and the ever-present possibility of an unexpectedly early ovulation combine to make the first postmenstrual 'infertile' phase appropriate for use chiefly by 'spacers', i.e. those who would accept a pregnancy earlier than planned; those wishing to limit their families are generally best advised to restrict intercourse to the postovulatory infertile phase with the use of abstinence (or a condom, according to choice) until the clinical indicators (see pages 213–214) signal the start of that phase.

While the motivation and modification of sexual behaviour required for the successful practice of NFP may initially present a problem to some couples many partners find the discipline enhances their sexual relationship and dialogue. Whatever the motivation, more and more couples today seem happier to be in autonomous control of their bodies and their fertility.

References

1. FORD, K. Recent changes in contraception practice among American couples: Results from the 1976 National Survey of Family Growth. *National Centre for Health Statistics 1978*, USA (1978)
2. MOORE, E. C. *Women and Health*. United States Public Health Reports: Sept–Oct 1980. United States Government Printing Office (1980)
3. OGINO, K. Ovulationstermin und Konzeptionstermin. *Zentralblatt fur Gynakologie*, **54**, 464 (1930)
4. KNAUS, H. Die Periodische Frucht – und Unfruchtbarkeit des Weibes. *Zentralblatt fur Gynakologie*, **57**, 1393 (1933)
5. WORLD HEALTH ORGANIZATION/BLAT Centre for Health and Medical Education. *Family Fertility Education*. A Resource Package for Teachers of Natural Family Planning: Education Handbook, p. 51 (1983)
6. BARRETT, J. C. and MARSHAL, J. The risk of conception on different days of the menstrual cycle. *Population Studies*, **23**, 455 (1969)
7. SCHWARTZ, N. B. and HOFFMAN, J. C. Ovulation: basic aspects. In: *Reproductive Biology*. (ed H. Balin and S. Glasser, Exerpta Medica, Amsterdam, p. 438 (1972)
8. KELTZKY, O. A., NAKAMURA, R. M., THORNEYCROFT, I. H. and MISHELL, D. R. Log distribution of

gonadotrophins and ovarian steroid values in the normal menstrual cycle. *American Journal of Obstetrics and Gynecology*, **121**, (5), 688–694 (1975)

9. GUERRERO, R., ROJAS, O. and CIFUENTES, A. Natural family planning methods. In: *Human Ovulation: Mechanisms, Prediction Detection and Induction* (ed. E. S. E. Hafez), North Holland Publishing, New York, pp. 477–490 (1979)
10. MARSHALL, J. R. Prediction and detection of ovulation as related to fertility and contraception. In: *Proceedings of the Congress of Italian Obstetricians and Gynaecologists* (Bari, Italy) (14 pages) (1980)
11. ORTIZ, M. E. and CROXATTO, H. B. Observations on the transport, ageing and development of ova in the human genital tract. In *Recent Advances in Reproduction and Regulation of Fertility* (ed. G. P. Talwar), (Proceedings of the Symposium, New Delhi, India, 1978) Elsevier/North Holland Biochemical Press, New York, pp. 307–317 (1979)
12. HARTMAN, G. G. *Science and the Safe Period*, Williams and Wilkins, Baltimore, Ch. 28, pp. 226–234 (1962)
13. VOLLMAN, R. F. The phases of the menstrual cycle. In: *The Menstrual Cycle* (ed. E. A. Friedman, W. B. Saunders, Philadelphia, pp. 91–149 (1977)
14. FLYNN, A. M., DOCKER, M., MORRIS, R. *et al.* The reliability of women's subjective assessment of the fertile period relative to urinary gonadotrophins and follicular ultrasonic measurements during the menstrual cycle. In *Studies in Fertility and Steriligy. Research in Family Planning* (eds. J. Bonnar, W. Thompson and R. F. Harrison), MTP Press, Lancaster, pp. 3–11 (1984)
15. KEEFE, E. F. Self-observation of the cervix to distinguish days of possible fertility. *Bulletin of the Sloane Hospital for Women*, **8**, 129–136 (1962)
16. BILLINGS, J. J. *The Ovulation Method.* Advocate Press, Melbourne, Australia (1964)
17. FLYNN, A. M., LYNCH, S. S., DOCKER, M. and MORRIS, R. Clinical hormonal and ultrasonic indicators of returning fertility after childbirth. Fertility and Sterility. In *Proceedings of the XIth World Congress on Fertility and Sterility* (Dublin, 1983) (eds R. F. Harrison, J. Bonnar and W. Thompson), MTP Press, Lancaster p. 325 (1984)
18. MARSHALL, J. A field trial of the basal body temperature method of regulating births. *Lancet*, **2**, 8–10 (1968)
19. RICE, F. J., LANCTOT, C. A. and GARCIA-DEVESA, C. Effectiveness of the sympto-thermal method of natural family planning: An international study. *International Journal of Fertility*, **26**, 222–230 (1981)
20. WORLD HEALTH ORGANIZATION. Task force on methods for the determination of the fertile period. Special programme of research, development and research training in human reproduction. A prospective multi-center trial of the ovulation method of natural family planning. 2 Effectiveness phase. *Fertility and Sterility*, **36**, 591–598 (1981)
21. PEREZ, A., ZABALA, A., LARRAIN, A. *et al.* The clinical efficiency of the ovulation method (Billings). *Revista Chilena de Obstetrica y Ginecologia*, **48** (2) 97 (1983)
22. BARBATO, M., BERTOLOTTI, G. Natural methods for fertility control prospective study. *Proc. 4th Europ. Congress IFFLP/FIDAF*, Vienna, Austria, 16–24 May 1987, pp 14–26
23. FRANK-HERMANN, P., BREMME, M., ROSMUS, T., KUNKEL, W. The use-effectiveness of a symptothermal method in Germany. *Proc. 4th Europ. Congress IFFLP/FIDAF*, Vienna, Austria, 16–24 May 1987, pp 27–45
24. MARSHALL, J. and ROWE, B. The effect of personal factors on the use of the basal body temperature method of regulating births. *Fertility and Sterility*, **23**, 417 (1972)
25. KLAUS, H. Natural family planning: A review. *Obstetrical and Gynecological Survey*, **37**, 128 (1982)
26. JOHNSTON, J. A., ROBERTS, D. B. and SPENCER, R. B. A survey evaluation of the efficiency and efficacy of natural family planning services and methods in Australia. *Report of a Research Project*. St Vincent's Hospital, Sydney. 440 pages (1978)
27. MARSHALL, J. The prevalence of mucus discharge as a symptom of ovulation. *Journal of Biosocial Science*, **7**, 49–55 (1975)
28. PEREZ, A. Natural family planning: Post partum period. *International Journal of Fertility*, **26**, 219–221 (1981)
29. BONNAR, J. Natural family planning. In *Ethical Issues in Reproductive Medicine* (ed. M. Reidy), Gill and MacMillan, Dublin, pp. 53–73 (1982)
30. BONNAR, J. Biological methods of identifying the fertile period. Fertility and sterility. In *Proceedings of the XIth World Congress on Fertility and Sterility* (Dublin, 1983) (eds R. F. Harrison, J. Bonnar and W.

Thompson), MTP Press, Lancaster, p. 77 (1984)

31. BAKER, T. S., HOLDSWORTH, R. J. and COULSON, W. F. The dual analyte assay for the detection of the fertile period in women. In *Research in Family Planning* (eds J. Bonnar, W. Thompson, and R. F. Harrison), MTP Press, Lancaster, pp. 45–52 (1984)
32. KLAUS, H. and FAGAN, M. U. Use effectiveness, couple satisfaction and progression to autonomy with the Billings ovulation method. *Journal of the American Medical Women's Association,* **37**(9), 231–241 (1982)
33. JOHNSTON, J. A. An analysis of continuity-discontinuity in natural family planning: an Australian factor analysis. *International Journal of Fertility*, **26**, 23 (1981)
34. DOLACK, L. Study confirms value of the ovulation method. *Hospital Progress,* **59,** 64–73 (1978)
35. BERNARD, C. Impact of natural family planning in six dioceses in Tamil Nada. In *The Dignity of Man and Created Love.* (Selected Papers from the Congress for the Family of Americas, Guatemala, July 1980) (eds J. Santamaria, R. Richards and W. Gibbons), Knights of Columbus, New Haven, Connecticut, pp. 28–36 (1980)
36. WEISSMANN, M. C., FOLIAKI, L., BILLINGS, E. L. and BILLINGS, J. J. A trial of the ovulation method of family planning in Tonga. *Lancet*, **2,** 813–816 (1972)
37. JONGBLOET, P. H. The intriguing phenomenon of gametopathy and its disastrous effects on human progeny. *Maandschrift voor Kindergeneeskunde*, **37**, 261–285 (1970)
38. OECHSLI, F. W. *Studies of the Consequences of Contraceptive Failure.* (Final Report, Berkeley, California. University of California, Berkeley, April 1976). (Contract No I – HD–5–28–6) (1976)
39. BRACKEN, M. B. and VITA, K. Frequency of non-hormonal contraception around conception and association with congenital malformations in offspring. *American Journal of Epidemiology*, **117**, 281–291 (1983)
40. GRAY, R. H. Contraception. Aged gametes, adverse pregnancy outcomes and natural family planning. An epidemiological review. *Contraception*, **30**, 297–309 (1984)
41. SHORT, R. V. Lactation – The central control of reproduction. In *Breast Feeding and the Mother.* Ciba Foundation Symposium 45: (New Series), pp. 73–86 (1976)
42. MCNEILLY, A. C. Effects of lactation on fertility. *British Medical Bulletin,* **35,** 151 (1979)
43. MCNEILLY, A. G., GLASIER, A. and HOWIE, P. N. Fertility after childbirth. Abstract 36 In *Proceedings of the XIth World Congress on Fertility and Sterility* Dublin, 1983 (eds R. F. Harrison, J. Bonnar and W. Thompson), MTP Press, Lancaster, (1984)
44. GROSS, B. A. Breast feeding and the return to fertility. *International Review of Natural Family Planning,* **8,** 102–120 (1984)
45. DIAZ, S., PERALTA, O., JUEZ, G. *et al.* Fertility regulation in nursing women: I. The probability of conception in full nursing women living in an urban setting. *Journal of Biosocial Science*, **14**, 329–341 (1982)
46. ISMAIL, M., ARSHAT, H., PULCRANO, J., ROYSTON, P. and SPEILER, J. An evaluation of the Bioself 110 fertility indicator. *Contraception,* **39**, 53–71
47. LABRECQUE, M., BROUIN, J., RIOUX, J., GINGRAS, S. and SPIELER, J. Validity of the Bioself 110 fertility indicator. *Fertility and Sterility*, **52**, 604–608 (1989)
48. BROWN, J. B., BLACKWELL, L. F., HOLMES, J. and SMYTH, K. New assays for identifying the fertile period. *Int. J. Gynecol. Obstet.*, Supp. 1: 111–122 (1989)
49. FLYNN, A. M., MCCARTHY, A. M., DOCKER, M. and ROYSTON, J. P. The temporal relationship between vaginal fluid volumes obtained with the Rovumeter vagina aspirator and the fertile phase of the cycle. *Human Reproduction*, **3**, 201–205 (1988)

Chapter 12

Contraception for the older woman

Peter Bowen-Simpkins

Hormonal contraception using the combined oestrogen-progestogen pill provides excellent contraception and, in theory, the ideal method up to and beyond the menopause. However, the Royal College of General Practitioners' oral contraception study [1] made it clear that for women who smoke cigarettes or have other risk factors such as hypertension, diabetes, or abnormal lipid levels there is a significant rise in morbidity and mortality over the age of thirty-five. In practice, therefore, many women need to look for other acceptable methods of family planning for fifteen years or more at the end of their reproductive life.

Declining fertility and reduced coital rates increase the effectiveness of non-hormonal methods, but the psychological problems of unwanted pregnancy in the 35+ age group increase, and the risks of pregnancy both to mother and fetus favours the choice of a method whose success rate approaches 100%.

Risks to mother and fetus

Most women are aware of the increased risk of chromosomal abnormalities associated with age. In practice this risk is largely confined to Down's syndrome and does not present a significant problem until the latter part of the fourth decade. With increasing use of fetal karyotyping, either by amniocentesis after 16 weeks of gestation or by chorionic villus sampling in the first trimester, a reliable diagnosis can be made and termination of pregnancy offered to the patient. To many patients this presents a moral or ethical dilemma that they could do without, and increases their desire for effective contraception. Spontaneous abortion rates of 12% are reported in the early twenties, and these increase to 26% in the 40–49 years age group [2]. Similarly, perinatal mortality rates double as the maternal age doubles (Figure 12.1) [3]. More worrying is the very sharp increase in the incidence of maternal mortality, being as much as fourfold in the fifth decade as compared with the third (Figure 12.2) [4]. The Office of Population Censuses and Surveys (1981) [5] show a steep reduction in live births in the fifth decade with a rising stillbirth rate and a legal abortion rate considerably in excess of the percentage for all ages (Table 12.1). This implies much emotional trauma for the women and families involved.

Coital frequency and age

Coital frequency is strongly and inversely associated with age reducing by 50%

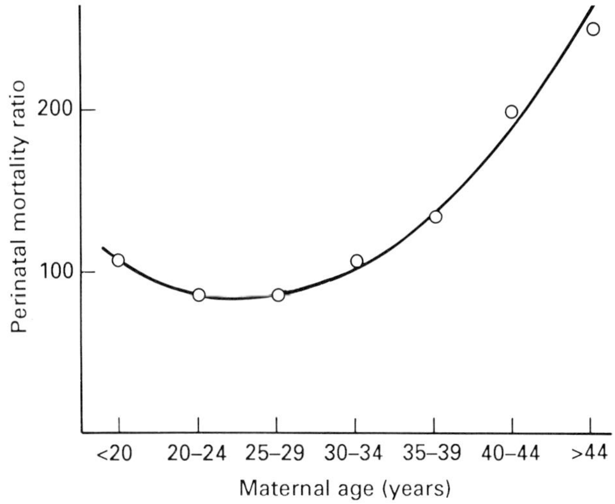

Figure 12.1. Perinatal mortality ratio plotted against maternal age in years.

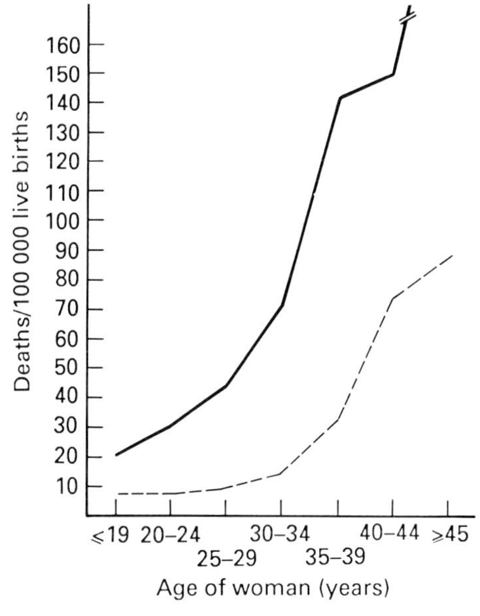

Figure 12.2. Maternal mortality rate by age of woman; United States 1974–1978. Solid line indicates black women, dashed line indicates white women. (After Buehler *et al.*, 1986 [4].)

Table 12.1 Births above age 40, 1981. (Office of Population Censuses and Surveys) [5]

Age (years)	*Live births*	*Stillbirths*	*(% of total births)*	*Legal abortions*	*(% of conceptions*)*
40–44	6 170	89	(1.4)	4 835	(43.6)
45–49	640	10	(1.5)	549	(45.8)
50+	50	1	(2.0)	15	(22.7)
All ages	634 492	4 207	(0.7)	128 581	(16.8)

* Excluding spontaneous abortions

between age 20 and the early 40s. Trussell and Westoff [6] demonstrated this in three surveys conducted in 1965, 1970 and 1975 as is shown in Figure 12.3. However, the mean coital frequency for all ages increased by 19% between 1965 and 1970 and by 5% between 1970 and 1975. This might be thought to be due to the changing age composition of the sample, but when the responses for each date are standardized on the 1970 distribution, the results are much the same. There is an increase in the mean coital frequency rate of 22% in the 10-year study period. The major increase was in the 1965–1970 period, and this increase is largely attributable to a shift to more effective forms of contraception at that time. Further increases may have been due to a more permissive attitude toward sex that developed in Western countries in the 1970s.

A major change seen in society over the past 20 years has been towards divorce. Over 30% of first marriages now end in divorce. For the majority of divorced couples, a new relationship is formed and this leads to an increase in coital frequency, especially in the early years of the new partnership. Inevitably the risk of conception increases, especially when a method of contraception related to coitus is used [7].

Fecundity in older women

The decrease in fecundity with increasing age is generally acknowledged [8]. 'Fecundity' is here used to denote the *capacity* for procreation rather than actual procreation. In a study of 2193 nulliparous women undergoing artificial insemination, success rates for those of 25 years and under and for those of 26–30 years were very similar. However, they differed significantly from the two older age groups of 31–35 years and those over 35 (Figure 12.4). The probability of success of artificial insemination after twelve cycles was 74% for those under 30 years, but dropped to 61% in the 31–35 year group and to 54% in those over 35 years. This large decrease was not simply due to inclusion of women over 40 years, since the sub-group 36–40

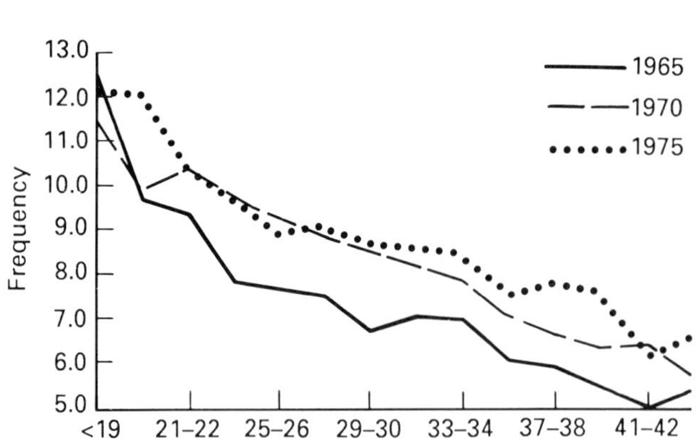

Figure 12.3. Mean frequency of intercourse in the 4 weeks before interview (by age); 1965, 1970, and 1975. (Reprinted with permission from J. Trussell and C. F. Westhoff, Contraceptive practice and trends in coital frequency. *Family Planning Perspectives*, **12,** 246–249 (1980) © 1980 by the Alan Gottmacher Institute)

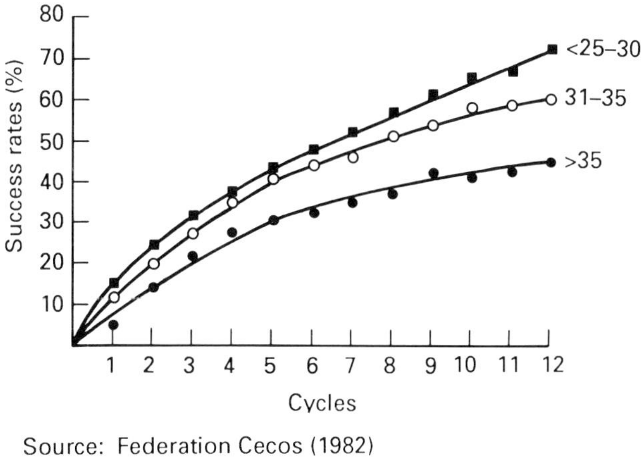

Figure 12.4 Pregnancy and artificial insemination by donor (AID), cumulative success rate (Federation CECOS (1982) [8].)

years had the same lower probability of success. For the older woman wishing to practise contraception, these fertility rates are still high.

Is there any way in which a woman who is perimenopausal can answer the question 'Am I still fertile?' Only a guarded reply can be given. Metcalf [9], reporting a study of 139 New Zealand women between 40 and 55 years, showed that the incidence of ovulation is associated with the regularity of menstruation. Among those women who reported no change in menstrual frequency, 95% ovulated in every cycle, whereas among those who reported recent oligomenorrhoea, only 34% ovulated consistently. Increasing cycle length was associated with a diminishing incidence of ovulation, but for those whose cycles were between 21 and 35 days, 93% appeared to ovulate. However, pregnancy rates remain low in this group, possibly due to an increase in shortened or inadequate luteal phases. Disordered ovum transport and delayed implantation may also impair fertility [10–12]. More disturbing was a report showing that some amenorrhoeic patients with flushes, high FSH levels, and low oestrogen levels subsequently menstruated [13]. Their FSH levels returned to normal, and pregnanediol excretion suggested ovulation. On several occasions high oestrogen levels were encountered even in the presence of high FSH levels.

It is clear therefore that exact advice cannot be given to the patient. As a rule of thumb any woman, whatever her age, who is regularly menstruating must be regarded as regularly ovulating. Women of over 45 years who have amenorrhoea for over twelve months can consider themselves contraceptively safe. During this 'waiting period' coitally related methods of contraception are safe.

Menstrual patterns that are erratic or prolonged or more frequent may occur as much as 10 years prior to the menopause [14]. This may lead some women to throw caution to the winds in the misguided belief that their reproductive capabilities have come to an end. Unfortunately their medical advisors sometimes fall into the same trap, and inadequate or no contraception is advised. It is nevertheless true that because of the decline in fertility, most methods of contraception are nearly 100% effective, if used carefully. Paradoxically the woman who is least likely to conceive – the one with increasing oligomenorrhoea – is the one who is repeatedly terrified that she has become pregnant. It is this group who would benefit most from some form of safe, cyclical hormonal contraception giving regular cycles and relief from menopausal symptoms.

Hormonal contraception

Combination of oestrogen and progestogen

The combined oral contraceptive provides many desirable features up to and during the climacteric. However, its use has to be discontinued at a certain age because of its acknowledged association with cardiovascular disease [15] (Table 12.2).

It must be stressed that for the non-smoking, normotensive women with no other cardiovascular risk factors, taking the combined pill up to the age of 45 is safer than the risk to life of an unwanted pregnancy. The risk to the woman over 45 is still less than that to a 35-year-old woman who is a habitual smoker, and less than the overall maternal mortality in the USA [4]. Sadly this fact has failed to get through to patients and, more regrettably, to many of their medical advisors.

The desirable features of combined hormonal contraception have been summarized by Guillebaud [3] (Table 12.3). A major advantage for the older woman is cycle control, associated with an overall reduction in hospital admissions for diagnostic curettage, laparoscopy, and hysterectomy. At present the woman in her 40s may be

Table 12.2 Circulatory deaths: excess deaths in ever-users each year [15]

Age	*Smokers*	*Non-smokers*
15–24	1 in 10 000	Nil
25–34	1 in 10 000	1 in 50 000
35–44	1 in 2 000	1 in 6 600
45+	1 in 550	1 in 2 500

Table 12.3 Desirable features of contraception up to and during the climacteric

1. Effective in this age group
   (a) perceived effectiveness and reassuring period pattern;
   (b) not being an intercourse-related method;
   (c) oestrogenic slowing of skin ageing, improved body image and libido, treatment of vaginal dryness
3. Controls climacteric symptoms (especially vasomotor and psychological symptoms, and the urethral syndrome)
4. Controls symptoms of 'normal' cycle (especially the premenstrual syndrome, and irregular, heavy or painful periods)
5. Reduces incidence or manifestations of gynaecological pathology. (This potential benefit applies to pelvic infection, extrauterine pregnancy, fibroids, dysfunctional haemorrhage, endometriosis, functional ovarian cysts and carcinoma of the ovary and uterus. There is a consequent reduction in the risks of treatment for these conditions, especially hysterectomy)
6. Oestrogenic protection against osteoporosis*
7. Absence of masking of the menopause
8. Absence of systemic adverse effects
   (a) known serious conditions such as hypertension and arterial cardiovascular disease;
   (b) possible effect on other serious conditions, for example breast cancer, especially with long duration of use

NB Only a combination of oestrogen and progestogen is capable of providing all the above desirable features (except 7 and 8). The remaining options chiefly act as contraceptives, without a positive benefit and sometimes with a deleterious effect, on the conditions shown.
* Now shown to be provided to some degree premenopausally by the combined pill as well as by oestrogen replacement therapy [16].

subjected to prolonged usage of high-dose progestogens, particularly norethisterone, in doses of up to 15 mg/day, or continuous use of danazol, the safety of which has not been established by prolonged epidemiological studies such as are available for the combined pill. It is now clear that progestogens are implicated in the cardiovascular risks to the older woman, and long-term use of high-dose progestogens may be dangerous [15]. Kay [15a] concludes it is reasonable to assume that if a woman uses combined preparations, with the lowest doses of progestogen, the risks to the non-smoker would be even lower than shown in Table 12.2. This is in addition to using the lowest acceptable dose of oestrogen, which is also advisable [16a].

Perhaps the strangest paradox is that marketed cyclical therapies for menopausal symptoms containing both oestrogens and progestogens do not confer the benefit of fully reliable contraception, yet the total dose of ingested progestogen in a given cycle often exceeds that found in low-dose contraceptive pills (Table 12.4). Clinicians are therefore left in a situation where they prescribe preparations with no certain contraceptive effect for hormone replacement therapy, yet these preparations are potentially more hazardous than the combined pill which the patient was advised to stop because of her age. Progestogens are added to cyclical hormonal replacement preparations to protect the endometrium from the risk of malignant change induced by unopposed oestrogens, yet the disease accounts for only 34 deaths per million women per year aged 45–55, compared with 705 from ischaemic heart disease and stroke (OPCS 1982) [5].

This problem must be resolved soon. (See pages 89–90.)

Magos *et al.* [17] have looked at continuous use of conjugated equine oestrogens combined with a progestogen-only pill taken one, two or three times daily to prevent breakthrough bleeding. This regimen may be ideal for the postmenopausal woman (particularly in the first postmenopausal year when additional contraception may be needed) but for the premenopausal woman, cyclical regimens would need to be adopted to provide regular menses. At present we have no proof that such regimens would be effective as contraception, would confer good cycle control, or would be safe from a cardiovascular standpoint.

Table 12.4 Mean daily progestogen doses in current combined preparations used for hormone replacement therapy

	Progestogen	*Total in 28 days* (μg)	*Equivalent per day* (μg)
Prempak-C	Levonorgestrel (75 μg × 12 days)	900	32
Prempak	Levonorgestrel (250 μg × 7 days)	1 750	62.5
Cyclo-Progynova	Levonorgestrel (250 μg × 10 days)	2 500	89
Trinordiol, Logynon*	Levonorgestrel (3 phases, 21 days)	1 925	69
Trisequens	Norethisterone acetate (1000 μg × 10 days)	10 000	357
Menophase	Norethisterone (3 phases, 13 days)	15 000	536
Brevinor, Ovysmen *	Norethisterone (500 μg, 21 days)	10 500	375

* Oral contraceptive preparations

Greenblatt in 1982 [18] was the first to indicate a possible answer to the dilemma with his use of the natural oestrogen oestradiol 17β in pellet form. Pellets are implanted into the anterior abdominal wall under local anaesthesia, using a special trocar and cannula. The method is quick and virtually painless; each implant dose is 100 mg and is combined with a suitable progestogen. Greenblatt used medroxyprogesterone acetate 10 mg or norethisterone acetate 5 mg for 5–7 days in every 28 days to produce a withdrawal bleed. In the light of present evidence about progestogens this is possibly too high a dose for too short a time, and a more suitable regimen would use a progestogen-only pill (e.g. levonorgestrel 30 mg or norethisterone 350 mg) for at least 10–12 days of the cycle. The implant may be supplemented with testosterone 100 mg if there is loss of libido. The initial dose of oestradiol is reduced (in 25 mg steps) every 6 months from 100 mg to 50 mg or even 25 mg. In some women menopausal symptoms may return, and in these circumstances the dose must be titrated against symptoms.

Magos *et al.* [19] have confirmed that 100 mg oestradiol implants plus norethisterone 5 mg for 7 days in each 28, as given by Greenblatt, suppresses cyclical ovarian activity, but they found that the action is not immediate in all cases. Magos [1987 Personal communication] suggests that an additional method of family planning be used for the first three cycles, a second 100 mg implant inserted after 3 months, and that the target 6-monthly maintenance dose should probably be 50 mg. These recommendations require full confirmation.

However Greenblatt's less cautious regimen nevertheless seemed effective in his population of 144 women aged 35–50 years studied for 7009 cycles. There was only one pregnancy (a Pearl index of 0.17 per 100 woman-years), which aborted in the first trimester. The use of natural oestrogens is believed to change clotting factors, particularly antithrombin III, far less than synthetic oestrogens [20–22]. Similarly, synthetic oestrogens have been shown to increase platelet aggregation but no comparable effect was shown with natural oestrogens [23]. Plasma triglyceride and lipid levels also show unfavourable changes with synthetic preparations compared with natural oestrogens. No cardiovascular morbidity occurred in Greenblatt's study over a period of 10 years, although numbers were small, and additional more extensive trials are warranted. Hopefully the near future will bring us a low-dose natural oestrogen–progestogen regimen (whether pill, implant, or using the transvaginal or transdermal routes) that will fulfil most of the criteria set out in Table 12.3.

The progestogen-only pill

This preparation has been associated with the older woman for many years. Unfortunately, the fact that it is a hormone in pill form has lead many practitioners to believe that the contraindications to its use are similar to, if not the same as, those for the combined preparations. However, the POP has very few side-effects and its efficiency as a contraceptive has been shown to be as good in this age group as that for the combined pill among women in their twenties [24]. It has several disadvantages. It must be taken on a regular basis with a leeway of no more than 3 h beyond a fixed time each day. The preparation relies mainly upon its effect on cervical mucus, which it renders hostile to sperm.

However, it commonly has a more direct effect on the hypothalamo–pituitary–ovarian axis, leading to irregular menses [25] and intermenstrual bleeding. In older women this may necessitate diagnostic curettage and make the method unacceptable. In a few, amenorrhoea may develop due to suppression of ovulation. In these patients it may be difficult to reassure them that they are not only not pregnant but are far more effectively protected than if they were seeing their periods regularly. In others amenorrhoea may be due to the menopause. In these, raised FSH levels would suggest ovarian failure and the patient should either continue with the POP for up to one year, or use a non-hormonal method for a similar period of time – unless further FSH levels permit earlier cessation of contraception. Guillebaud [3] mentions abdominal discomfort as a not uncommon side-effect. His studies showed an increase in the incidence of functional ovarian cysts demonstrated by ultrasound. The pain is usually mild, but some women may require laparoscopy to exclude tubal pregnancy, itself more common in POP takers.

Long-term systemic effects are of even less frequency than the low rate with combined oestrogen–progestogen preparations, but some studies [26,27] have suggested that there may be minimal metabolic changes threatening the cardiovascular system. Therefore it is sensible to be cautious in prescribing to older patients who have known risk factors such as smoking, hypertension, or obesity, although Vessey [24] feels that even these women can have every confidence in the method. It is believed that ovarian follicular activity produces enough natural oestrogen in most women to balance the minimal metabolic effects of the progestogen.

The POP provides an excellent and safe form of contraception for most women over the age of 35 years and its use by a total of 290 000 women in the UK represents poor publicity of its advantages rather than a vote against it because of its side-effects. The preparation has the advantages that it is highly efficient for the older woman, has few if any metabolic effects, avoids all the side-effects in which synthetic oestrogens are implicated, and minimizes any side-effects in which higher dose progestogens are implicated. The minor symptoms of the combined pill such as nausea, loss of libido, and weight gain are not a problem. Premenstrual symptoms and dysmenorrhoea are often improved and its effect on cervical mucus may protect against pelvic infection.

Injectable progestogens

The administration of steroids by injection has had considerable appeal for some time and depot medroxyprogesterone acetate (DMPA) has been used for over twenty years. Together with norethisterone oenanthate (NET-OEN), it is estimated that 1.5 million women around the world are using them [28]. The injectable contraceptives have largely been used in developing countries, and amongst women of low socioeconomic classes. As such, their use has come under suspicion for largely political reasons, and much adverse and sometimes ill-informed criticism has been unjustly levelled at them.

Amenorrhoea occurs in over 35% of patients using DMPA and between 10% and 20% with NET-OEN, and this may cause anxiety about pregnancy and the onset of the menopause. DMPA has an initial inhibitory effect on proliferation of the endometrium, with subsequent secretory effect. After about 20 days the endometrium becomes atrophic [29]. This may be of considerable benefit to women whose endometrium shows unopposed oestrogen activity, common at the climacteric. Unfortunately, irregular bleeding that may occur with injectables will need further gynaecological investigation in the over 40s. When heavy bleeding develops, a further injection of the progestogen, one month after the initial dose, often suffices to induce amenorrhoea.

Metabolic effects include a reduction in HDL-C levels of about 20% [30], although this has not been associated with any increase in cardiovascular disease. Initial anxiety about its association with breast disease, based on work on the beagle dog, has been dispelled. Firstly, the use of the beagle bitch as an appropriate model for human comparison has been seriously questioned because of the increased incidence of breast tumours that this breed is prone to. The effect of large doses of progestogens on the animal appears to be species specific.

Secondly, a recent WHO report [31], although based on small numbers, fails to demonstrate any relationship between DMPA use and breast disease. Similarly, a further WHO report [32] fails to show any statistically significant increased incidence in cervical invasive neoplasia in patients using injectable progestins.

Other progestogen delivery systems rely upon either subcutaneous or vaginal placement of the matrix from which the progestogen is slowly released. These have been fully reviewed by Fotherby [33]. They include non-biodegradable systems such as Silastic rods containing levonorgestrel, biodegradable systems such as polymer steroid complexes containing norethisterone (Chronomer or Alzamer), or microspheres of dipolylactic acid in which micronized norethisterone is homogeneously dispersed, and vaginal rings releasing either oestradiol and a progestogen or a progestogen alone. Like other progestogen systems, disadvantages include disruption of the menstrual cycle and a slightly increased rate of ectopic pregnancies, although the latter is proportionately smaller in the older woman. (See also chapter 7.)

Non-hormonal reversible contraception

Intrauterine devices (IUD)

The IUD would appear, at face value, to be the most attractive of the non-hormonal reversible methods of contraception. Apart from the initial fitting, no motivation is required, although users should be encouraged to check the presence of the device by feeling for the strings after each period. Pregnancy rates, expulsions, perforations, and infection are all lower in the older woman. Removal for bleeding or pain remains constant throughout the age groups studied by Tietze and Lewit [34]. This suggests good counselling, because prior to insertion a major consideration is the woman's pre-existing menstrual cycle. Menorrhagia and prolonged bleeding (i.e. in excess of 7 days) are obvious contraindications. Uterine myomata are more common in the older woman, but when encroaching on the uterine cavity (submucous) are likely to lead to menstrual problems. If the menstrual pattern is normal, but bimanual examination indicates the presence of fibroids, careful sounding of the uterus to exclude deformities of the cavity is essential prior to the insertion of a device. Ultrasound examination is probably more reliable.

The risk of infection in the woman over 35 years is lower than for younger age groups, even when fitted in the nulliparous woman [35]. This may signify a marked reduction in multiple-partner sexual exposure in the older woman. Intermenstrual or postcoital bleeding in a patient with an IUD may be acceptable, if only occasional, in the younger woman, but for any woman over the age of 35 with similar symptoms, gynaecological investigation is essential. This must include cervical cytology (Papanicolaou smear) and some form of endometrial biopsy after removal of the device.

Choice of type of IUD for the older woman should be the same as for younger age groups. Plastic inert devices which tend to be larger than the copper-bearing devices are no longer recommended, although there is no reason, if they have already been fitted, for them to be removed until one year after the menopause, unless complications intervene. Because of declining fertility in the fifth decade, copper-bearing devices may be left *in situ* for considerably longer than officially approved.

Much interest has been shown in a new generation of T-shaped devices containing levonorgestrel or 3-keto-desogestrel in the main limb. Initial studies in Western Europe [36] suggest that there is a lower pregnancy rate and fewer menstrual problems. The progestogen affects the cervical mucus, rendering it hostile to sperm, and possibly also helps to prevent ascending infections. For the woman at the climacteric, anovulatory cycles become more common and there may be associated hyperplastic changes of the endometrium. These should be prevented by such a device, and in theory, it may protect against endometrial carcinoma. Hormone replacement therapy could then be given during these troublesome years, combining all the advantages of such treatment with excellent contraception (and without the need for systemic progestogen).

Further research along these lines is needed. Intermenstrual bleeding has been reported and the appropriate action, as outlined above for other IUDs, must be taken.

Barrier methods

Although barrier methods still remain the most popular method of contraception throughout the world, doctors are often loath to recommend them to their patients because of the supposed low effectiveness rates. In fact, pregnancy rates in the older woman fall dramatically, particularly because of reasons already stated such as declining fertility and coital frequency, but also because of more proficient use. The Oxford/Family Planning Association study looked at two age groups of women whose partners had used the condom for 4 years or more. The failure rate in women over 35 years was 0.7 per 100 couple-years compared to 3.6 in the younger age group (25–34 years) [37].

Barrier contraception offers many advantages to couples, particularly a profound reduction in risk of sexually transmitted diseases, and possible protection against the development of abnormal cervical cytology and carcinoma of the cervix. Condoms in recent years have been lubricated with spermicide, but it is still good practice to recommend that a vaginal spermicide be used in conjunction with the condom, particularly at mid-cycle. The method is remarkably free of side-effects; but the use of condoms may lead to or exacerbate psychosexual problems, especially erectile impotence, particularly in the older age group. For this small group the condom is obviously contraindicated. Rarely, allergies may develop to the latex, and non-allergic sheaths are available.

Female barrier methods

The diaphragm was used by 10% of women in the 1960s but, following the widespread introduction of IUDs and hormonal methods, only 2–3% of British couples now use the method [38]. It is more popular amongst the older group where contraindications to other methods are more common.

The insertion of a diaphragm requires premeditation, some couples find the method messy, and the diaphragm may be uncomfortable. Vaginal and uterine prolapse and retroversion may make satisfactory fitting difficult, but the arcing diaphragm, widely used in the USA, largely overcomes these anatomical difficulties.

Cervical caps of various designs may be making a come-back [39,40]. (See also Chapter 10).

The Collatex sponge (Today) has been marketed in the USA since 1983 and is approved for sale in many other parts of the world. The sponge is made of polyurethane foam impregnated with 1 g nonoxynol-9 and can be left *in situ* for up to 24 h. Initial trials suggest a high failure rate [38], but there may be a useful place for the woman who is 45 years old or older, particularly with irregular cycles or needing contraception in the year following cessation of menstruation. Rare cases of toxic shock syndrome have been reported, and details about this are now included in the manufacturer's literature in the package.

Spermicides are available in a variety of forms. As a sole method of contraception, they are not recommended except in patients who are menopausal. The creams and foams have the advantage of increasing vaginal lubrication, and this may be of some benefit to the menopausal woman suffering from the effects of oestrogen depletion and the early changes of vaginal atrophy.

Natural family planning methods

These methods currently rely upon the use of basal body temperature charts, cervical mucus assessment, and calculations based on the length of the menstrual cycle. For those who menstruate regularly and who can accept the modifications of sexual behaviour that a fertile period imposes, the method has very obvious advantages, and with declining fertility and coital rates there is a low failure rate. However, for those with irregular periods and who are approaching the menopause, interpretation of temperature charts becomes very difficult. Similarly, cervical mucus changes become less dependable and at present the method has little place in women of older age, unless there are religious or ethical objections to the use of other methods.

This could change with the development of a simple method of predicting infrequent ovulations from appropriate changes in a body fluid such as urine or saliva, and doing this far enough ahead to allow for sperm survival. (See Chapter 11.)

Coitus interruptus (withdrawal)

In a recent survey of women seeking termination of pregnancy, almost 25% of those over the age of 35 years were using withdrawal as their sole method of contraception [Bowen–Simpkins, 1985, Unpublished data]. Failure of the method led over 80% to request an irreversible method after termination of the pregnancy.

The psychological strain placed upon such a woman whose partner relies upon this method is enormous, particularly if periods become delayed towards the menopause, and the method has nothing to commend it.

Postcoital contraception

The indications and contraindications for this method are precisely the same as for younger age groups. The Yuzpe method, using four tablets of a 50 μg levonorgestrel-containing combined oral contraceptive pill may be given, even in patients over the age of 45 in a high-pregnancy-risk case, because the exposure to the high dose of hormone is so short-lived. However, caution must be exercized in the woman with a past history of deep-vein thrombosis or severe hypertension.

Insertion of an IUD may often be preferable, as it solves the immediate problem and at the same time confers continuing contraception.

Irreversible methods

Female sterilization

This is now becoming one of the most popular forms of contraception for the woman of over 35 years of age. Considerable changes in the method of sterilization have largely accounted for this increase in popularity, the introduction of laparoscopy being the major innovation. Tubal occlusion by laparotomy is still practised in a number of centres, but is associated with a longer stay in hospital and increased morbidity. Laparoscopic methods, often performed as a day-case under local or general anaesthesia, include bipolar tubal electrocoagulation, the application of Silastic bands (Falope rings) or occlusive clips (Hulka Clemens, or Filshie).

Initial worries that menstrual disorders may be induced have not been supported by recent studies [41]. Lu and Chun [42] proposed a mechanism for increased menstrual loss following tubal ligation. They suggested that there was interruption of the utero-ovarian circulation due to occlusion of the terminal branches of the uterine arteries. It has been proposed that this is more likely with tubal division than with occlusion by clips or rings, and that this is the explanation for improved results with laparoscopic methods. However, Alderman [43] conducted a prospective trial of patients undergoing Pomeroy-type tubal ligation and failed to show any increase in menstrual loss. Electrocoagulation similarly would be expected to destroy utero-ovarian circulation, yet a comparative study of this method with occlusive Silastic rings or spring-loaded clips failed to show any significant difference in menstrual loss [44].

Careful counselling of the woman, and wherever possible her partner, is mandatory. The method must be considered irreversible, and this must be explained. The increased number of patients seeking reversal of sterilization emphasizes the need for thorough counselling, the commonest reason for reversal being change of partner. However, these requests are less commonly seen in patients in the latter part of their reproductive life.

Consideration of gynaecological problems, especially of a menstrual type, must play a part in the final decision as to whether a patient should undergo sterilization or a more major procedure such as hysterectomy. The morbidity and mortality for the latter is far in excess of any tubal operation and must be borne in mind when advising a patient. Hysterectomy should never be considered primarily as a sterilization procedure, although this is often recommended by those who still mistakenly believe that sterilization subsequently leads to menstrual disturbances.

Male sterilization

Vasectomy, like female sterilization, has become popular over the last decade. The operation is safe, easy, and effective, can be carried out under local anaesthetic, and is usually an outpatient (office) procedure. In the UK, there has been a shift in age groups seeking the operation. In McEwan's survey between 1970 and 1973 [45], 52% of patients were over 35 years of age, whereas only 38.6% were of the same age range in Newton's study of 1979–1982 [46]. The most significant reason for this was the publication of reports on the side-effects of oral contraception [47,48] and the subsequent unwillingness of women to continue oral contraception over the age of 35. However, completion of the family, most commonly for financial reasons, remains the most prominent reason for seeking vasectomy. Reversibility of vasectomy is a relatively easy procedure, but up to 50% of vasectomized men develop sperm autoantibodies, leading to sperm clumping or reduced motility and subsequent poor fertility rates.

The topic of men taking their share in overcoming some of the problems of fertility control in this age-group seems an appropriate note on which to end this chapter.

Postscript

On October 26, 1989, after the first printing of this book, the Fertility and Maternal Health Drugs Advisory Committee of the United States Food and Drug Administration (FDA) decided to remove the upper age limit on oral contraceptive use for *healthy non-smoking women* (*i.e. free of all CVS risk factors*). This statement strongly reinforces the opinion in this chapter and also in Chapter 5 that the combined pill may be used up to the age of 45; but it also makes it possible to use the method till the time of the menopause in selected women. This enormously simplifies contraception for many women, though not of course for smokers who should still discontinue the combined pill at the age of 35. The optimal COC to choose would, where available, use one of the modern 'lipid-friendly' progestogens (for example gestodene or desogestrel), combined with no more than 30 mcg and preferably only 20 mcg of ethinyloestradiol [49].

References

1. Royal College of General Practitioners' Oral Contraceptive Study. Further analysis of mortality in oral contraceptive users. *Lancet*, **1**, 541–546 (1981)
2. JANSEN, R. P. Fertility in older women. *IPPF Medical Bulletin*, **18**, 4–6 (1984)
3. GUILLEBAUD, J. Contraception for the older woman. *Journal of Obstetrics and Gynaecology*, **5** [suppl. 2], 570–577 (1985)
4. BUEHLER, J. W., KANNITZ, A. M., HOGUE, C. J. R. *et al.* Maternal mortality in women aged 35 years or older: United States. *Journal of the American Medical Association*, **255**, 53–56 (1986)
5. Office of Population Censuses and Surveys (OPCS). *Statistics for Fertility and Mortality 1981 and 1982.* HMSO, London (1984)
6. TRUSSELL, J. and WESTOFF, C. F. Contraceptive practice and trends in coital frequency. *Family Planning Perspectives*, **12**, 246–249 (1980)
7. BARRETT, J. C. and MARSHALL, J. The risk of conception in different days of the menstrual cycle. *Population Studies*, **23**, 455–461 (1969)
8. Federation CECOS, SCHWARTZ, D., MAJAUX, M. J. Female fecundity as a function of age. *New England Journal of Medicine*, **306** 404–406 (1982)
9. METCALF, M. G. Incidence of ovulatory cycles in women approaching the menopause. *Journal of Biosocial Science*, **11**, 39 (1979)
10. Editorial. Have I stopped ovulating yet? *Lancet*, **1**, 477–478 (1979)
11. DÖRING, G. K. The incidence of anovular cycles in women. *Journal of Reproductive Fertility* [Suppl.], **6**, 77–81 (1969)
12. FRANCIS, W. J. A. Reproduction at the menarche and menopause in women. *Journal of Reproductive Fertility*, [Suppl] **12**, 89 (1970)
13. METCALF, M. G. and DONALD, R. A. Fluctuating ovarian function in peri-menopausal women. *New Zealand Medical Journal*, **89**, 45–47 (1979)

14. BOWEN-SIMPKINS, P. Contraception for older women (Editorial). *British Journal of Obstetrics and Gynaecology*, **91**, 513–515 (1984)

15. KAY, C. The Royal College of General Practitioners' Oral Contraception Study: Some recent observations. *Clinics in Obstetrics and Gynaecology*, **11** (3) 759–786 (1984)

15a. LAROSA, J. C. Effect of estrogen replacement therapy on lipids: implications for cardiovascular risk. *Journal of Reproductive Medicine*, 30 (Suppl. 10), 811–813 (1985)

16. LINDSAY, J., TOHME, J., KANDERS, B. The effect of oral contraceptive use on vertebral bone mass in pre- and post-menopausal women. *Contraception*, **34**, 333–340 (1986)

16a. STADEL, B. V. Oral contraceptives and cardiovascular disease. New England Journal of Medicine, **305**, 612–618, 672–671 (1981)

17. MAGOS, A., BRINCAT, M., STUDD, J. *et al.* Amenorrhea and endometrial atrophy with continuous oral estrogen and progestogen therapy in postmenopausal women. *Obstetrics and Gynecology*, **65**, 496–499 (1985)

18. GREENBLATT, R. B. Contraception for middle-aged women. In *Recent Advances in Fertility Research*. (Part A. Developments in Reproductive Endocrinology). (eds T. G. Muldoon, V. B. Mahesh and B. Perez Ballester), Alan Liss, New York, pp. 287–300 (1982)

19. MAGOS, A. L., COLLINS, W. P. and STUDD, J. W. Effects of subcutaneous oestradiol implants on ovarian activity. *British Journal of Obstetrics and Gynaecology*, **94**, 1192–1198 (1987)

20. THOM, M., DUBIEL, M., KAKKAR, V. V. and STUDD, J. W. W. The effect of different regimes of estrogens on the clotting and fibrinolytic systems of postmenopausal women. *Frontiers of Hormone Research*, **5**, 192 (1978)

21. DAVIES, J. A. Workshop Report: Estrogens and clotting factors. In: *Consensus on Menopause Research* (eds. P. A. van Keep, R. B. Greenblatt and M Albeaux–Fernet), MTP Press, Lancaster, pp. 55–58 (1976)

22. NOTELOVITZ, M. Coagulation, oestrogen and the menopause. *Clinics in Obstetrics and Gynaecology*, **4**, 107–128 (1977)

23. EL KELES, R., HAMPTON, J. and MITCHELL, J. Effect of human oestrogen on platelet behaviour. *Lancet*, **2**, 315 (1968)

24. VESSEY, M. P. Progestogen only oral contraception. Findings in a large prospective study with special reference to effectiveness. *British Journal of Family Planning*, **10**, 117–121 (1985)

25. LANDGREN, B. M. and DICZFALUSY, E. Hormonal effects of 300 μg norethisterone (NET) minipill. *Contraception*, **21**, 87–113 (1980)

26. SPELLACY, W. N. Carbohydrate metabolism during treatment with estrogen, progestogen and low dose oral contraceptives. *American Journal of Obstetrics and Gynecology*, **142**, 732–734 (1982)

27. WYNN, V. and NITHTHYANANTHAN, R. The effect of progestins in combined oral contraceptives on serum lipids with special reference to high density lipoprotein. *American Journal of Obstetrics and Gynecology*, **142**, 766–772 (1982)

28. FRASER, I. S. and WEISBERG, E. A comprehensive review of injectable contraception with special emphasis on depomedroxy progesterone acetate. *Medical Journal of Australia*, **1**, [Special Supplement1], 1–20 (1981)

29. ROBERTS, D. K., HORBELT, D. V. and POWELL, L. C. The ultrastructural response of human endometrium to medroxy progesterone acetate. *American Journal of Obstetrics and Gynecology*, **123**, 811–818 (1975)

30. KRAMER, J., DE BRUIJN, H. W. A. and HINDRICKS, F. R. Serum high density lipoprotein cholesterol levels in women using a contraceptive injection of Depomedroxy progesterone acetate. *Contraception*, **22**, 359–367 (1980)

31. WHO Collaborative Study of Neoplasia and Steroid Contraceptives. Breast cancer and depomedroxy progesterone acetate. *Bulletin of the World Health Organization* **63**, 513–519 (1985)

32. WHO Collaborative Study of Neoplasia and Steroid Contraception. Invasive cervical cancer and depomedroxy progesterone acetate. *Bulletin of the World Health Organization*, **63**, 51 (1985)

33. FOTHERBY, K. A new look at progestogens. *Clinics in Obstetrics and Gynaecology*, **11**, 701–722 (1984)

34. TIETZE, C. and LEWIT, S. Evaluation of intrauterine devices: 9th progress report of the Cooperative Statistical Program. *Studies in Family Planning*, **1** (1970)

35. ORY, H. W. A review of the association between intrauterine devices and acute pelvic inflammatory disease. *Journal of Reproductive Medicine*, **20**, 200 (1978)

36. NYGREN, K. G. New intrauterine devices. In *23rd British Congress of Obstetrics and Gynaecology*.

Summaries N. 110, Royal College of Obstetricians and Gynaecologists, London p. 145 (1983)
37. VESSEY, M. P., LAWLESS, M. and YEATES, D. Efficacy of different contraceptive methods. *Lancet*, **1**, 841–842 (1982)
38. MILLS, A. Barrier contraception. *Clinics in Obstetrics and Gynaecology*, **11**, 641–660 (1984)
39. KOCH, J. P. The Prentif contraceptive cervical cap: acceptability aspects and their implications for future cap design. *Contraception*, **25**, 161–163 (1982)
40. BOEHM, D. The cervical cap: effectiveness as a contraceptive. *Journal of Nurse Midwifery*, **28** (1), 3–6 (1983)
41. VESSEY, M. P., LAWLESS, M., MCPHERSON, L. and YEATES, D. Tubal sterilization: findings in a large prospective study. *British Journal of Obstetrics and Gynaecology*, **90**, 203–209 (1983)
42. LU, T. and CHUN, D. A long term follow up of 1055 cases of post partum tubal ligation. *Journal of Obstetrics & Gynaecology of the British Commonwealth*, **74**, 875–880 (1967)
43. ALDERMAN, B. Menstrual loss after tubal ligation. *Lancet*, **2**, 1039 (1975)
44. BHIWANDIWALA, P. P., MUMFORD, S. D. and FELDBLUM, P. J. Menstrual pattern changes following laparoscopic sterilisation with different occlusion techniques. *American Journal of Obstetrics and Gynecology*, **145**, 684–694 (1983)
45. MCEWAN, J., NEWTON, J. R., YATES–BELL, A. and HOY, J. Hospital family planning; a vasectomy service. *Contraception*, **9**, 177–192 (1974)
46. NEWTON, J. R. *The Changing Pattern of Male and Female Sterilization*. Birth Control Trust, London, pp. 5–14 (1982)
47. VESSEY, M. P., DOLL, R., PETO, R. *et al.* A long term follow-up study of women using different methods of contraception – an interim report. *Journal of Biosocial Science*, **8**, 373–427 (1976)
48. KAY, C. Mortality among oral contraceptive users. RCGP. Study. *Lancet*, **2**, 727–731 (1977)
49. FORTNEY, J. A. Oral contraceptives for older women. *IPPF Medical Bulletin*, **24**, 3–4 (1990)

Chapter 13

Cervical ripening prior to termination of pregnancy

G. M. Filshie, G. Robinson and C. C. Welch

Mechanical dilatation of the cervix during termination of pregnancy is potentially hazardous, both in the perioperative period and the long term. Cervical injury is directly related to the mechanical process necessary for the procedure, especially during the latter part of the first and the early part of the second trimester [1,2]. Other complications may possibly be related to insufficient or difficult dilatation, i.e. haemorrhage or incomplete evacuation [3].

In the long term, cervical incompetence leading to increased fetal loss in the middle or early third trimester has also been related to previous vaginal termination of pregnancy [4–6]. The procedure for mechanical dilatation involves the application of substantial tensile force along the cervical canal. It has been suggested by Hulka *et al.* [7] and Liu *et al.* [8] that dilatation beyond 9 mm may represent actual tearing of the internal os, rather than true dilatation. The overall incidence of cervical damage has been estimated at between 0.4% and 4.8% [2,6,9]. This has led many workers to attempt to develop drugs or techniques which will achieve gradual dilatation of the cervix in order to allow easier evacuation of uterine contents, thus minimizing trauma to the cervix. In order to quantify the results of dilating agents, many machines have been developed which will record the force required to overcome cervical resistance [7,8,10–17]. Most devices measure changes in longitudinal forces transmitted by the attached dilator to a transducer, which are then relayed either mechanically or electronically to a recording monitor. Johnstone [18] devised an instrument to measure the internal diameter of the cervix.

Several preoperative dilating agents have been tested, the main ones being prostaglandins and their analogues; *Laminaria digitata*; Lamicel, a synthetic hydrophilic tent, and Dilapan, a hydrogel polymer.

Prostaglandins

Over a decade ago, it was noted by the early workers with prostaglandins that when prostaglandin-induced abortion failed, it was commonly found that the cervix had dilated sufficiently to allow easy evacuation of the uterine contents with little or no surgical dilatation [19–21]. This observation led Beguin [22] and Haspels and Neth [23] to suggest that surgical evacuation of late first-trimester pregnancies (11–13 weeks) could be facilitated with preoperative administration of a prostaglandin by either the vaginal or extra-amniotic route. Wiqvist and colleagues [24] injected 250–750 μg $PGF_{2\alpha}$ or 25–75 μg PGE_2 at intervals of 1–4 h into the extraovular space, for a maximum of 8 h in ten patients at 12 weeks gestation. At evacuation, the cervix was found to be sufficiently dilated for easy insertion of the curette. The only side-effect noted by these authors was vomiting in three patients. Haspels and Neth [23] administered a single extra-amniotic dose of 0.5 mg. $PGF_{2\alpha}$ to 11 women (gestation 7–13 weeks; parity 0–5) 4.5–20 h prior to evacuation. Varying degrees of cervical dilatation were noted in most women, but side-effects occurred in almost half, i.e. two cases of nausea, three cases of vomiting, and one with hypotension.

Three studies utilizing vaginal administration of $PGF_{2\alpha}$ or PGE_2 for cervical dilatation have been reported. Craft [25] inserted two 100 mg $PGF_{2\alpha}$ pessaries on two occasions within 24 h before vaginal termination of pregnancy in ten subjects. Gestational age ranged from 9–12 weeks, and parity from 0–9. Adequate cervical dilatation and vacuum aspiration was achieved in only two cases. Side-effects included headaches and flushing (five), diarrhoea (five) and difficulty in breathing and rectrosternal discomfort (one). All patients had uterine cramps.

In a controlled study reported by by Brenner and colleagues [26], 40 nulliparous women were given 50 mg $PGF_{2\alpha}$ in the form of vaginal pessaries 3 h prior to vacuum aspiration, 20 nulliparae served as controls. Fifty-five per cent of the treatment patients were dilated sufficiently to perform suction curettage, compared with 5% of the control group. Those $PGF_{2\alpha}$ subjects needing further dilatation and evacuation required less than their controls for similar gestational age. Side-effects including vomiting and diarrhoea (43%), severe uterine cramps requiring analgesia (13%), and mild cervical trauma was observed in one treated patient and in three of the control group.

Ostergaard [27] attempted to extend the application to the non-pregnant cervix. Twenty-milligram PGE_2 pessaries were inserted and the cervical dilatation pre- and post-pessary compared. The drug had little or no effect, but all patients suffered severe side-effects including rigor (five), nausea (four), pyrexia above 38°C (four), abdominal cramps (four), vomiting (three), diarrhoea (two) and hypotension (one).

The overall impression from these early trials was that although effective in producing cervical dilatation, the response was by no means uniform in all and that side-effects really made their use unpleasant for patients, who could be subjected to these unwanted symptoms for many hours. The major problem was due to the inherent chemical instability of natural prostaglandins. This problem has been overcome by commercial formulations. The addition of methyl groups at the 15 and/or 16 position of the prostaglandin molecule prevents rapid metabolism by enzymes in the lung, thus lengthening its duration of activity.

Analogues have been developed which enable easy local application, ensuring uniform efficacy in a short time with a minimum of side-effects for use in both the out-patient and in-patient situation. The following five analogues have received the most attention by workers in the field:

1. 15-methyl $PGF_{2\alpha}$ methylester;
2. 16-phenoxy-ω-tetranor PGE_2 methylsulphonylamide (i.m.);
3. 16-16 dimethyl-trans-Δ_2 PGE_1 methylester (vaginal);
4. 9-deoxo-16-16-dimethyl-9-methyline PGE_2;
5. 16-16-dimethyl-PGE_2-*p*-benzaldehyde semicarbazone ester (i.m./vaginal).

The degree of preoperative cervical dilatation using the first four of these analogues has been the subject of a recent large trial by Christensen and colleagues [28]. Although not a purely random study of a homogeneous group, they showed quite clearly that the mean cervical dilatation following pretreatment with an analogue for

3 h was significantly greater than that following the use of a medium-sized laminaria tent for the same period of time.

The degree of cervical dilatation was measured as that achieved by the easy passage of the largest Hegar dilator. The longer the application, particularly of the E series, the greater was subsequent cervical dilatation. However, the longer the application, the more frequent became the side-effects such as a significant increase in the frequency of abortion prior to schedule, and the need for analgesic injections, as well as gastrointestinal side-effects. Similar findings were published in an earlier multicentre study by WHO [29].

The overall conclusion reached was that using equivalent dose schedules, the E analogues were more efficacious than a medium-sized laminaria tent in producing cervical dilatation, and the side-effects were both dose and time related. A 3 h schedule, although not producing the maximum cervical effect possible (both in the analogue and laminaria groups), produced enough cervical dilatation to reduce the mechanical stress required to perform vacuum aspiration by a significant amount. This allowed use in both the out-patient and in-patient situation without upsetting established clinic procedures. Welch and Elder [15] in an open study of 25 nulliparae comparing 16-16 dimethyl-trans-Δ_2 PGE_1 methylester vaginal pessaries 3 h pretermination with 18 similar patients receiving no preoperative treatment, actually measured the force required to dilate the cervix, using a spring-gauge which could be attached to the handle of the Hegar dilators used. They assessed cervical resistance by determining the maximum diameter of the Hegar dilator that could be passed with a force of less than 0.3 kg (the lowest reading on the spring-gauge). They also recorded the force required to insert the largest dilator needed in both groups. Measurement of both parameters showed a significant reduction in cervical resistance in the treatment group. Side-effects occurred solely in the treated group. Fifty-four per cent experienced mild or moderate pain and bleeding which began between 20 min and 3 h post-insertion. Three patients reported nausea, but only one reported vomiting. Postoperatively, 64% experienced pain, whilst 20% vomited, compared with 55% of the control group, in which there were no patients who vomited.

The conclusion drawn was that this analogue was very effective in reducing cervical resistance but was troubled by a few annoying side-effects in some patients. It was suitable for use in in-patients, being easy to insert and manage and not associated with unnecessary change in clinical practice. As with all prostaglandin analogues, it has to be stored in a refrigerator prior to use which, it was noted, could be inconvenient and perhaps preclude its use in some third-world countries.

Recently, Fisher and Taylor [30] in New Zealand in a randomized double-blind placebo-controlled study, compared the effects of the same analogue with a placebo pessary in a group of 110 consecutive primigravid patients. All the terminations were to be done on an out-patient basis under local anaesthesia, and due to the constraints of the clinic, the insertion-to-procedure interval was only 2 h. The change in cervical resistance was not measured, but the amount of dilatation was determined by the ability to pass the largest Hegar dilator and the subsequent subjective ease with which the required mechanical dilatation occurred. The mean dilatation in the treated group was 5.8 mm (SD 1.4), and 4.9 mm (SD 1.3) in the placebo group ($P < 0.001$). Mechanical dilatation as required in 49 women of the treated group and in 54 of the placebo group. There was a significant statistical difference between the two groups ($P < 0.05$) in the ease of dilatation. Operative blood loss appeared to be significantly less in the treated group. Preoperative abdominal cramps were reported in 25 patients in the treated group ($P < 0.001$), but actual pain occurred in only six. No pain relief was needed preoperatively. These authors reported no difference in the amount of nausea or vomiting between the two groups, which is probably a reflection of the short insertion–procedure interval.

They concluded that the analogue facilitated easy therapeutic termination of pregnancy by cervical dilatation with relatively few side-effects [30].

Laminaria digitata

In medical parlance a tent is any material, usually hygroscopic, which is placed in a sinus or canal to maintain patency or cause dilatation. Laminaria (*Laminaria digitata*, seatangle) is a species of seaweed, the stem (stipe) of which is, when dried, quite hygroscopic and capable of dilatating to 3–4 times its original diameter. Other materials used in the past include various cloth, sponges, types of wood (slippery elm) and Turpelo (*Nyssa uniflora*) as well as dried corn stalk. Of these, the most popular has been laminaria. Reports of its use appeared frequently in American literature in the 1860s and 1870s. Special instruments were developed for insertion and various sizes and shapes were experimented with. A hollow version allowed uterine drainage, and curved varieties made introduction into the flexed uterus easier. Medicated laminaria were covered in wax which released absorbed antiseptics as they melted. Recommended uses included treatment of primary dysmenorrhoea, cervical stricture causing infertility, vaginal atresia, and for cervical ripening prior to the induction of labour, missed abortion, or death-in-utero. It was not long before adverse reports of its use began to appear. Boer in 1882, described a death due to sepsis following the use of a laminaria tent, which had been ordered to dilate the cervix of a patient with prolonged metrorrhagia.

Other reports followed, citing infection as a major serious complication of its use. This was especially true of land-derived plants in which clostridia spores were found which, because of the rather primitive methods of sterilization, could not be deactivated. *Laminaria digitata*, however, grows in cold northern seas, and since marine bacteria are relatively non-pathogenic to man these were less likely to produce problems. However, poor handling and packaging as well as increased pollution of coastal sites gradually rendered this relative safety factor invalid. The combination of mounting complications including retention, perforations, lacerations, and developing interest in medical gadgetry for cervical dilatation led to the disappearance of laminaria tents in American literature by 1910, although it continues to remain popular in parts of Europe and the Far East to the present day.

Renewed interest in laminaria was shown by workers in America, particularly in the 1960s and early 1970s. Olsen and colleagues [31] in a large series of therapeutic abortions in Denmark between 1961 and 1968 noted that 'stipes laminaria with evacuation the following day was used in a considerably smaller number of cases [than dilatation with Hegars (2159 vs 8684)] but with a lower rate of complications, particularly fever.' There were only three recorded perforations of the uterus compared with 73 in the Hegar-dilated group, and there were no ruptures of the cervix compared with 15 with the Hegars [31].

Newton [32], in his report of 500 consecutive patients in whom laminaria had been used prior to termination of pregnancy, noted no known uterine perforations and an incidence of cervical damage of 0.6%. Cervical dilatation was adequate to perform the evacuation in over 99% of patients. The primary complication was infection, the rate attributable to laminaria being 2.2%. This compared with 5% in a series of 246 suction abortions without laminaria. It was suggested that if new tents were used and then discarded the rate would be considerably lower [32]. Hale and Pion [33] in their review of 887 abortions reported similar rates of complications. They also encountered other minor problems including difficulty in insertion in eight cases, expulsion of the device in 12 cases and difficulty in removing the tents in four cases. Twenty to thirty per cent of their patients complained of slight uterine cramps prior to surgery, and a mucoid, purulent discharge was recorded in 10%.

The need to leave the tent *in situ* for up to 24 h must be considered an added disadvantage which has deterred clinicians in the past. The drive has been to find a similar mode of cervical dilatation but in a shorter time, to fit in with modern clinic procedures [33].

Lamicel

Having renewed interest in non-pharmacological cervical dilatation by laminaria, a search began for a synthetic equivalent which would hopefully be as effective in a shorter time and yet not be troubled by the more serious complications associated with the use of seaweed. Lamicel [17,34,35] is a polyvinyl alcohol polymer sponge impregnated with 450 mg magnesium sulphate. It is hydrophilic and acts as a cervical osmotic dilator. The sponge is compressed to form a thin cylindrical tent (75 mm long and 3–5 mm diameter) and when inserted in the endocervical canal and left in position, the Lamicel absorbs and retains fluid from the cervical tissues because of its hygroscopic properties. The tents swells to 3–4 times its original diameter and is converted from a hard object into a soft sponge.

Nicolaides and colleagues [35] showed that Lamicel was an effective cervical dilator. In their study, 60 nulliparae admitted for termination of pregnancy were allocated to various treatment groups, in whom the Lamicel was left in situ for different lengths of time prior to operation. A comparable non-treatment group was used as a control. An electronic machine was developed specifically to record both pressure trace and peak pressure achieved during cervical dilatation with Hegar dilators, which were attached to the specially designed handle [18]. The results showed firstly that the pressure recordings of the controls, compared with the treatment groups, were significantly different ($P < 0.001$). Therefore, the tent was effective and, indeed, became so in a relatively short time; peak reduction in resistance occurred at 2 h with a further mild decrease up to 6 h. Figure 13.1 shows change in cervical resistance with time of insertion.

It was also noted that as well as cervical dilatation, a degree of softening and change in consistency of the cervical stroma also occurred, very similar to that reported by clinicians using laminaria tents. Side-effects were few, mainly lower abdominal discomfort (33%) which resolved spontaneously in all patients within 5 min. In 90% of patients insertion of the larger size tent was easily accomplished, and in all but two of the rest the smaller size was used. Despite being unable to negotiate the internal os in two patients, the cervix was still affected by Lamicel. There were no problems with lacerations or perforations and no evidence of infection [35].

A further study to attempt to elucidate the mechanism of action of Lamicel by Nicolaides and colleagues [34] showed that the changes in the cervix were not associated with alterations in circulating levels of prostanoids and steroids or, indeed, with levels of prostanoids and steroids in amniotic fluid. Further, the observed cervical dilatation did not appear to be due to increased uterine activity as measured

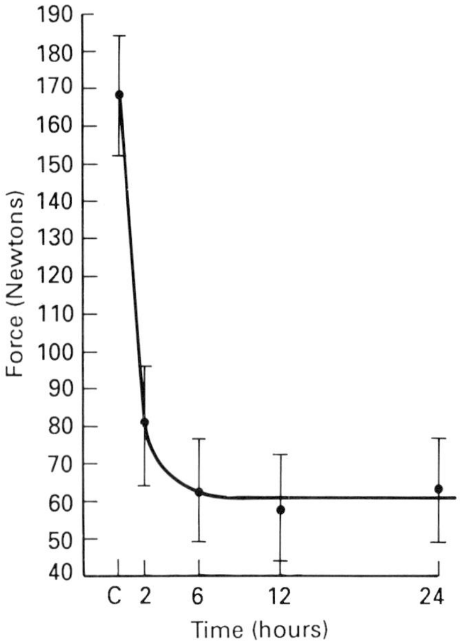

Figure 13.1. A graphic representation of the mean forces (±SD) required to dilate the cervix up to Hegar 10, following Lamicel treatment. C=control; 2, 6, 12 and 24 represent the duration of treatment with Lamicel prior to the operation.

by changes in intrauterine pressures. The serum levels of magnesium sulphate did not change significantly, suggesting that its tocolytic properties were of no consequence. Lamicel, unlike laminaria, is soft when used and does not exert a high mechanical pressure on the cervix. This finding, however, does not exclude a local effect by Lamicel. If cervical and uterine circulations have relatively large concentrations of magnesium sulphate, prostanoids, and steroids, then they might all act together to produce the observed local effect with no change in values in the general circulation. Indeed, Ellwood [36] suggested that prostanoids and steroids are involved in a cascade system of hormonal interactions with the collagenous framework and matrix of the cervix, converting it from hard and rigid to soft and distensible.

Histologically, changes in the mast cell population and an increase in ground substance, oedema, and sulphated mucopolysaccharides all suggest an allergic phenomenon in both laminaria and Lamicel. More research is required to understand their mechanisms of action. However, Lamicel provides a potent, acceptable vehicle for producing preoperative cervical dilatation which is associated with few if any significant side-effects.

Dilapan

Dilapan is a synthetic hygroscopic dilator made from a polacrylate-based hydrogel. Like laminaria, it not only extracts water from the cervix but also applies a radial force to the cervical canal as it swells. One reported advantage of Dilapan over other synthetic dilators is the speed at which it expands. Darney [37] has reported that a 4 mm dilator expands to 8 mm in 30 min, to 12 mm in 1 h and to 20 mm in 4 h. Little published information regarding the clinical use of Dilapan is available at the present moment. However, Filshie [unpublished observations] has shown that it produces effective atraumatic dilatation, and Blumenthal [38] has shown that for induction of abortion the average time to induction was shorter in patients pretreated with Dilapan than in patients treated with laminaria.

Mechanisms involved in dilatation with hygroscopic dilators

Since their introduction it has been assumed that hygroscopic tents produce dilatation by extracting water from the cervical stroma and, in the case of laminaria and Dilapan, also exert a radial force as the device swells during uptake of the extracted water [37,39]. The question of whether or not the extraction of water produces dilatation by solely causing a shrinkage of the cervix or by effecting a remodelling of the connective-tissue stroma, as occurs at term, was not answered. However, the report that Lamicel produces cervical softening would seem to indicate that a remodelling of the connective tissue stroma is involved [34]. In order to study the dilatation and cervical softening produced by hygroscopic dilators, Robinson and colleagues [40,41] examined samples of cervixes from patients who had been treated with either Lamicel, Dilapan, or laminaria prior to total abdominal hysterectomy for benign conditions. These light and electron microscope studies showed that the changes in the cervical connective tissue were pronounced following treatment with all three dilators, and that irrespective of the device employed, the principal histopathological changes following treatment were similar. Initially in the superficial stroma there was oedema, vascular dilatation and separation of the fibres within the collagen bundles. As treatment time progressed these changes became more widespread and increased in magnitude. In particular, in sections stained for polymerized collagen at the light-microscope level, there was a decrease in staining intensity with increasing treatment time. At the fine structural level, a progressive disorganization, disruption, and dissolution of the collagen fibres was noted (Figures 13.2 and 13.3). Concomitant with this loss of collagen was an increase in the connective-tissue

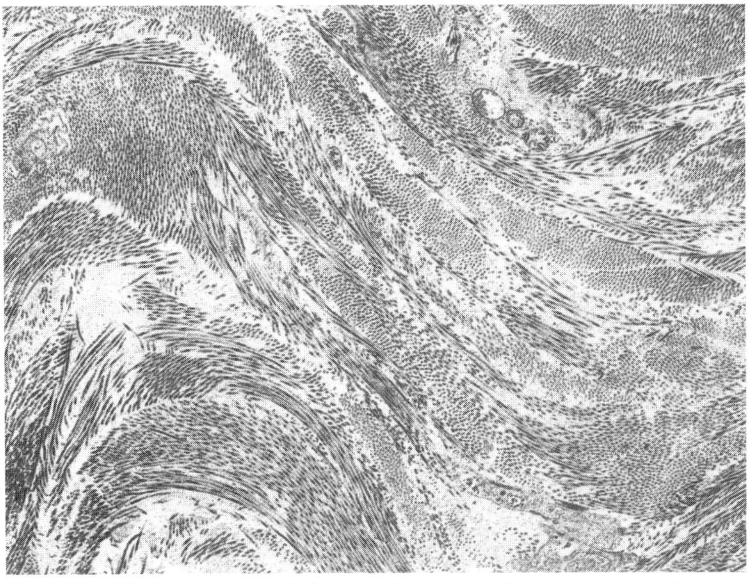

Figure 13.2. Electron micrograph showing the dense collagenous stroma of normal cervix × 3850.

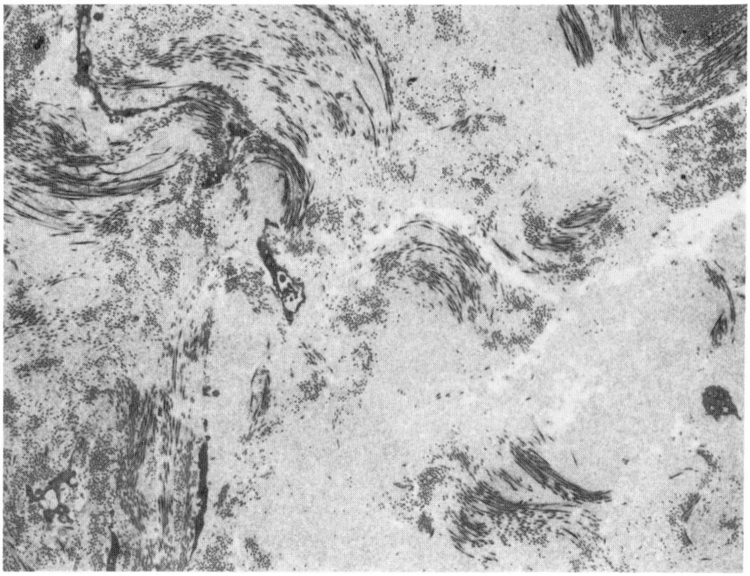

Figure 13.3. Electronic micrograph showing collagen dissolution in the stroma of a cervix treated with Dilapan for 3 h × 3850.

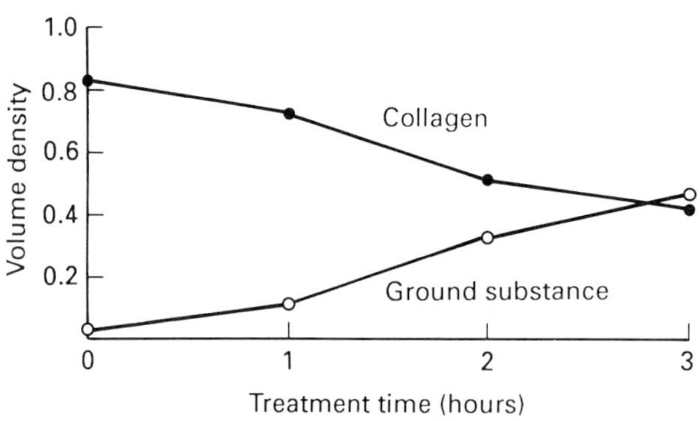

Figure 13.4. Volume density (i.e. mm^3 of component/mm^3 of stroma) for collagen and ground substance in Lamicel-treated cervices.

ground substance. The collagen remaining subsequent to treatment with Lamicel and Dilapan was quantified using stereological analysis, and the results showed that both dilators produced a progressive and statistically significant decrease in the amount of polymerized collagen (Figure 13.4).

It would appear, therefore, that the three most popular hygroscopic dilators in use at the present time initiate a process which is similar in outcome to the as yet unknown process which produces ripening of the cervix at term. Although neither study elucidated the mechanism or mechanisms involved, it is self-evident that the changes produced by the dilators must be explained in terms of cellular mechanisms operating within the cervical stroma itself. Although it may be possible that the extraction of water from the helical hyaluronic molecules within the connective-tissue stroma is solely responsible for the breakdown that occurs, as collagen degradation is reported to require the activity of collagenase [42], the possibility exists that the extraction of water (or some other stimulus provided by the dilators) initiates a cascade of events similar to that occurring at term.

Conclusions

For a hundred years, clinicians have been attempting to overcome the natural barrier to surgical exploration of the uterine cavity, the cervix. In modern medicine the consensus of opinion agrees that forcible cervical dilatation, particularly in termination of pregnancy, is harmful and may affect subsequent reproductive ability.

There are at present two approaches to the problem. The use of pharmacological agents which change cervical dilatation by a combination of uterine activity and local alteration in cervical composition, and the use of hygroscopic tents which act either by exerting pressure on the cervix in combination with local changes or, probably act locally in total. Both types of agent appear to be effective and it is a question of tolerable side-effects, local facilities or cost as to whether one regimen or another, is used. Prostaglandins and their analogues are easily manufactured and can be used with little or no medical supervision. They act in a short time, but are associated with unwanted although relatively minor side-effects. However, the need for storage of the analogue pessaries at 4°C limits their potential use in third-world countries. Products like laminaria, Lamicel and Dilapan are equally effective, but require medical supervision to insert and monitor. Laminaria, although fallen into disrepute, provides an easy, effective method of cervical dilatation, being limited by the length of time necessary to gain maximum benefit. Lamicel and Dilapan appear to be equally as effective with few or no significant side-effects. They can be used in a day-case situation and are suitable for the world market.

Welch and colleagues [43] in a recent study compared the efficacy of Cervagem (16-16 demethyl-trans-Δ^2 PGE_1 methylester), and Lamicel. They were both found to be equally effective in reducing cervical resistance to forceful mechanical dilatation. Lamicel was associated with fewer side-effects. Thus, on the evidence that exists, it is recommended that some effort be made by clinicians to reduce the possible damage to cervical tissue through mechanical dilatation, whilst we await the outcome of prospective long-term trials, to assess the proposed benefit of those procedures.

References

1. KOTASEK, A. Artifical termination of pregnancy in Czechoslovakia. *International Journal of Gynaecology and Obstetrics*, **9**, 118–119 (1971)
2. STALLWORTHY, J. A., MOOLGAOKER, A. S. and WALSH, J. J. Legal abortion: a critical assessment of its risks. *Lancet*, **2**, 1245–1249 (1971)
3. EDELMAN, D. A., BRENNER, W. E. and BERGER, G. S. The effectiveness and complications of abortion by dilatation and vacuum aspiration versus rigid metal curettage. *American Journal of Obstetrics and Gynecology*, **119**, 473–481 (1974)
4. WRIGHT, C. S. W., CAMPBELL, S. and BEAZLEY, J. Second trimester abortion after vaginal termination of pregnancy. *Lancet*, **1**, 1278–1279 (1972)
5. RICHARDSON, J. A. and DIXON, G. Effects of legal termination on subsequent pregnancy. *British Medical Journal*, **1**, 1303–1304 (1976)
6. HILLIER, K., MACKENZIE, I. Z. Experiences and advances in the use of prostaglandins in obstetrics and gynaecology in the United Kingdom. In *Proceedings of the Asian Federation of Obstetrics and*

Gynaecology. (ed S. M. M. Karim). International Congress, 1976. Obstetrics and Gynaecological uses of prostaglandins. MTP Press, Lancaster, p. 83–104 (1976)

7. HULKA, J. S., LESTER, H. T., JR. ANGLONE, A. and LACHENBRUCK P. A. A new electronic force monitor to measure factors influencing cervical dilation for vacuum curettage. *American Journal of Obstetrics and Gynecology*, **120**, 166–173 (1974)
8. LIU, D. T. Y., BLACK, H. M. M., MELCHER, D. H. *et al.* Dilatation of the parous non-pregnant cervix. *British Journal of Obstetrics and Gynaecology*, **82**, 246–251 (1975)
9. TIETZE, C. and LEWITT, S. Joint program for the study of abortion (JPSA): early medical complications of legal abortion. *Studies in Family Planning*, **3**, 97–122 (1972)
10. ATIENZA, M. F., BURKMAN, R. T. and KING, T. M. C. Forces associated with cervical dilation at suction abortion. In *Dilation of the Uterine Cervix*, (ed. F. Naftolin and R. G. Stubblefield), Raven Press, New York pp. 343–354 (1980)
11. DINGFELDER, J. R., BRENNER, W. E., HENDRICKS, C. H. and STAVROVSKY, L. G. Reduction of cervical resistance by prostaglandin suppositories prior to dilatation for induced abortion. *American Journal of Obstetrics and Gynecology*, **122**, 25–30 (1975)
12. BLACK, M. M., MELCHER, D. H., MELVILLE, H. A. H. and ALDERMAN, B. Developments in cervical dilatation including the use of vibrating techniques. *Clinics in Obstetrics and Gynaecology*, **2**, 173–201 (1975)
13. CARTER, L., BLACK, M. M., MELCHER, D. H. and MELVILLE, H. A. H.. A vibrating and force measuring cervical dilator. In *Physical Science Techniques in Obstetrics and Gynaecology*, (eds. M. M. Black and H. J. English), Pitman Medical, Tunbridge Wells, pp. 100–113 (1977)
14. FISHER, J., ANTHONY, G. S., MCMANUS, T. J. *et al.* Use of force measuring instrument during cervical dilatation. *Journal of Medical Engineering and Technology*, **5** (4), 194–195 (1981)
15. WELCH, C. C. and ELDER, M. G. Cervical dilation with 16-16 dimethyl transΔ^2 PGE_1 methylester pessaries before surgical termination of first trimester pregnancies. *British Journal of Obstetrics and Gynaecology*, **89**, 849–852 (1982)
16. FILSHIE, G. M., BHIWANDIWALA, P., HESLIP, M. Nouvelle methode d'interruption de la grossesse. In *Le Controle de Fertilité*. (eds. M. Shelli, M. Kharouf and R. M'Rad Daly), Societé Tunisienne de Gynaecologie et Obstetrique, Tunis, pp 401–405 (1981)
17. CRAWFORD, A. J., PLANT, G. R., FILSHIE, G. M. *et al.* A force sensor and peak-reading recorder for measurement of cervical dilatation force. *Journal of Biomedical Engineering*, **6**, 289–292 (1984)
18. JOHNSTONE, F. D., BEARD, R. J., BOYD, I. E. and MCCARTHY, T. G. Cervical diameter after suction termination of pregnancy. *British Medical Journal*, **1**, 68–69 (1976)
19. NAFTOLIN, F., KIRSHEN, E. J. and RYAN, K. J. Therapeutic abortion utilising local application of Prostaglandin $F2_\alpha$. In *The Prostaglandins – Clinical Applications in Human Reproduction*. (ed. E. M. Southern), Futura, Mount Kisco, NY, pp. 423–431 (1972)
20. PION, R. J., HALE, R. W. and REICH, L. Vaginal administration of prostaglandins and early abortion. In *The Prostaglandins – Clinical Applications in Human Reproduction*. (ed. E. M. Southern), Futura, Mount Kisco, NY, pp. 367–372 (1972)
21. WENTZ, A. C., BURNETT, L. S., ATIENZA, M. F. and KING, T. M. Experience with intra-amniotic prostaglandin $F2_\alpha$ for abortion. *American Journal of Obstetrics and Gynecology*, **117**, 513–521 (1973)
22. BEGUIN, F., BYGDEMAN, M., TOPPOZADA, M. and WIQVIST, N. The response of the mid-pregnant human uterus to vaginal administration of prostaglandin suppositories. *Prostaglandins*, **1**, 397–405 (1972)
23. HASPELS, A. A. and NETH, F. Induction of abortion (I) by intravenous (II) intra-uterine administration of PGF_α (extra and intra-amniotic). *Advances in the Biosciences*, **9**, 515–524 (1973)
24. WIQVIST, N., BYGDEMAN, M., BIGUIN, F., FERNSTROM, I. and TOPPOZADA, M. Induction of abortion by extra-amniotic prostaglandin administration. *Prostaglandins*, **1**, 37–53 (1972)
25. CRAFT, I. The use of prostaglandin pessaries prior to vaginal termination. *Prostaglandins*, **3**, 377–381 (1973)
26. BRENNER, W. E., DINGFELDER, J. R., STAVROSKY, L. G. and HENDRICKS, C. H. Vaginally administered $PGF_{2\alpha}$ for cervical dilation in nulliparae prior to suction curettage. *Prostaglandins*, **4**, 819–836 (1973)
27. OSTERGAARD, D. R. The cervical relaxant properties of postaglandin E2 in non-pregnant subjects. *Prostaglandins*, **4**, 701–702 (1973)
28. CHRISTENSEN, N. S., BYGDEMAN, M. and GREENE, K. Comparison of different prostaglandin analogues and laminaria for pre-operative dilatation of the cervix in late first trimester abortion. *Contraception*, **27**, (1) 51–61 (1983)

29. WHO Prostaglandin task force. Vaginal administration of 15 methyl $F_{2\alpha}$ methylester for pre-operative cervical dilation. *Contraception*, **23**, 251–257 (1981)
30. FISHER, P. R. and TAYLOR, J. H. Controlled study of 16, 16-dimethyl-trans$^{\Delta 2}$ PGE_1 methylester vaginal pessaries prior to suction termination of first trimester pregnancies. *British Journal of Obstetrics and Gynaecology*, **9**, 1141–1144 (1984)
31. OLSEN, C. T., NIELSON, H. B. and OSTERGAARD, E. Complications in therapeutic abortions. *International Journal of Obstetrics and Gynaecology*, **8**, 823–829 (1970)
32. NEWTON, B. W. Laminaria tent: relic of the past or modern medical device? *American Journal of Obstetrics and Gynecology*, **113**, 442–448 (1972)
33. HALE, R. W. and PION, R. J. Laminaria: An under-utilised clinical adjunct. *Clinical Obstetrics and Gynecology*, **15**, 829 (1972)
34. NICOLAIDES, K. H., WELCH, C. C., KOULLAPIS, E. N. and FILSHIE, G. M. Cervical dilatation by Lamicel: studies on the mechanism of action. *British Journal of Obstetrics and Gynaecology*, **90**, 1060–1064 (1983)
35. NICOLAIDES, K. H., WELCH, C. C., MACPHERSON, M. B. A. *et al.* Lamicel – a new technique for cervical dilatation before first trimester abortion. *British Journal of Obstetrics and Gynaecology*, **90**, 475–479 (1983)
36. ELLWOOD, D. A. The hormonal control of connective tissue changes in the uterine cervix in pregnancy and at parturition. *Biochemical Society Transactions*, **5**, 662–667 (1980)
37. DARNEY, P. D. Preparation of the cervix: hydrophilic and prostaglandin dilators. *Clinics in Obstetrics and Gynaecology*, **13**, 43–15 (1986)
38. BLUMENTHAL, P. D. Comparison of Dilapan and laminaria for pre-treatment of the cervix in mid trimester abortion. In *Abortion Services: a Contribution to the Nation's Health*, (ed. G. P. Bagley), National Abortion Federation, Washington, pp. 6–7 (1987)
39. MACKENZIE, I. Z. Clinical studies on cervical ripening. In *The Cervix in Pregnancy and Labour* (eds D. A. Ellwood and A. B. M. Anderson) Churchill Livingstone, Edinburgh, pp. 163–186, (1981)
40. ROBINSON, G., FILSHIE, G. M., POWELL, M. C. and JOHNSON, I. R. Alteration in collagen organisation during Lamicel-mediated dilatation of the cervix. *Journal of Pathology*, **142**, A43 (1984)
41. ROBINSON, G., BENHAM, M., FILSHIE, G. M. *et al.* Histopathological changes in the human cervix subsequent to dilation with Dilapan. In *Abortion Services: a contribution to the Nations health.* (ed G. P. Bagley) National Abortion Federation, Washington, pp. 8–10 (1987)
42. ELLWOOD, D. A., ANDERSON, A. B. M., MITCHELL, M. D. *et al.* Prostanoids, collagenase and cervical softening in sheep. In *The Cervix in Pregnancy and Labour* (eds D. A. Ellwood and A. B. M. Anderson), Churchill Livingstone, Edinburgh, pp. 57–73, (1981)
43. WELCH, C. C., MACPHERSON, M. B. A., JOHNSON, I. R. *et al.* Pre-operative dilatation of the first trimester cervix: a comparison between Lamicel and 16-16 dimethyl-trans-Δ^2 PGE_1 methylester pessaries. *American Journal of Obstetrics and Gynecology*, **149** (4), 400–402 (1984)

Chapter 14

Abortion

G. M. Filshie

Introduction

Abortion is a universal phenomenon which has been recorded since ancient times and in all levels of society. It may be defined as the loss of a pregnancy before the 28th week of intrauterine life as calculated by menstrual age. The pregnancy loss may be spontaneous or induced. The incidence of spontaneous abortion reported to the physician is approximately 1 per 5–10 recorded pregnancies. This incidence is fairly constant, as pregnancy failure includes those caused by blighted ovum, congenital fetal abnormalities, uterine abnormalities, and maternal ill health [1,2]. Induced abortion, however, has a variable reported incidence which is lower in communities which do not attach stigmata to unplanned pregnancies or pregnancies out of wedlock, and a higher incidence when social and economic pressures result from that pregnancy [3]. Historical finds of vaginal speculae and instrumentation suitable for abortion have been recovered from Hippocrates' time and before. Unwanted pregnancies have always been conceived; attitudes towards abortion have always been varied and fluctuant.

Until 50 years ago the operation was associated with a moderately high mortality, as techniques were poor and antibiotics were not available. In 1930, 432 deaths were reported in England because of induced abortion. This can be compared with six reported deaths in 1986 [4]. It is not surprising, therefore, that before 1930 there was a lot of resistance to accepting abortion as recommended practice.

Even today, the British public appear polarized into a pro-abortion lobby and an anti-abortion lobby, the basis being a combination of religious and political views. Nevertheless, whatever legislation exists, abortion occurs either legally or illegally. Although patients choose to have an abortion for personal reasons, it is recognized that abortion is an important influence on societies' birth rates and population size [5,6]. Tietze in 1983 [7] estimated that there are approximately 50 million induced abortions performed throughout the world every year, giving an overall incidence of 70 per thousand known pregnancies. In Latin America alone in 1974 five million abortions were estimated, giving an incidence of 65 per thousand pregnancies. This was despite the fact that induced abortion was illegal in those countries. Higher abortion rates have been recorded in the Soviet Union and in some parts of China [8].

The current world growth rate is approximately 1.8% [9] which represents a doubling of the population every 39 years. Some countries have a natural growth rate much higher than that, for example Kenya, which has a growth rate of 3.95, and Nigeria which has a growth rate of 3.2% [6,9]. These countries are doubling their population every 17–15 years. It is of interest to note that these countries have a low contraceptive prevalence and a low abortion incidence.

It is the relentless increase in the world's population which poses a threat to the stability of the world. In 1977 the World Bank's president, Robert MacNamara was quoted as saying 'short of thermo-nuclear war itself, it is the gravest issue the world faces over the decades ahead . . . Indeed in many ways rampant population growth is an even more dangerous, if subtle, threat to the world than thermo-nuclear war for it is intrinsically less subject to rational safeguards and less amenable to organised control' [10].

History of abortion and the law

Both the Romans and the ancient Greeks tolerated abortion. Both Plato and Aristotle were in favour of abortion for eugenic reasons, as they encouraged it for women over 40 and for women who had completed their family. Only fit men and women were encouraged to reproduce [11]. Early Christians were profoundly pronatalist and regarded abortion as taking life and equal to murder. St Augustine in the 4th and 5th century promoted the attitude that sex within marriage but without procreation was wrong. This attitude was to remain for almost 1000 years [11]. Although abortion was practised at this time, the distinction was made between early abortion and late abortion. Late abortion was defined as after quickening. This distinction was reaffirmed by Pope Gregory IX. Abortion at this time was partially condoned to save the woman's life. However, in 1869 Pope Pius XI concluded that the distinction between early and late abortion did not exist and abortion was therefore prohibited [12–14]. Both abortion and contraception were generally prohibited, even by Protestants until 1930 when contraception was conditionally approved, and was more readily accepted in 1958.

The date 1803 represents the basis of modern British legislation: in an attempt to rationalize the law the Lord Ellenborough's Act [15] included clauses relating to 'attempting to discharge loaded firearms, stabbing, cutting, wounding, poisoning and the malicious using of means to procure a miscarriage of women and the malicious setting fire to buildings'. Abortion was therefore among a long list of felonies which originally qualified for the death penalty. If a woman was not quick with child, the offence was not classified as a capital offence but warranted the pillory or transportation. A number of modifications to the Act occurred in 1828 and 1837 which generally altered the penalties. A major change occurred when the 1861 Offences Against the Person Act became established. Section 58 deals with abortion:

Section 58

Every woman being with child, who, with intent to procure her own miscarriage, shall unlawfully administer to herself any poison or other noxious thing, or shall unlawfully use any instrument or other means whatsoever with the like intent, and whosoever, with the intent to procure the miscarriage of any woman, whether she be or be not with child, shall unlawfully administer to her or cause to be taken by her any poison or other noxious thing, or shall unlawfully use any instrument or other means whatsoever with the like intent, shall be guilty of felony.

(Section 59 makes it a misdemeanor to supply noxious things and instruments for those purposes.)

This law was the basis of the British abortion laws for over 100 years, and although in 1837 it was suggested that abortion be legal to preserve the life of the woman, this was not incorporated into the Act until the Infant Life Preservation Act of 1929, which made a proviso that 'no act shall be punishable when done in good faith with the intent to save the life of the mother'.

There was the celebrated case of Mr Alec Bourne, a senior gynaecologist in London, when in 1938 he was presented with the plight of a 14-year-old girl who had been lured into a guards barracks by some soldiers who promised to show her a horse with a green tail. She went inside only to be raped by several of the guardsmen. She was in such a state both mentally and physically that she was admitted to hospital and observed for several days. Mr Bourne subsequently performed what was probably a D and C to procure an abortion. He informed the Director of Public Prosecutions and was immediately arrested and sent for trial. The case was contested and at the conclusion Mr Bourne was acquitted. Although the conclusion was that abortion could be performed under very special circumstances and depended on the interpretation of 'life', the law was still generally unclear.

Although abortion was often performed there was still an air of uneasiness among surgeons. In an attempt to clarify the law many parties, including the Abortion Law Reform Association (ALRA), put pressure on the government. After much debate the present law, promoted by David Steel, was passed in 1967 and remains the essence of the law today.

The 1967 Act permits abortion under the following clauses:

1.. '... that the continuance of the pregnancy would involve risk to the life of the pregnant woman ... greater than if the pregnancy were terminated.'

Interpretation. The spirit of this clause is that if a woman is seriously ill, e.g. with severe heart or kidney disease, termination of pregnancy would be less dangerous than continuing the pregnancy to full term. The operation is therefore to save or preserve life. However, under the law, this clause may be interpreted to mean that below 12 weeks gestation the risk of termination is substantially less than the risk of a full-term pregnancy. It could therefore be argued that it would be safer to terminate that pregnancy than to allow it to go to term. Any abortion under 12 weeks could thus be interpreted as being legal.

2.. '... that the continuance of the pregnancy would involve risk ... of injury to the physical or mental health of the pregnant woman greater than if the pregnancy were terminated.

Interpretation. This clause is very difficult to interpret precisely. It relates particularly to the patient who, for various reasons, cannot face continuing with the pregnancy and develops a reactive depression. This may proceed to mental or physical deterioration, and if abortion were considered likely to reverse this process, it is clearly justified.

3.. '... that the continuance of the pregnancy would involve risk ... or injury to the physical or mental health of ... any existing children of the family greater than if the pregnancy were terminated.'

Interpretation. If another baby would substantially affect the mental or physical health of the existing child or children then termination of pregnancy would be legal.

4.. '... that there is a substantial risk that if the child were born it would suffer from such physical or mental abnormality as to be seriously handicapped.'

Interpretation. This covers cases of possible fetal abnormality, e.g. following maternal rubella or where congenital abnormality such as Down's syndrome, spina bifida or sex-linked disease has been identified.

The operation should take place in NHS premises, and prior to the operation the green form HSA 1 should be signed by two registered practitioners. Following the abortion the buff form HSA 4 should be completed and sent to Alexander Fleming House within 7 days. (A fact worth considering is that with the present work-load of hospital doctors, ward clerks, and secretaries, together with the accepted second-class postage arrangements, to get the forms back at the appropriate time is nothing short of a miracle).

Abortion used to be permitted up to 28 weeks' gestation, but legal difficulties emerged if the fetus was born alive and subsequently died. The Human Fertilization and Embryology Bill of 1990 now permits abortion up to 24 weeks' gestation, but no upper limit has been set for termination of abnormal fetuses.

When abortions are performed within the private sector, special conditions must be fulfilled. The premises must be approved and regularly vetted by the DHSS. A local consultant gynaecologist and haematologist must be appointed to supervise treatment, and this includes making available anti-D to those patients where it is appropriate. Only a small number of special clinics have been appointed to abort gestations between 20 and 24 weeks (neonatal resuscitation facilities must be available in these premises). Some private hospitals are not allowed to perform day-case procedures, despite the government giving encouragement for day-case facilities in the National Health Service [17].

Abortion has been made legal in eastern Europe since the mid-fifties. However, it was subsequent to the 1967 Abortion Act that abortion laws in many western European countries were clarified such that abortions under various circumstances are permitted in most European countries.

Effect of the Abortion Act in Britain

Since the introduction of the 1967 Abortion Act all legal abortions have been documented. The number of cases has risen and has continued to rise until this date. In 1968 23 000 procedures were reported, and in 1987 198 000 procedures were reported. Although approximately one-third of these were performed on women from overseas, the figures represent a disappointment. Demographic trends from eastern Europe show that after a period of some 15–20 years following liberalization, the abortion numbers decline. This has not happened in England. The abortion rate, however, has not substantially altered, suggesting that numerically more females are available to become pregnant. In 1968 25% of all patients were aborted in the second trimester, and most had hysterotomies. In 1987 this went down to approximately 13%, showing an encouraging trend of having terminations of pregnancy performed earlier. Unfortunately, some patients who are referred for termination of pregnancy early do not obtain their abortions until late because of poor administrative communication [18].

Despite 20 years of the abortion law there is still an inequality in terms of the services which are provided. In the Tyneside area and the Devon area over 94% of all abortions are performed within the National Health Service, whereas in Leicestershire the figure is only 13% [19]. Second-trimester abortions have become much safer as hysterotomy and hypertonic saline have been replaced by prostaglandins and, in a few expert hands, dilatation and evacuation.

There has been a great deal of reluctance on behalf of some doctors and administrators to rationalize the National Health Service abortion services. Instead of having purpose-provided abortion clinics, patients seeking abortions are still often seen in routine gynaecological clinics and operations are still performed on routine gynaecological lists. All too frequently do we find infertility patients lying alongside patients who are having an abortion. This is an inhumane and abhorrent practice.

Counselling

Counselling is a process of discussion between the pregnant woman and the counsellor directed towards helping the woman make the right decision. The discussion should be informed, non-directive, non-judgemental, and should preferably take place in a relaxed, informal setting. A woman with an unwanted pregnancy is usually in a dilemma. To continue the pregnancy may present what appears to be insoluble and impractical problems, whereas to have an abortion may seem equally abhorrent. The pressures involved in either course of action are substantial and the woman may not be entirely objective under the strain of her predicament. Therefore, sympathetic counselling is often required for the woman to reach the right decision. On the other hand, by the time the woman sees the doctor, she may be so certain of her decision that she rejects any offer of counselling advice and wishes an immediate referral to an appropriate gynaecologist or agency. Counselling begins with the first professional contact and may involve and include the family practitioner, the clinic doctor or nurse. More detailed counselling may be carried out by those trained in such techniques, who may be doctors, nurses, social workers or even lay-persons. It is often helpful to discuss the problem with someone who is not involved with the final decision-making process of whether or not to proceed with an abortion.

Counselling assistance is available from a number of charitable pregnancy advisory services including the British Pregnancy Advisory Service; the British Advisory Service; the Brook Advisory Centre, and Marriage Guidance Services. Counselling services are also available from Lifeline and from the Right to Life Society. However, this counselling is usually directed towards helping the woman continue with her pregnancy. It is helpful to interview the partner or parents to help build a more comprehensive picture of the problem and also to assess the relative extent of external pressures which may be operating on the woman.

Objectives of abortion counselling

The counselling interview should aim to help the woman:

1. To decide the best course of action.
2. To ascertain what her real wishes are.
3. To help her to take the ultimate responsibility for her decision.
4. To help avoid serious regrets subsequently.
5. To understand how the woman came to be in her present predicament so as to avoid the same situation again [20].

The counsellor should also ensure that:

1. The circumstances conform to the legal requirements of the law.
2. The patient is not ambivalent or unsure.
3. Informed consent is obtained before embarking on the termination of pregnancy. The woman should understand what an abortion entails.

It is important to develop a rapport with the patient seeking abortion. Many patients are very worried about discussing all aspects of their problem freely. Other patients feel aggressive and demanding while yet others are singularly mute, making it very difficult to understand what true feelings exist. Many questions need to be asked as to why the pregnancy is unwanted. Is an unwanted pregnancy just another symptom of an inadequate personality? What were the circumstances of conception? Who was the partner and is he supporting the woman? Is the woman concerned as to how her family or friends will react? Has she a problem with contraception?

To help reach the appropriate decision the patient must be advised on the following matters:

1. The alternatives to abortion. The three choices are adopting, fostering, or keeping the baby herself. There is an abundance of help available for any of these choices. Information on maternity leave, pay, grants, housing priorities and other benefits are available from any local social services officer. Many women cannot conceive the idea of relinquishing their baby after delivery, which is why there are so few babies available for adoption today.

2. What does an abortion entail? The patient should have the appropriate procedure explained to her. The method of termination of pregnancy depends upon gestation, and the training of the gynaecologist. The woman should be told what anaesthetic will be used and what overall risks are present.

3. How long will she stay in the hospital? Early abortions may be performed as day-cases. However, the DHSS sometimes make it mandatory for the patient to stay overnight in some private hospitals.

4. The importance of reaching a decision without too much delay, as well as of leaving adequate time to consider all the implications of her decision. The earlier the termination of pregnancy request is referred to a doctor, the earlier the procedure is performed and less complications, either mental or physical, will occur. The woman should always be given the opportunity to delay the procedure if she wishes for more time to come to her decision.

5. The cost. This is free if the operation is carried out within the National Health Service. If the patient is referred for a private procedure, then the full costs should be made known to the woman.

6. When does normal menstruation occur? The patient should be informed that blood-loss will occur for a week to 10 days following the procedure and that her normal periods will resume approximately 4–5 weeks later.

7. How would a termination of pregnancy affect her future fertility? An early termination does not impair future fertility, provided the procedure is uncomplicated and that no undue force is exerted on the cervix during dilatation. Repeated termination of pregnancy and postoperative infections (e.g. chlamydia) are factors which could impair fertility.

8. What future contraception should be adopted? This is a very important issue, as most unplanned and unwanted pregnancies are associated with either no contraception or poor use of contraception. Under these circumstances the whole issue is that

of resolving a major contraceptive problem. Resolution of this problem lies in the termination of pregnancy followed by adequate contraceptive practice. Provided that no contraindications exist, the combined contraceptive pill may be started immediately after a termination of pregnancy. She could have an intrauterine contraceptive device fitted at the time of the procedure. Sterilization may also be performed at the time of termination of pregnancy. It is important that the decision is well understood prior to the procedure as regret rates after tubal ligation are often increased when associated with a termination of pregnancy.

Some of this information may be incorporated into a leaflet which could be distributed to each woman [21].

High-risk cases

The following women need careful counselling, and if the pregnancy is terminated often require support afterwards:

1. *Teenage girls.* Special attention should be paid to this group, particularly if the patients are under 16 years of age. Here, the parents or the legal guardian need to sign the consent form unless the operation is urgent and needs to be performed to save her life (which is very rare). Many of these young girls become pregnant again within a year of their termination. It is therefore prudent to spend extra time discussing the benefits of contraception in order to avoid this unfavourable situation. It must also be borne in mind that many girls become pregnant as a result of sex abuse.
2. *Women requiring a late termination of pregnancy.* Many of these women present late because of ambivalence. At first there may be a personal denial of the situation. Ambivalence is a very worrying factor. These women may regret subsequently their termination of pregnancy and may well need extra counselling prior to their decision. They may need support afterwards.
3. *Women who have underlying psychiatric or personality disorders.* These patients may well benefit from a psychiatric opinion prior to making a decision.
4. *Patients who have repeated terminations of pregnancy.* Although relatively uncommon, these patients require extra counselling. These women often have personality disorders and are often inadequate. One must remember that the second unwanted pregnancy is just as unwanted as the first.
5. *Patients who have a termination of pregnancy on medical or genetic grounds or because of the risk of other fetal abnormalities.* These patients tend to blame themselves for their situation and need special support. There are self-help groups for such women and it is helpful to give the appropriate information to them.
6. *Women who have been raped or sexually abused.* These women need extra support, and if paternity testing is required, products of conception should be collected for genetic 'finger-printing' (genetic satellite profile).

Assessment

This is by the usual history, examination, and special investigations. After the history the patient should be examined to assess the gestation of the pregnancy. In early pregnancy a routine pregnancy test is only reliable 10–14 days after the missed period. A vaginal examination should always be performed to assess gestation. This procedure is always difficult when there is associated obesity or a retroverted uterus. Particular attention should be paid to performing a cervical smear test, and checking to see whether there is any concomitant vaginal infection, e.g. chlamydia or sexually transmitted disease. Appropriate swabs should always be taken if a discharge is found, and where necessary treatment should be instigated prior to the termination. An ultrasound examination should always be performed when there is doubt as to the actual gestation. This is particularly important if the patient is around 13–14 weeks gestation or if she is on the upper limit of the time an abortion can be performed (this is 20 weeks in most hospitals or 24 weeks in some specially selected nursing homes).

Techniques for termination of pregnancy

A number of techniques are available for terminating pregnancies. Important factors to consider are the duration of the pregnancy and, to a lesser degree, the preference of the gynaecologist who is to be responsible for the procedure. The techniques are described in three main groups.

Very early termination of pregnancy

This is an abortion carried out up to the 7th week after the last menstrual period. The method is also euphemistically known as menstrual regulation, menstrual extraction, or menstrual induction. In some countries abortion may be illegal, but as a standard pregnancy test may not be reliable or conclusive during this period, menstrual regulation is accepted.

Medical techniques

There is a great demand for a simple method of 'hindsight' family planning. When a patient misses her period unintentionally she immediately becomes highly motivated to seek advice. Such a patient often requests a simple pill or pessary which will bring back and restore menstruation. In response to this demand, many research workers have tested various types, routes, and doses of prostaglandins in an endeavour to achieve the patient's expectation. The method is largely experimental but the following results are worth noting.

The first report of menstrual induction came from Karim in 1971 [22]. He reported the administration of PGE_2 and $PGF_{2\alpha}$ as a vaginal preparation to induce menstruation in 12 women whose periods were delayed from 2 to 7 days. Success was achieved in eleven of these women. The side-effects included nausea, vomiting, menstrual cramps and a heavy menstrual flow. Similar trials were undertaken using suppositories or solutions by other research workers [23–25]. The high incidence of side-effects was discouraging. Nevertheless, the study promoted the evaluation of a number of different routes of administration and a number of different analogues of prostaglandins in the hope of finding a more acceptable mode of treatment. The subcutaneous and intramuscular routes of naturally occurring prostaglandins were painful and were associated with unaceptable side-effects. The intrauterine route (impact dose) was described by Csapo *et al.* in 1972 [26] and was further evaluated by Karim in 1973 [27]. This was a very effective method but the side-effects, especially severe uterine cramps, needed substantial medication to relieve the discomfort. Since prostaglandins were inserted into the cavity of the uterus, this method must be regarded as a combination of medical and surgical techniques.

The use of a large number of synthetic analogues has been recorded by many

Table 14.1 Very early first-trimester abortion induced by prostaglandin analogues

Prostaglandin analogue	*No of women*	*Period of gestation (weeks)*	*Route*	*Success rate % effective (complete)*
16-phenoxy-PGE$_2$ methylsulphonylamide				
Karim *et al.* [28]	240	5–6	Extraovular	95
Csapo and Pulkkinen [29]	10	<6	Intramuscular	100
Caspo *et al.* [30]	90	7	Intramuscular	96
Fleischer *et al.* [31]	19	<7	Vaginal suppository	95
Bygdeman *et al.* [32]	34	<7	Intramuscular	94
16,16-dimethyl-PGE$_2$ MacKenzie *et al.* [33]	34	<4	Vaginal suppository	100
16,16-dimethyl-PGE$_1$ methylester				
Karim *et al.* [34]	50	<6	Vaginal suppository	92
Bygdeman *et al.* [32]	63	<7	Vaginal suppository	92
9-methylene-PGE$_2$ Bygdeman *et al.* [32]	101	<7	Vaginal suppository	92–98

investigators. The most popular and promising analogues have been methylesters of 15-methyl-PGE$_2$ or F$_{2\alpha}$, 16-16-dimethyl-trans-Δ^2-PGE$_1$ methylester and 16,16-dimethyl-PGE$_2$ and 16-phenoxy-ω-tetranor-PGE$_2$ methylsulphonamide. The results of these clinical trials [28–34] have been summarized by Bygdeman [32]. The intrauterine route is more effective and needs substantially less prostaglandin than the vaginal route, but the vaginal route may be self-administered. These analogues are demonstrating fewer and more tolerable side-effects. However, the efficacy is still only about 90%–95% on average. A summary of these analogues is given in Table 14.1.

Anti-progesterone compounds

Progesterone is vital to the maintenance of pregnancy. It is often referred to as the 'hormone of pregnancy'. Progesterone is produced by the corpus luteum, and this luteal production of progesterone is vital, firstly to prepare the endometrium for implantation and secondly to contain the pregnancy until the placenta takes over production from about the ninth week of gestation. There are two types of antiprogesterone preparation. One of the first used was Trilostane [35] which is a progesterone-synthesis inhibitor. The second group comprises progesterone-blocking compounds and includes Mefipristone (RU486) [36]. Both these groups of drugs have been used to terminate early pregnancy. Side-effects are few and a mild suppression of adrenocortical hormones has been observed. The efficiency, however, is only about 70%.

Combinations of Antiprogesterone preparations and prostaglandins

By first administering Mefipristone in doses of 400–600 mg and following this by the administration of Gemprost (a vaginal pessary), the success rate is over 95%, which makes the technique a highly possible therapeutic approach [37,38].

Before medical techniques can be made freely available a number of practical considerations must be overcome. The first is that the gestation must be early, i.e. 4–7 weeks menstrual age. If the treatment is given when the gestation is too advanced an incomplete abortion will be inevitable, requiring an evacuation of the uterus. The legal aspects of the treatment are still unclear, as at present treatment must conform to the regulations concerning therapeutic abortion. The treatment therefore cannot be administered at home. However, as most patients experience bleeding not dissimilar to a normal period, it becomes nonsensical to keep a patient in hospital whilst she menstruates.

Surgical methods for very early termination of pregnancy

Techniques for evacuating the uterus using suction have been known for decades. In 1927 Bykow [39], a Russian gynaecologist, described a suction technique using a syringe as a vacuum source and a cone-shaped tube which was introduced into the uterine cavity. Bykow recommended this treatment 5–7 days before menstruation as the safest form of contraception available. Nearly half a century passed during which time there was little interest in this field. It was not until the advent of plastics and the pioneering work of Harvey Karman, an American psychologist, that this method was reintroduced and popularized. The curette designed by Karman has now been used extensively for terminating early pregnancies of up to 12 weeks gestation as an out-patient procedure under local anaesthesia [40]. For very early termination of pregnancy, i.e. up to 7 weeks, a syringe kit may be used. Beyond this, the portable Karman suction equipment [41] or an electrical suction pump may be used as a vacuum source.

Up to 7 weeks of amenorrhoea the technique is usually referred to as menstrual extraction or menstrual regulation. Once the patient has been counselled and the pregnancy has been confirmed, the procedure is similar to that taken for any patient requesting a termination of pregnancy.

Patients are not premedicated or shaved and lie on a gynaecological bed in the lithotomy position. The vulva is cleansed, a speculum is inserted into the vagina and the cervix cleansed, preferably with povidone-iodine solution. A local anaesthetic, 0.5–1% lignocaine (5 ml), is injected intracervically at the 12 o'clock position. The anterior of the cervix is then grasped with a tenaculum and a further 5 ml of local anaesthetic is injected at the 3, 6 and 9 o'clock positions. Lewis [41] recommends that the injection sites should be at the 12, 4 and 8 o'clock positions. A 4-mm Karman curette attached to a 50-ml syringe is introduced through the cervical canal into the uterus. The plunger of the syringe is withdrawn until it locks on the catch. The vacuum so obtained is in the order of 67–80 kPa (500–700 mmHg). The curette is then gently moved up and down and rotated around the uterine cavity until a characteristic grating sensation is felt on all the internal surfaces. The uterus is now empty and the curette may be withdrawn. The curettings should be collected and sent for histological examination.

Occasionally the curette will not pass through the cervix, which then has to be dilated. A 5–6 mm curette is sometimes necessary to complete the procedure. No oxytocic drugs are necessary. Patients who are rhesus negative with no antibodies should receive an injection of anti-D immunoglobulin postoperatively. For pregnancies of more than 7 weeks duration and up to 12 weeks duration the procedure is essentially similar.

A critical evaluation of menstrual extraction was performed by Stringer *et al.* [42] when 424 patients were studied. No analgesics or anaesthetics were used in 136 of these patients, and an intracervical block was used for the remainder. The pain or discomfort experienced was much less in the treated group. Twenty-nine per cent of patients were found not to be pregnant on histological examination and only 3% required a dilatation prior to curettage. The time taken for the whole procedure was 3–4 min without an anaesthetic and 7–8 with an anaesthetic. The mean time taken for the curettage itself was 2 min for pregnant patients and 2 min 20 s for non-pregnant patients. The mean volume of aspirate was 16.34 ml for pregnant patients and 3.8 ml for non-pregnant patients. An aspirate of 60 ml or more was suggestive of a pregnancy greater than 6 weeks gestation. Side-effects included nausea and vomiting in 10.4%, faintness in 3.7%, and tinnitus or dizziness in 16.5%. Complications included pyrexia in 3.4%, retained products of conception in 2.8%, and a continuing pregnancy rate of 2.6%. A laparoscopy was performed to exclude ectopic pregnancy in three patients, and minor psychological disturbances were recorded in 18%. Ninety-six per cent of the patients would not consider the method as an alternative to contraception.

First-trimester termination of pregnancy

Termination of pregnancy up to 13 weeks gestation (first trimester) is performed using suction curettage. This method is similar to menstrual extraction and may be performed under local or general anaesthesia. Dilatation is more frequently required, and a suction pump is employed as a vacuum source. The following aspects of the technique demand special consideration.

Anaesthesia

General anaesthesia is emotionally kinder to the patient but it does subject her to the small but definite risk of general anaesthesia. The time interval between the operation and discharge can be delayed. As the operation is of short duration, quick-acting general anaesthetics are used. Most general anaesthetics tend to depress uterine activity and may potentiate uterine haemorrhage. Halothane relaxes the uterus and should not be used. Ketamine, however, contracts the uterus and is therefore a useful anaesthetic agent [43]. Although oxytocics have been used routinely for patients having a general anaesthetic, it is not necessary for early gestations. Intravenous ergometrine will contract the uterus, but it makes the patient feel very nauseated.

Local anaesthetic is becoming very popular. Early reports from Lewis *et al.* 1971 [44] and subsequently by Filshie and Sanders, 1977 [45] have supported this method. The technique is suitable for pregnancies up to 12 weeks gestation. However, reports from Beekhuizen *et al.* 1982 [46] have shown that a termination of pregnancy may be performed safely up to 18–20 weeks gestation using local anaesthetic only. An intracervical block using 20 ml 0.5–1% lignocaine is used as previously described. In addition the author recommended the insertion of 5–8 ml of 0.5% lignocaine into the extraovular space to reduce the discomfort of the curette on the internal surface of the uterus [45]. Adrenaline 1:200 000 may be used with the lignocaine. This has been used by Beekhuizen *et al.* [46], who give multiple injections of local anaesthetic into the cervix and up to the internal os.

If the cervix has been prepared with cervical softening agents, less local and general anaesthetic is required.

Dilatation of the cervix

Dilatation of the cervix is usually required. This may be achieved by medical or mechanical means. Dilatation is more often required by primigravid patients than multigravid patients [45]. Too much dilatation, however, is neither necessary nor safe for the patient. Dilatation should only be performed to the size of the appropriate curette. A 6–7-mm curette is suitable for an 8-week gestation and an 8–9 mm curette is suitable for a 10-week gestation. A 10-mm curette is suitable for a 12-week gestation and a 12-mm curette for a 13–14 week gestation. Mechanical dilatation is with parallel-sided dilators (Hegar) or tapered dilators (Pratt or Hawkins–Ambler). The force needed to overcome cervical resistance is reduced using tapered dilators compared with the parallel-sided design [47]. However, tapered dilators can perforate the uterus with less force than can Hegar dilators. The tapered dilators are therefore more suited to the experienced surgeon.

Non-mechanical methods of dilating the cervix are becoming more popular, as such dilators make the procedure simple, quick, and safer for the patients, particularly primigravid patients. Cervical incompetence following traumatic cervical dilatation has been described by Kotasek [48], Stallworthy *et al.* [49], Wright *et al.* [50] and Richardson and Dixon [51]. This is thought to have been responsible for the high incidence of fetal wastage in subsequent pregnancies. Prostaglandins have been known to stimulate the upper segment of the uterus and relax the lower segment [52]. This latter property has been evaluated extensively for preoperative dilatation of the cervix (Chapter 13). Although naturally occurring prostaglandins have been used both vaginally and extra-amniotically, the analogues of prostaglandins appear to be more effective, with fewer side-effects. Cervagem, the 16, 16-dimethyl derivative is now commercially available for softening the cervix.

Laminaria tents (*Laminaria japonicum* (*digitata*)) has been traditionally used for years to dilate cervices. It absorbs water from the cervix, and swells. It has been used predominantly for dilating the cervix prior to second-trimester dilatation and evacuation of the uterus [53,54].

More recently two synthetic hygroscopic dilators have been made available, namely Lamicel and Dilapan. These are much cheaper than Cervigem. Lamicel is composed of a compressed polyvinyl alcohol sponge impregnated with 450 mg magnesium sulphate. Dilapan is made of a hygroscopic polymer and physically expands. The mechanical action of these dilators is dealt with in Chapter 13. In practice, the cervical softening agents are administered approximately 2 h prior to the operation.

Curettage

Originally the uterine cavity was curetted with a sharp curette. Fortunately, this practice has been superseded by the use of the vacuum curette. This was used in Russia by Bykow [39] and in China by T'sai [55] and Wu and Wu [56] for years before it became accepted in the United Kingdom. Thanks to Kerslake and Casey in 1967 [57] this method was introduced into the West. The original vacuum curettes were metal or glass and were reusable (Beierer and Kerslake). Now, disposable curettes are popular and are either of the flexible type (Karman) or the rigid type (Berkley). They both come in a range of sizes up to 14 mm. The curettes are introduced into the uterine cavity and are attached to the vacuum source. A negative pressure of 67–80 kPa (500–700 mmHg) is used. The products may be visualized as they pass down the curette and disposable clear tubing. The end-point of the procedure is when a grating feeling is present on all internal surfaces of the uterus. It is the recommended practice of some gynaecologists to inspect the products of conception to ensure that the abortion is complete.

Second-trimester termination of pregnancy

This term is used for patients who are in excess of 13 weeks gestation at the time of the abortion. It accounted for approximately 30% of all cases in 1967, but this figure had dropped to 14% in 1982 and is now falling only slowly. Less than 2% of all abortions are performed at 20 weeks gestation or over. Governmental concern over the large number of second-trimester terminations of pregnancy prompted them to ask the Royal College of Obstetricians and Gynaecologists to review the situation. The response resulted in a publication entitled *Late Abortion in England and Wales* published in 1984 [58]. This publication highlights the problems encountered by patients before, during, and after the procedure. The reasons for late abortion are many. Some patients refuse to accept the situation. Ignorance and ambivalence are other factors, as are problems of diagnosing congenital fetal abnormality.

It is a sad fact that many patients request a referral for an abortion before 12 weeks but are aborted much later because of deficiencies in the provision of services [18]. Nationally there is a widely differing acceptance of late abortions. Provisions of services range from over 87% within the National Health Service in the north to 20% in the west Midlands. The private sector compensates where provisions of services are lacking in the National Health Service.

Techniques of performing second-trimester termination of pregnancy are as follows:

Hysterotomy or hysterectomy

An abdominal hysterotomy was commonly practiced until nearly 15 years ago when prostaglandins became more readily available. The two types include the classical incision or the lower transverse incision (lower segment). As with a caesarean section, the classical scar is weaker than the transverse lower-segment incision as far as future pregnancies are concerned. The classical incision (a vertical incision of the anterior part of the uterus) is recommended only if a concomitant sterilization is performed. The lower transverse approach is safer, as the bleeding is reduced and the scar is retroperitoneal and therefore is less likely to be associated with subsequent adhesions. The technique should be very similar to a mini-caesarean section. Subsequent pregnancies have an outcome similar to those following a traditional caesarean section [59]. A few surgeons employ a vaginal hysterotomy technique. This could be useful if the abdomen is known to have multiple adhesions from previous operations or infections. The vaginal hysterotomy entails an anterior midline incision through the cervix, up through the internal os, and through to the upper segment for a small way after reflecting the bladder away. Products may be evacuated with forceps and the cavity subsequently curetted.

Maternal mortality is high with hysterotomy, and represents 48 per 100 000 women between the ages of 10 and 29 and 70 per 100 000 for women of 30–49 [60].

Hysterectomy is only rarely performed. Indications are mainly those of coexistant large fibroids or cervical carcinoma.

Intravenous prostaglandins

Karim and Filshie first used prostaglandins $F_{2\alpha}$ and E_2 intravenously for therapeutic termination of pregnancy [61,62]. Similar results were obtained by others [63–69]. The method is associated with a high incidence of side-effects such as nausea, vomiting, and diarrhoea. Because of the side-effects the intra-amniotic or extraovular routes have been used. The dose of $PGF_{2\alpha}$ is 50 μg/min and of PGE_2 is 5 μg/min. The method is occasionally used when other routes have failed and when the patient has a missed abortion.

Intra-amniotic injections

Hypertonic saline. This method was popular prior to the advent of prostaglandins and is still relatively popular in the USA. The method is preferably used when the gestation is 16 weeks or more, as before this the amniotic sac is difficult to enter and the volume of amniotic fluid is insufficient for transfer [70]. The technique involves insertion of a Tuohy needle into the amniotic sac using local anaesthesia. This is achieved by choosing a point midway between the fundus of the uterus and the symphysis pubis. Lignocaine 1% (5 ml) is injected subdermally and through the layers of the abdomen into the uterus. A Tuohy 16 French gauge needle is inserted vertically into the amniotic sac. Two hundred millilitres of amniotic fluid is withdrawn using a 50 ml syringe via a three-way tap. Ensuring a constant reflux of amniotic fluid, 200 ml 22.5% hypertonic saline is slowly instilled, and the Tuohy needle is removed. Alternatively, an epidural catheter can be placed into the amniotic cavity and the hypertonic saline slowly injected with a pump over several hours.

Throughout the infusion the patient should be observed, to check that the hypertonic saline has not been inadvertently misdirected into the placenta, myometrium, or peritoneal cavity. If the hypertonic saline is absorbed systematically, the patient may compalin of continuous abdominal pain, feeling a salty taste on her tongue, and may experience palor and tingling of the extremities. If any of these symptoms occur the infusion should be immediately discontinued and 5% dextrose infused intravenously. The intra-amniotic infusion should also be discontinued if reflux does not occur or if the tap becomes bloody. The induction/abortion interval can be reduced by giving intravenous oxytocin, although care must be taken to avoid water intoxication [71].

The hypertonic saline has a substantial effect on the patient. There is an increase in amniotic fluid [72–74] and the placenta becomes oedematous, and widespread thrombosis and infarction occurs. The fetus usually dies *in utero*. Maternal deaths have been reported from Japan [75] and the UK [76]. Most of these are due to inadvertent injection of saline into the wrong place. Cerebral infarction is the cause of death.

In large comparative studies in the USA between intra-amniotic prostaglandins and hypertonic saline, very little difference was observed between the two methods [77]. Fever, endometritis and retained products of conception were noted to be higher in the prostaglandin group than in the saline group, but there was no difference in in-patient hospital time. Endocrine changes appeared to be similar in both groups.

In New York State, Berger (1974) [78] reported 11 deaths in 56 274 hypertonic saline procedures (19.5 per 100 000), which was 8 times that reported from suction or sharp curettage.

Intra-amniotic prostaglandins. Intra-amniotic injections of prostaglandins are appealing because of their simplicity of use and reduction of side-effects. Intra-amniotic $PGF_{2\alpha}$ and PGE_2 have been used extensively since 1971 [79–97] and have eclipsed the use of hypertonic saline in the USA.

Intra-amniotic injections may be performed with any needle suitable for amnocentesis (18–20 French gauge). One of the drawbacks of the method, however, is the failed tap, i.e. when an unsuccessful attempt has been made to enter the amniotic cavity, which occurs in approximately 5% of cases. As with hypertonic saline, patients can be mobilized without an intravenous infusion. Both naturally occurring prostaglandins and their analogues are used.

Side-effects of prostaglandins are very much less than with the intravenous route. Following the injection, the uterus enters a phase of hypertonus which occasionally results in premature rupture of the membranes and loss of fluid and medication. The abortion then has to be completed by using either intramuscular or intravenous injections of prostaglandins. If the abortion has not occurred after 12–24 h, a repeat intra-amniotic injection may be given. Intravenous oxytocin may also be given to shorten the induction–abortion interval. The dose of prostaglandins used are: $PGF_{2\alpha}$: 15 mg [84], 40–50 mg [80,82–84] or 100 mg [87–98]. The dose of PGE_2 is 5–10 mg. The 15-methyl analogue of $PGF_{2\alpha}$ and E_2 is from 2.5–5 mg [99–102].

Other intra-amniotic injections. In an attempt to reduce the dangers of hypertonic saline, hypertonic urea has been used [103–105]. The induction–abortion interval is 30–100 h, and oxytocin is also recommended. Care must be taken to avoid water intoxication. Glucose [106–108], alcohol [109], fructose and mannitol [104] have all been tried and found to be less effective than the prostaglandins; they are also associated with a higher infection rate.

Extraovular instillation

The extraovular route is one of the oldest routes used and has been used both legally and illegally (e.g. Higginson's syringe and soapy water!). More recently, soft soaps and pastes (Utas paste) have been used by Barns [110] and Lachelin [111]. Sood [112], however, reported a high incidence of infection and one death due to a ruptured uterus. This fact, together with the risk of embolus, has put the method into disrepute. Ethacridine lactate (Rivanol), is safer and has been used extensively in Japan [113] and Sweden [114] with very favourable results. One hundred and fifty millilitres of 0.1% solution is instilled slowly via a Foley catheter, and repeated when necessary. Intravenous oxytocin helps to reduce the induction–abortion interval. As Rivanol is a mild antiseptic the incidence of infection is reduced. Hypertonic saline has also been given by the extraovular route. This method is not as effective as the intra-amniotic route [115].

Prostaglandins. Wiqvist and Bygdeman [116] report that side-effects of prostaglandins could be dramatically reduced if the prostaglandins could be positioned close to the target organ. Similar reports were made by Embrey and Hillier [117] and Lauersen and Wilson [118,119]. The prostaglandins were instilled by Foley catheter and infused at a rate of 100–200 μg of PGE_2/h or 375 μg $PGF_{2\alpha}$/h. Alternatively, a bolus dose can be injected every 2 h if an infusion pump is not available. Midwinter *et al.* [120] recommended an infusion rate of 66.5 μg/h. $PGF_{2\alpha}$ appeared to produce more side-effects than PGE_2 [121].

The 15-methyl analogue $PGF_{2\alpha}$ has been used by Bygdeman *et al.* [122] and by the WHO task force [123,124]. The action of the analogue is prolonged and the mean induction–abortion interval is 14.5 h (range 6.3–27.7 h) [122].

A new combination of prostaglandin E_2 and oxytocin has been used for years in Nottingham, with favourable results. The addition of the oxytocin to the infusion avoids the necessity of a routine intravenous drip.

The value of the extraovular route is that it is an easily mastered technique, and it is also likely that over a period of time the presence of a foreign body in the cervix may augment the procedure. However, to have a foreign body in cases of a prolonged induction–abortion interval may well promote infection and endometritis [119].

Intravaginal route. In 1971 Karim and Sharma [125] reported the successful use of prostaglandins vaginally for second-trimester termination of pregnancy. Both PGE_2 and $PGF_{2\alpha}$ were used. Bolognese and Corson [126] and Lauersen *et al.* [127] confirmed these results. This route seems satisfactory for intrauterine fetal death [128,129]. More recently Cervagem [130] has been used for mid-trimester termination of pregnancy [131,132].

Intramuscular route. The intramuscular route using naturally occurring prostaglandins is painful and ineffective. However, the analogues, including the 15-(S)-15-methyl PGE_2 or $E_{2\alpha}$ [133–139] and 16-phenoxy-ω-17,18,19,20-tetranor PGE_2 methyl sulphonylamide [140–142] have been used successfully. The 15-(S)-15-methyl $PGF_{2\alpha}$ was given in doses of 100–200 μg injections every 2–4 h, and the 16-phenoxy-ω-17,18,19,20 tetranor PGE_2 methyl sulphonylamide in doses of 0.5–1 mg 4–8-hourly. The intramuscular route is particularly useful when premature rupture of membranes occurs, whether spontaneously or with either the intra-amniotic or the extraovular route.

Dilatation and evacuation

This method, which is also known as aspirotomy [46], entails dilating the cervix up to at least 10–12 Hegar and evacuating the uterine contents. This method has been used up to 20 or more weeks gestation. Adequate dilatation of the cervix is essential, and this can be achieved by the use of laminaria tents, Lamicel or Dilapan preoperatively. The operation can be performed under local or general anaesthesia. A paracervical or an intracervical block with local anaesthesia is recommended; adrenaline 1:200 000 can help to cut down the blood loss. The technique involves first rupturing the membranes and draining off the liquor. The umbilical cord usually prolapses at this stage and can be cut, thus exsanguinating the fetus. The placenta can then be evacuated by aspirotomy forceps. Finally, the fetus is evacuated piecemeal. The caput is the most difficult part to expel. Most centres who perform aspirotomy have ultrasound to check that the uterus is empty at the end of the procedure. The technique has been well reviewed by Hern [143], Beekhuizen *et al.* [46], Grimes *et al.* [144] and Stubblefield [145].

Comparative studies in the United States by the Joint Program for the Study of Abortion (Center for Disease Control, 1977) [146] have shown that when correctly performed this method has a very low complication rate (0.69 per hundred cases as compared with 1.81 and 2.9 for hypertonic saline and intra-amniotic $PGF_{2\alpha}$ respectively).

The method has many advantages for the patient. It is quick and safe. However, it is an unpleasant procedure for the physician, who is therefore not overenthusiastic to learn the technique.

Complications of abortion

Generally speaking abortion is a relatively safe procedure when performed correctly.

The morbidity and mortality increase with the gestation of pregnancy, the highest mortality being when hysterectomy is employed which is fortunately only rarely. The more experienced the surgeon, the fewer the complications [21]. This may be one of the reasons that complications in the private sector, where experienced surgeons operate, are fewer than in the National Health Service, where operations are performed by all grades of training gynaecologists. The overall mortality has been reduced to less than 2 per 100 000. Nevertheless, morbidity can occur, and may be either early or late.

Early complications

Retained products of conception. These present as a heavy vaginal blood loss, associated with lower abdominal pain. The incidence varies from 0.4% to 2.9% [147–150] in the first trimester, and may be as much as four times this after 12 weeks gestation [148]. The rate of retained products can be reduced by scanning the patient at the end of the procedure, but this practice is rarely performed. The treatment is by repeating the curettage. It is good practice to cover the procedure by a broad-spectrum antibiotic.

Haemorrhage. This may be due to cervical trauma, uterine perforation, or uterine atony. Blood loss increases with gestation, and a loss of 500 ml is regarded as significant. It has been reported as 1 out of 400 procedures by Stone *et al.* [149] and as 6% by Loung *et al.* [150]. Uterine atony can be treated by intravenous oxytocin or ergometrine. Sometimes the uterus fills up with blood and needs re-evacuating. Oxytocin and bimanual compression may also be required. Mortality from haemorrhage is approximately 0.21 per 100 000. If bleeding is persistent, a laparotomy should be performed and the internal iliac arteries ligated. A hysterectomy should be performed if this fails.

Andolsek *et al.* [151] showed that postoperative heavy bleeding over the following 7 days occurred in 2.5% of patients in Singapore and 8.5% in Ljubljana.

Uterine perforation. The incidence of uterine perforation varies between 0.04% and 1.7% [49,152,153], although in this condition there is an element of under-diagnosing and therefore the incidence may well be higher. The pregnant uterus is soft, and perforation occurs easily. Perforation may be caused by a uterine sound, which is not recommended with this procedure. Cervical dilators or the evacuating curette may also perforate the uterus. The main problem is to recognize the event and to ensure that the uterus is empty. A simple perforation may be managed conservatively by more frequent observations of the pulse and blood pressure following the operation. An intravenous line should be installed in case fluid replacement is required. If the perforation is complicated, for instance by curetting bowel or by withdrawing the bowel with ovum forceps, then a laparotomy is indicated. The damaged bowel should be repaired or resected and the uterine rent oversewn. where doubt exists as to whether any internal damage has been done, a laparoscopy should be performed. Care should be taken to ensure the uterus is empty at the end of the procedure.

Cervical trauma. The epithelium over the cervix is often traumatized during dilatation, and may require a suture to control the bleeding. Laceration of the substance of the cervix from overzealous dilatation is also a frequent occurrence, particularly with young primigravid patients. These tears are usually at the 3 and 9 o'clock positions, and occur in 7% of cases [154]. This type of trauma can be reduced by the use of preoperative cervical ripening agents. When laceration is recognized it should be repaired.

The cervix may also be traumatized by creating a false passage through its substance and into the myometrium. In rare cases the uterus has been ruptured into the posterior fornix and the products of conception expelled through the rent. This happens particularly when prostaglandin or hypertonic saline installations have been used in combination with oxytocin [155–158]. Uterine rupture is a very unusual event following the extraovular technique used in association with a Foley catheter.

Sepsis. Approximately 5% of all patients having an early termination of pregnancy have sepsis as a complication [48]. This figure increases to approximately 10% in the second trimester. Most cases of pelvic sepsis are due to retained products of conception. The treatment is to give a broad-spectrum antibiotic and to re-evacuate the uterus. Endometritis may still occur in the absence of retained products of conception, in which case the organisms responsible may be those residing in the vagina and include, in some patients, *Neisseria gonorrhoeae*, *Escherichia coli*, *Chlamydia trachomatis*, *Bacteroides* and rarely *Clostridium welchii*, all of which may be present in the vagina or cervical canal. Most of these patients will respond to antibiotics, but in severe infections intravenous antibiotics, e.g. ampicillin and streptomycin with intravenous fluids and oxygen will be required. Anti-clostridium serum may also be needed where appropriate. Occasionally a hysterectomy may be required to remove a gangrenous organ.

Failed termination of pregnancy. Very occasionally, particularly if the procedure is undertaken at a very early gestation [42], the decidua only may be evacuated, and the conceptus not dislodged. Such a patient may continue her pregnancy for many months and may either abort spontaneously or continue to term. It is for this reason that all women undergoing abortion should have a follow-up check that the pregnancy has indeed been terminated [159].

Long-term sequelae following termination of pregnancy

Cervical incompetence. This results in future mid-trimester abortions or premature labour [48–51]. These problems were reported in a recent study from the Royal College of General Practitioners and the Royal College of Obstetricians [160]. The problem is particularly common in primigravid patients. The complication could be eliminated if cervical softening agents were used prior to termination, although long-term studies are yet to be conducted to confirm the hypothesis.

Chronic pelvic inflammatory disease and subfertility. This may occur without obvious symptoms. The incidence has been recorded as 25%, although this appears particularly high [48]. Other studies have shown the incidence to be more like 2.5% [161]. These patients may have a low-grade infection which is only recognized later when they attend the subfertility clinic. Damaged tubes may be diagnosed at subsequent laparoscopy and hydrotubation. Intrauterine adhesions may cause subfertility and may be diagnosed by hysterosalpingography [162].

Subsequent light-for-dates infants. Subsequent pregnancies have a higher incidence of being light for dates [163]. The cause of this phenomenon is not clear.

Rhesus Isoimmunization. This may occur in rhesus negative patients. Anti-D has substantially eliminated this problem.

Ectopic pregnancy. A higher incidence of ectopic pregnancy is reported after a termination [164]. This is thought to be a consequence of subsequent pelvic inflammatory disease, which occurs in a number of patients. The incidence of ectopic pregnancy appears to be rising [165].

Psychiatric sequelae. The decision to have a termination of pregnancy is usually harrowing for the patient. It is often the only appropriate solution to her problem, even though it may be the lesser of two difficult situations. The feeling of guilt is almost universal and some patients experience a form of postabortion depression. However, long-term psychiatric sequelae necessitating hospital admission is very rare [166]. The problem may be minimized if pretermination counselling is performed sympathetically and adequately. A sympathetic attitude should be adopted by both the nursing and the medical staff on the ward. It is clearly undesirable for a patient to be seen in a gynaecological clinic or on a gynaecological ward, side by side with infertility patients. A specially designed termination clinic with adequate counselling facilities and sympathetic staff is to be recommended. A postoperative abortion counselling service should be available, e.g. Abortions Anonymous where the patients can discuss their feelings and fears.

References

1. JAMES, W. H. The incidence of spontaneous abortion. *Population Studies*, **24**, 241 (1970)
2. POTTER, R. G., WYON, J. B., NEW, M. and GORDON, J. E. Fetal wastage in 11 punjab villages. *Human Biology*, **37**, 262 (1965)
3. DEVEREUX, G. A typological study of abortion in 350 primitive, ancient and pre-industrial societies. In *Abortion in America* (ed. H. Rosen), Beacon Press, Boston, pp 97–152 (1967)
4. GODBER, G. Recent progress and future aims in obstetrics. *Journal of Obstetrics and Gynaecology of the British Commonwealth*, **78**, 193 (1971)
5. DAVID, H. *Abortion Research: International Experience*. Lexington DC Health, pp. 109–226 (1974)
6. MUMFORD, S. D. and KESSEL, E. Role of abortion in control of global population growth. *Clinics in Obstetrics and Gynaecology*, **13** (1), 19–31 (1986)
7. TIETZE, C. *Induced Abortion: A World Review*, 5th edn., Population Council, New York, pp. 116 (1983)
8. TIEN, H., WAN, X. I. and SHAO. How China meets its population problem. *International Family Planning Perspectives*, **6**, 65–69 (1980)
9. ANONYMOUS. *The Global 2000 Report to the President Entering the 21st Century*. US Government Printing Office, Washington DC, p. 1 (1980)
10. MCNAMARA, R. *Address to the Massachusetts Institute of Technology* April 1977. World Bank, Washington DC (1977)
11. CHANDRASEKHAR, S. Abortion in a crowded world. University of Washington Press, Seattle, p. 184 (1974)
12. CALLAHAN, D. *Abortion Law: Choice and Mortality*. McMillan, New York, p. 524 (1970)
13. MOHR, J. *Abortion in America. The Origins and Evolution of National Policy 1800–1900*. Oxford University Press, New York, p. 343 (1978)
14. DAVID, H. P. The abortion decision: national and international perspectives. In *Abortion Parley* (ed. J. P. Burchael), Andrew and McMeel, Kansas City, pp. 57–98 (1980)
15. 43 Geo IIIc 1803
17. *Day Case Abortion and the National Health Service* (eds. D. Cossey and P. Diggory), Birth Control Trust, London (1980)
18. ALBERMAN, E. and DENNIS, K. J. *Later Abortions in England and Wales. Report of a National Confidential Study*, Royal College of Obstetricians and Gynaecologists, Chameleon Press, pp. 29–35 (1984)
19. OPCS Statistics.
20. SIMS, M. *Report on Non-Medical Abortion Counselling*, Birth Control Trust, London (1973)
21. HULL, M. G. R., GORDON, C. and BEARD, R. W. Organisation and results of a pregnancy termination service in a National Health Service Hospital. *Journal of Obstetrics and Gynaecology of the British Commonwealth*, **81**, 173–181 (1974)

22. KARIM, S. M. M. Once a month administration of prostaglandin E_2 and $F_{2\alpha}$ for fertility control. *Contraception*, **3**, 173–181 (1971)
23. CORLETT, R. C., SRIBYATTA, B., MISHELL, D. R. *et al.* Termination of early gestation with vaginal prostaglandin $F_{2\alpha}$. *Prostaglandins*, **2**, 453–464 (1972)
24. BOLOGNESE, R. J. and CORSON, S. L. Abortion of early pregnancy by the intra-vaginal administration of prostaglandin $F_{2\alpha}$. *American Journal of Obstetrics and Gynecology*, **117**, 246–250 (1973)
25. FREID, N. D., TREDWAY, D. R. and MISHELL, D. R. Termination of early pregnancy with prostaglandin E_2 vaginal suppository. *Contraception*, **8**, 255–263 (1973)
26. CSAPO, A. I., RUTTNER, B. and WIEST, W. G. First trimester abortion induced by a single extra-ovular injection of prostaglandin $F_{2\alpha}$. *Prostaglandins*, **1**, 365–371 (1972)
27. KARIM, S. M. M. Intrauterine prostaglandins for out-patient termination of very early pregnancy. *Lancet*, **2**, 794 (1973)
28. KARIM, S. M. M., RAO, R., RATNAM, S. S. *et al.* Termination of early pregnancy (menstrual induction) with 16-phenoxy-ω-tetranor-PGE_2 methylsulfonylamide. *Contraception*, **16**, 377–381 (1977)
29. CSAPO, A. I. and PULKKINEN, M. G. The mechanism of action of prostaglandin action on the early pregnant human uterus. *Prostaglandins*, **18**, 479–490 (1979)
30. CSAPO, A. I., PESKIN, E. G., SAUVAGE, J. P. *et al.* Menstrual induction in preference to abortion. (Letter). *Lancet*, **1**, 90–91 (1980)
31. FLEISCHER, A., SCHULMAN, H., BLATTNER, P. *et al.* Early pregnancy-abortion model using sulprostone. *Prostaglandins*, **23**, 643–655 (1983)
32. BYGDEMAN, M., CHRISTENSEN, N. J., GREEN, K. *et al.* Termination of early pregnancy: future development. *Acta Obstetricia et Gynecologica Scandinavica* [Suppl.] **113**, 125–129 (1983)
33. MACKENZIE, I. Z., EMBREY, M. P., DAVIES, A. J. and GUILLEBAUD, J. Very early abortion by prostaglandins. *Lancet*, **1**, 1223–1226 (1978)
34. KARIM, S. M. M., RATNAM, S. S. and ILANCHERAN, A. Menstrual induction with vaginal administration of 16,16 dimethyl transΔ^2-PGE_1 methyl ester (ONO-802). *Prostaglandins*, **14**, 615–616 (1977)
35. WRIGHT, C. Trilostane for the medical induction of first trimester abortion. In *Inyanga (Proceedings of C.T. ISO Anniversary Meeting, University of Capetown* (ed. J. Taylor), Medical Students' Council, Capetown, pp. 119 (1979)
36. BAULIEU, E. E. Contragestion by anti-progestin: A new approach to fertility control. In *Abortion: Medical Progress and Social Implications.* Ciba Foundation Symposium 115, Pitman Publishing, London, pp. 192–206 (1985)
37. CAMERON, I. T., MICHIE, A. F. and BAIRD, D. T. Therapeutic abortion in early pregnancy with antiprogestogen RU486 alone or with a prostaglandin analogue (Gemprost). *Contraception*, **34**, 459–468 (1986)
38. SWAHN, M. L. and BYGDEMAN, M. Menstrual regulation. *Prostaglandin Perspectives*, **2** (1), 6–8 (1985)
39. BYKOW, E. Aspiration of the gravid uterus. *Vrachebnoe Delo*, **9**, 21 (1927)
40. KARMAN, H. and POTTS, M. Very early abortion using a syringe as a vacuum source. *Lancet*, **1**, 1051–1052 (1972)
41. LEWIS, S. C. Vacuum termination of pregnancy. *British Medical Journal*, **4**, 365 (1971)
42. STRINGER, J., ANDERSON, M., BEARD, R. W. *et al.* Very early termination of pregnancy (Menstrual extraction). *British Medical Journal*, **3**, 7–9 (1975)
43. OATS, J. J. N., VASEY, D. D. and WALDRON, B. A. The effect of ketamine on the pregnant uterus. *British Journal of Anaesthesia*, **51** (12), 1163–1166 (1979)
44. LEWIS, S. C., LAL, S., BRANCH, B. and BEARD, R. W. Out-patient termination of pregnancy. *British Medical Journal*, **4**, 606–610 (1971)
45. FILSHIE, G. M. and SANDERS, R. R. Out-patient termination of pregnancy. *British Journal of Obstetrics and Gynaecology*, **84** (7), 509–513 (1977)
46. BEEKHUIZEN, W., VAN SCHIE, K. J., VAN LITH, D. A. F. *et al.* Aspirotomy for out-patient termination of pregnancy in the second trimester. In *Second Trimester Pregnancy Termination*, (ed. M. J. Kierse, N. L. Bennebrok, J. Gravenhurse *et al.*), London University Press, The Hague, pp. 52 (1982)
47. HULKA, J. F., LEFLER, H. T. JR., ANGLONE, A. and LACHENBRUCH, P. A. A new electronic force monitor to measure factors influencing cervical dilatation for vacuum curettage. *American Journal of Obstetrics and Gynecology*, **120** (2), 166–173 (1974)

48. KOTASEK, A. Artificial termination of pregnancy in Czechoslovakia. *International Journal of Gynaecology and Obstetrics*, **9**, 118–119 (1971)

49. STALLWORTHY, J. A., MOOLGAOKER, A. S. and WALSH, J. J. Legal abortion: a critical assessment of its risks. *Lancet*, **2**, 1245–1249 (1971)

50. WRIGHT, C. S. W., CAMPBELL, S. and BEAZLEY, J. Second trimester abortion after vaginal termination of pregnancy. *Lancet*, **1**, 1278–1279 (1972)

51. RICHARDSON, J. A. and DIXON, G. Effects of legal termination on subsequent pregnancy. *British Medical Journal*, **1**, 1303–1304 (1976)

52. NAJAK, Z., HILLIER, K. and KARIM, S. M. M. The action of prostaglandins on the human isolated non-pregnant cervix. *Journal of Obstetrics and Gynaecology of the British Commonwealth*, **77**, 701 (1970)

53. GRIMES, D. A., SCHULZ, K. F., CATES, W. JR. and TYLER, C. W. Mid-trimester abortion by dilatation and evacuation: a safe and practical alternative. *New England Journal of Medicine*, **296**, 1141–1145 (1977)

54. HERN, W. M. and OAKES, A. G. Multiple laminaria treatment in early mid-trimester out-patient suction abortion: a preliminary report. *Advances in Planned Parenthood*, **12**, 93 (1977)

55. TSAI, K. I. Application of electric vacuum suction in artificial abortions. 30 cases. *Chinese Journal of Obstetrics and Gynecology*, **6**, 445 (1958)

56. WU–YUAN–TAI and WU–HSEIN–CHEN. Suction curettage for artificial abortions. Preliminary report of 300 cases. *Chinese Journal of Obstetrics and Gynecology*, **6**, 447 (1958)

57. KERSLAKE, D. and CASEY, D. Abortion induced by means of the uterine aspiratoı. *Obstetrics and Gynecology (NY)*, **30**, 35 (1967)

58. Report of the National Confidential Study: Royal College of Obstetricians & Gynaecologists. (eds E. Alberman and K. J. Dennis), *Late Abortion in England and Wales 1984*. The Chameleon Press (1984)

59. CLOW, W. M. and CROMPTON, A. The wounded uterus: pregnancy after hysterotomy. *British Medical Journal*, **1**, 321–323 (1973)

60. Committee on the Working of the Abortion Act (1974). Report, I HMSO, London p. 45 (1974)

61. KARIM, S. M. M. and FILSHIE, G. M. Therapeutic abortion using prostaglandin $F_{2\alpha}$. *Lancet*, **i**, 157–159 (1970)

62. KARIM, S. M. M. and FILSHIE, G. M. Use of prostaglandin $F_{2\alpha}$ for therapeutic abortion. *British Medical Journal*, **3**, 198–200 (1970)

63. ROTH–BRANDEL, U., BYGDEMAN, M., WIQVIST, N. and BERGSTROM, S. Prostaglandins for induction of therapeutic abortion. *Lancet*, **1**, 190 (1970)

64. WIQVIST, N. and BYGDEMAN, M. Induction of therapeutic abortion with intravenous prostaglandin $F_{2\alpha}$. *Lancet*, **2**, 889 (1970)

65. BYGDEMAN, M. and WIQVIST, N. Early abortion in the human. *Annals of the New York Academy of Sciences*, **180**, 473–482 (1971)

66. WIQVIST, N., BYGDEMAN, M. and TOPPOZADA, M. Induction of abortion by the intravenous administration of prostaglandin $F_{2\alpha}$. A critical evaluation. *Acta Obstetricia et Gynecologica Scandinavica*, **50**, 381–389 (1971)

67. KINOSHITA, K., WAGATSUMA, T., HOGAKI, M. and SAKAMOTO, S. The induction of abortion by prostaglandin $F_{2\alpha}$. *American Journal of Obstetrics and Gynecology*, **111**, 855–858 (1971)

68. HASPELS, A. A. and LUIGIES, J. H. H. Induction of abortion by intravenous and intrauterine administration of prostaglandin $F_{2\alpha}$. In *The Prostaglandins*, (ed. E. M. Southern), Futura, Mount Kisco, NY, pp. 433–441 (1972)

69. WENTZ, A. C. and JONES, G. S. Intravenous prostaglandin $F_{2\alpha}$ for induction of menses. *Fertility and Sterility*, **24**, 569–577 (1973)

70. REISS, H. E. Methods and dangers of termination of pregnancy. *Proceedings of the Royal Society of Medicine*, **62**, 832–833 (1969)

71. LAUERSON, N. H. and BIRNBAUM, S. J. Water intoxication associated with oxytocin administration during saline induced abortion. *American Journal of Obstetrics and Gynecology*, **121**, 2–6 (1975)

72. GOCHBERG, S. H. and REID, D. E. Intra-amniotic injection of hypertonic saline for termination of pregnancy. *Obstetrics and Gynecology (NY)*, **27**. 648–654 (1966)

73. WAGNER, G. Intrauterine volume after intraovular instillation of hypertonic saline. *Acta Obstetricia et Gynecologica Scandinavica*, **50** [Supplement 9], 44 (1971)

74. KERENYI, T. D. and MUZSNAI, D. Volume and sodium concentration studies in 300 saline induced abortions. *American Journal of Obstetrics and Gynecology*, **121**, 590–595 (1975)

75. WAGATSUMA, T. Intra-amniotic injection of saline for therapeutic abortion. *American Journal of Obstetrics and Gynecology*, **93**, 743–745 (1965)
76. CAMERON, J. M. and DAYAN, A. D. Association of brain damage with therapeutic abortion induced by amniotic fluid replacement: report of two cases. *British Medical Journal*, **1**, 1010–1013 (1966)
77. LAUERSEN, N. H., WILSON, K. H., BELING, C. G. and FUCHS, F. Comparison of prostaglandin $F_{2\alpha}$ and hypertonic saline for induction of mid-trimester abortion. *American Journal of Obstetrics and Gynecology*, **120**. 875–889 (1974)
78. BERGER, G. S., TIETZE, C., PAKTER, J. and KATZ, S. H. Maternal mortality associated with legal abortion in New York State: July 1 1970–June 30 1972. *Obstetrics and Gynecology (NY)*, **43**, 315–326 (1974)
79. LAUERSEN, N. H. Investigation of prostaglandins for abortion. *Acta Obstetricia et Gynecologica Scandinavica*, [Suppl.], **81**, 1–36 (1979)
80. ANDERSON, G. G., HOBBINS, J. C., RAJKOVIC, V. *et al.* Mid-trimester abortion using intra-amniotic prostaglandin $F_{2\alpha}$. *Prostaglandins*, **1**, 147–155 (1972)
81. KARIM, S. M. M., SHARMA, S. D. and FILSHIE, G. M. Termination of second trimester pregnancy with intra-amniotic administration of prostaglandins E_2 and $F_{2\alpha}$. In *The Prostaglandins – Clinical Applications in Human Reproduction*, (ed. E. M. Southern), Futura, Mount Kisco, NY, pp. 403–416 (1972)
82. BERGSTROM, S. *Prostaglandins in Fertility Control (3)*, WHO Research and Training Centre on Human Reproduction, Stockholm (1973)
83. BRENNER, W. E., DINGFELDER, J. R., HENDRICKS, C. H. and STAUROVSKY, L. Induction of therapeutic abortion with a single dose of intra-amniotically administered prostaglandin $F_{2\alpha}$. *Prostaglandins*, **4**, 485–498 (1973)
84. BRENNER, W. E., HENDRICKS, C. H., FISHBURNE, J. I. JR. *et al.* Intra-amniotic prostaglandin $F_{2\alpha}$ dose twenty four hour abortifacient response. *Journal of Pharmaceutical Sciences*, **62**, 1278–1282 (1973)
85. CRAFT, I. Intra-amniotic prostaglandin E_2 and $F_{2\alpha}$ for induction of abortion: a dose-response study. *Journal of Obstetrics and Gynaecology of the British Commonwealth*, **80**, 46–47 (1973)
86. ROBERTS, G., GOMERSALL, R., ADAMS, M. and TURNBULL, A. C. Therapeutic abortion by intra-amniotic injection of prostaglandins. *Biosciences*, **9**, 555–560 (1973)
87. WIQVIST, N., BYGDEMAN, M. and TOPPOZADA, M. Intra-amniotic prostaglandin administration – a challenge to the currently used methods for induction of mid-trimester abortion. *Contraception*, **8**, 113–131 (1973)
88. CORLETT, R. C. JR. and BALLARD, C. A. The induction of mid-trimester abortion with intra-amniotic prostaglandin $F_{2\alpha}$. A single dose technique. *American Journal of Obstetrics and Gynecology*, **118**, 353–357 (1974)
89. LAUERSEN, N. H. and WILSON, K. H. Mid-trimester abortion induced with a single intra-amniotic instillation of prostaglandin $F_{2\alpha}$. *American Journal of Obstetrics and Gynecology*, **118**, 210–217 (1974)
90. BRENNER, W. E. The current status of prostaglandins as abortificients. *American Journal of Obstetrics and Gynecology*, **123**, 306–328 (1975)
91. KAJANOJA, P., JUNGER, G., SEPPALA, M. *et al.* Prostaglandin induction of mid-trimester abortions: three years' experience of 626 cases. *Acta Obstetricia et Gynaecologica Scandinavica*, [Suppl], **37**, 51 (1975)
92. ANDERSON, G. G. and STEAGE, J. F. Clinical experience using intra-amniotic prostaglandin $F_{2\alpha}$ for mid-trimester abortion in 600 patients. *Obstetrics and Gynecology (NY)*, **46**, 591–595 (1975)
93. BHATT, R. V., PATEL, N. F., PATHAK, CHAUHAN, L. and BHIWANDIWALA, P. Prostaglandins in mid-trimester termination of pregnancy – a comparative study. In *Obstetric and Gynecological Uses of Prostaglandins* (ed. S. M. M. Karim), University Park Press, Baltimore, pp. 171–174 (1976)
94. RAGAB, M. I. and EDELMAN, D. A. Mid-trimester abortion: a comparison of intra-amniotic prostaglandin $F_{2\alpha}$ and hypertonic saline. *International Journal of Obstetrics and Gynaecology*, **14**, 393–396 (1976)
95. WHO Task Force on the Use of Prostaglandins for the Regulation of Fertility. Prostaglandins and abortion 3. Comparison of single intra-amniotic injections of 15-methyl prostaglandin $F_{2\alpha}$ and prostaglandin $F_{2\alpha}$ for termination of second trimester pregnancy: An international multi-center study. *American Journal of Obstetrics and Gynecology*, **129**, 601–605 (1977)
96. KAJANOJA, P. Induction of abortion by prostaglandins in the second trimester of pregnancy. *Acta Obstetricia et Gynaecologica Scandinavica*, [Suppl.] **113**, 145–151 (1983)
97. LANGE, A. P. Prostaglandins as abortifacients in Denmark. *Acta Obstetricia et Gynaecologica Scandinavica*, [Suppl.] **113**, 117–124 (1983)

98. CORSON, S. L., BOLOGNESE, R. J. and MEROLA, J. Intra-amniotic prostaglandin to induce mid-trimester abortion. *American Journal of Obstetrics and Gynecology*, **117**, 27–34 (1973)
99. KARIM, S. M. M. and SHARMA, S. D. Second trimester abortion with single intra-amniotic injection of prostaglandins E_2 and $F_{2\alpha}$. *Lancet*, **2**, 47–48 (1973)
100. KARIM, S. M. M., SHARMA, S. D. and FILSHIE, G. M. Termination of pregnancy with 15-methyl analogues of prostaglandins E_2 and $F_{2\alpha}$. *Journal of Reproductive Medicine*, **9**, 383–391 (1972)
101. AMY, J. J., KARIM, S. M. M. and SIVASAMBOO, R. Intra-amniotic administration of prostaglandin 15(S)15 methyl-E_2 methyl ester for termination of pregnancy. *Journal of Obstetrics and Gynaecology of the British Commonwealth*, **80**, 1017–1020 (1973)
102. WIQVIST, N., BYGDEMAN, M. and TOPPOZADA, M. Intra-amniotic prostaglandin administration – a challenge to the currently used methods for induction of mid-trimester abortion. *Contraception*, **8**, 113–131 (1973)
103. GREENHALF, J. O. and DIGGORY, P. L. C. Induction of therapeutic abortion by intra-amniotic injection of urea. *British Medical Journal*, **1**, 28–29 (1971)
104. CRAFT, I. L. and MUSA, B. D. Induction of mid-trimester therapeutic abortion by intra-amniotic urea and intravenous oxytocin. *Lancet*, **2**, 1058–1060 (1971)
105. PUGH, M., KHUNDA, S. and BALDWIN, R. Induction of therapeutic abortion with urea. *British Medical Journal*, **1**, 345 (1971)
106. WOOD, C., BOOTH, R. T. and PINKERTON, J. H. M. Induction of labour by intra-amniotic injection of hypertonic glucose solution. *British Medical Journal*, **2**, 706–709 (1962)
107. MENZIES, D. N. and HAWKINS, D. F. Therapeutic abortion using intra-amniotic hypertonic solutions. *Journal of Obstetrics and Gynaecology of the British Commonwealth*, **75**, 215–218 (1968)
108. DROEGEMUELLER, W. and GREER, B. E. Saline versus glucose as a hypertonic solution for abortion. *American Journal of Obstetrics and Gynecology*, **108**, 606–609 (1970)
109. GOMEL, V. and CARPENTER, C. W. Induction of mid-trimester abortion with intra-uterine alcohol. *Obstetrics and Gynecology (NY)*, **41**, 455–458 (1973)
110. BARNS, H. H. F. Therapeutic abortion by means of soft soap pastes. *Lancet*, **2**, 825–827 (1947)
111. LACHELIN, G. C. L. and BURGESS, D. E. Therapeutic abortion using Utus paste. *Journal of Obstetrics and Gynaecology of the British Commonwealth*, **75**, 1173–1175 (1968)
112. SOOD, W. V. Some operative and post-operative hazards of legal termination of pregnancy. *British Medical Journal*, **4**, 270–273 (1971)
113. MANAGE, Y. Artificial abortion at mid-pregnancy by mechanical stimulation of the uterus. A review of 20 years' experience with current methods in Japan. *American Journal of Obstetrics and Gynecology*, **105**, 132–146 (1969)
114. INGEMANSON, C. A. Extra-amniotic ethacridine catheter technique (Rivanol). (Booerhaave Committee for Post-Graduate Medical Education. Second Trimester Pregnancy Termination, Faculty of Medicine) University of Leiden, pp. 55–57 (1980)
115. CHAUDRY, S. L., HUNT, W. B. II and WORTHMAN, J. Pregnancy termination in mid-trimester – review of major methods. *Population Reports, Series F*, **5**, 65–83 (1976)
116. WIQVIST, N. and BYGDEMAN, M. Therapeutic abortion by local administration of prostaglandin. *Lancet*, **2**, 716–717 (1970)
117. EMBREY, M. P. and HILLIER, K. Therapeutic abortion by intra-uterine instillation of prostaglandins. *British Medical Journal*, **1**, 588–590 (1971)
118. LAUERSEN, N. H. and WILSON, K. H. Continuous prostaglandin $F_{2\alpha}$ infusion for middle trimester abortion. *Lancet*, **1**, 1195 (1973)
119. LAUERSEN, N. H. and WILSON, K. H. Continuous extra-ovular administration of prostaglandin $F_{2\alpha}$ for mid-trimester abortion. *American Journal of Obstetrics and Gynecology*, **120**, 273–280 (1974)
120. MIDWINTER, A., SHEPHARD, A. and BOWEN, M. Continuous extra-amniotic prostaglandin E_2 for therapeutic termination and the effectiveness of various infusion rates and dosages. *Journal of Obstetrics and Gynaecology of the British Commonwealth*, **80**, 371–373 (1973)
121. MACKENZIE, I. Z., EMBREY, M. P. and HILLIER, K. Intra-amniotic prostaglandin for induction of abortion: an improved regime using prostaglandin E_2. *Journal of Obstetrics and Gynaecology of the British Commonwealth*, **81**, 554–557 (1974)
122. BYGDEMAN, M., BEGUIN, F., TOPPOZADA, M. *et al.* Intra-uterine administration of 15(S)-15 methyl prostaglandin $F_{2\alpha}$ for induction of abortion. *Lancet*, **1**, 1336–1337 (1972)
123. WHO Task Force on the Use of Prostaglandins for the Regulation of Fertility. Prostaglandins and

abortion. 2. Single extra-amniotic administration of 0.92 mg of 15-methyl prostaglandin $F_{2\alpha}$ in Hyskon for termination of pregnancies in weeks 10 to 20 of gestation: an international multi-center study. *American Journal of Obstetrics and Gynecology*, **129**, 597–600 (1977)

124. WHO Task Force on the Use of Prostaglandins for the Regulation of Fertility. Prostaglandins and abortion. 3. Comparison of single intra-amniotic injections of 15-methyl prostaglandin $F_{2\alpha}$ and Prostaglandin $F_{2\alpha}$ for termination of second trimester pregnancy: an international multi-center study. *American Journal of Obstetrics and Gynecology*, **129**, 601–606 (1977)
125. KARIM, S. M. M. and SHARMA, S. D. Therapeutic abortion and induction of labour by intra-vaginal administration of prostaglandin E_2 and $F_{2\alpha}$. *Journal of Obstetrics and Gynaecology of the British Commonwealth*, **78**, 294–299 (1971)
126. BOLOGNESE, R. J. and CORSON, S. L. Prostaglandin E_2 vaginal suppository as an early second trimester abortifacient. *Obstetrics and Gynecology (NY)*, **43**, 104–108 (1974)
127. LAUERSEN, N. H., SECHER, N. J. and WILSON, K. H. Mid-trimester abortion induced by intra-vaginal administration of prostaglandin E_2 suppositories. *American Journal of Obstetrics and Gynecology*, **122**, 947–954 (1975)
128. LAUERSEN, N. H. and WILSON, K. H. Induction of labour in patients with missed abortions and fetal death in utero with prostaglandin E_2 suppositories. *American Journal of Obstetrics and Gynecology*, **127**, 609–611 (1977)
129. SOUTHERN, E. M., GUTKNECHT, G. D., MOHBERG, N. R. and EDELMAN, D. A. Vaginal prostaglandin E_2 in the management of fetal intra-uterine death. *British Journal of Obstetrics and Gynaecology*, **85**, 437–441 (1978)
130. MARTIN, J. N., BYGDEMAN, M., RAMADAN, M. *et al.* Vaginally administered 16,16-dimethyl PGE_2 for the induction of mid-trimester abortions. *Prostaglandins*, **11**, 123 (1976)
131. SAKAMOTO, S., SATOH, K., KINOSHITA, K. *et al.* Application of ONO-802 for second trimester abortion – double blind controlled study. *Obstetrics and Gynecology (NY)*, **48**, 1681 (In Japanese) (1981)
132. SAKAMOTO, S., SATOH, K., NISHIYA, I. *et al.* Abortifacient effect and uterine cervix dilating action of 16,16-dimethyl-transΔ^2 PGE_1 methyl ester (ONO-802) in the form of a vaginal suppository. A randomized, double-blind controlled study in the second trimester of pregnancy). *Prostaglandins Leukotrienes and Medicine*, **9**, 349 (1981)
133. BRENNER, E. E., DINGFELDER, J. K., STAUROVSKY, L. G. *et al.* Intra-muscular administration of 15(S)-15-methyl prostaglandin E_2 methyl ester for induction of abortion. *American Journal of Obstetrics and Gynecology*, **120**, 833–836 (1974)
134. BRENNER, W. R., DINGFELDER, J. R., STAUROVSKY, L. G. *et al.* Intra-muscular administration of 15(S)-15 methyl prostaglandin E_2 methyl ester for induction of abortion. A comparison of two dose schedules. *Fertility and Sterility*, **26**, 369–379 (1975)
135. LAUERSEN, N. H. and WILSON, K. H. Mid-trimester abortion induced by serial intra-muscular injections of 15(S)-15 methyl prostaglandin $F_{2\alpha}$. *American Journal of Obstetrics and Gynecology*, **121**, 273–276 (1975)
136. BRENNER, W. E., GRUBER, W., STAUROVSKY, L. G. and DINGFELDER, J. R. Induction of abortion with intra-muscular administration of 15(S)-15 methyl PGE_2 and 15(S)-15 methyl $PGF_{2\alpha}$. In *Obstetric and Gynecological Uses of Prostaglandins* (ed. S. M. M. Karim), University Park Press, Baltimore, pp. 175–186 (1976)
137. DHALL, G. I., DEVI, P. K., GULATI, S. and DHALL, K. Induction of mid-trimester abortion with serial intra-muscular injections of 15(S)-15 methyl PGE_2. In *Obstetric and Gynecological Uses of Prostaglandins* (ed. S. M. M. Karim), University Park Press, Baltimore, pp. 199–204 (1976)
138. LANGE, A. P. and SECHER, N. J. Mid-trimester and missed abortion treated with intra-muscular 15(S)-15 methyl $PGF_{2\alpha}$. *Prostaglandins*, **14**, 389–395 (1977)
139. WHO Task Force on the Use of Prostaglandins for the Regulation of Fertility. Prostaglandins and Abortion. 1. Intra-muscular administration of 15-methyl prostaglandin $F_{2\alpha}$ for induction of abortion in weeks 10 to 20 of pregnancy. *American Journal of Obstetrics and Gynecology*, **129**, 593–596 (1977)
140. KARIM, S. M. M., CHOO, H. T., LIM, A. L. *et al.* Termination of second trimester pregnancy with intra-muscular administration of 16 Phenoxy-ω-17,18,19,20 Tetranor PGE_2 methyl sulfonylamide. *Prostaglandins*, **15**, 1063–1068 (1978)
141. WHO Task Force on the Use of Prostaglandins for the Regulation of Fertility. Termination of second trimester pregnancy by intra-muscular injection of 16-phenoxy-ω-17,18,19,20-Tetranor-PGE_2 methyl sulphonylamide. *International Journal of Obstetrics and Gynaecology*, **20**, 383–386 (1982)

142. KARIM, S. M. M., RATNAM, S. S. and LIN, A. L. Termination of second trimester pregnancy with laminaria and intra-muscular 16-Phenoxy-ω-17,18,19,20-Tetranor PGE_2 methyl sulfonylamide. *Prostaglandins*, **23**, 257–263 (1982)
143. HERN, W. M. *Abortion Practice*, J. B. Lippincott, Philadelphia (1984)
144. GRIMES, D. A. and CATES, W. J. Dilatation and evacuation. *Second Trimester Abortion. Perspectives After a Decade of Experience*, (eds. G. S. Berger, W. G. Brenner and L. G. Keith), John Wright, Boston, p. 119 (1981)
145. STUBBLEFIELD, P. G. Mid-trimester abortion by curettage procedures: an overview. In *Abortion and Sterilisation Medical and Social Aspects*, (ed. J. E. Hodgson), Grune and Stratton, New York, p. 277 (1987)
146. Center for Disease Control. *Abortion Surveillance 1975*, U.S. Department of Health, Education and Welfare, Public Health Service, Center for Disease Control, Atlanta, Georgia p. 49 (1977)
147. HODGSON, J. E. and PORTMAN, K. C. Complications of 10 453 consecutive first-trimester abortions: a prospective study. *American Journal of Obstetrics and Gynecology*, **120**, 802–807 (1974)
148. PAKTER, J., HARRIS, D. and NELSON, F. Surveillance of abortion program in New York City. *Bulletin of the New York Academy of Medicine*, **47** (8), 853–874 (1971)
149. STONE, M., MORRIS, N. and BLAIR, M. Factors influencing morbidity following termination of pregnancy. *European Journal of Obstetrics, Gynecology and Reproductive Biology*, **7**, 69–72 (1977)
150. LOUNG, K. C., BUCKLE, A. E. R. and ANDERSON, M. M. Results in 1000 cases of therapeutic abortion managed by vacuum aspiration. *British Medical Journal*, **4**, 477–479 (1971)
151. ANDOLSEK, L., CHENG, M., HERN, M. The safety of local anesthesia and out-patient treatment: a controlled study of induced abortion by vacuum aspiration. *Studies in Family Planning*, **8**, 118–124 (1977)
152. Centre for Disease Control. *Abortion Surveillance, Annual Summary, 1981*, Department of Health and Human Services, p. 13. (1985)
153. BERIC, B. and KUPRESANIN, M. Vacuum aspiration, using paracervical block, for legal abortion as an out-patient procedure up to the 12th Week of Pregnancy. *Lancet*, **2**, 619–621 (1971)
154. STRAUSZ, I. K. and SCHULMAN, H. 500 Out-patient abortions performed under local anesthesia. *Obstetrics and Gynecology (NY)*, **38**, 199–205 (1971)
155. WENTZ, A C., THOMPSON, B. H. and KING, T. M. Posterior cervical rupture following prostaglandin-induced mid-trimester abortion. *American Journal of Obstetrics and Gynecology*, **115**, 1107–1110 (1973)
156. LOWENSOHN, R. and BALLARD. G. A. Cervicovaginal fistula: an apparent increased incidence with prostaglandin $F_{2\alpha}$. **119**, 1057–1061 (1974)
157. DUENHOELTER, J. H. and GANT, N. G. Complications following prostaglandin $F_{2\alpha}$. induced mid-trimester abortion. *Obstetrics and Gynecology (NY)*, **46**, 247–250 (1975)
158. GOODLIN, R., NEWELL, J., O'HARE, J. and STURZE, H. Cervical fistula. *Obstetrics and Gynecology*, **40**, 82–84 (1972).
159. *Medical Defence Union Annual Report* (1979). London, England pp. 23 (1979)
160. FRANK, P. I., KAY, C. R., SCOTT, L. M., HANNAFORD, P. C. and HARAN, D. Pregnancy following induced abortion: maternal morbidity and neonatal death. *British Journal of Obstetrics and Gynaecology*, (1987)
161. LINDAHL, J. In: *Somatic Complications Following Legal Abortion*. Heinemann, London (1959)
162. MOMSE, K. Intra-uterine adhesions as seen with hysterosalpingography in relation to the intra-uterine instrumentation with pregnancy. In: *Harmful Effects of Induced Abortion* (ed. Koya), Family Planning Federation of Japan, Tokyo, pp. 45–48 (1966)
163. WYNN, M. and WYNN, A. *Some Consequences of Induced Abortion to Children Born Subsequently*. Foundation for Education and Research in Child-Bearing, London, pp. 30 (1972)
164. NOVAK, F. Effects of legal abortion on the health of mothers in Yugoslavia. In: *Changing Patterns in Fertility*. Excerpta Medica Foundation, New York pp. 223–224 (1963)
165. BERAL, V. An epidemiological study of recent trends in ectopic pregnancy. *British Journal of Obstetrics and Gynaecology*, 775–782 (1975)
166. BREWER, C. Incidence of post-abortion psychosis: a prospective study. *British Medical Journal*, 1, 476–477 (1977)

Chapter 15

Female sterilization and its reversal

Jacques-E. Rioux

Introduction

Sterilization is the most effective means of fertility regulation and worldwide also ranks as the most popular. Indeed, more than a hundred million couples have opted for sterilization as their method of permanent contraception. In the US alone, 750 000 female sterilizations are done every year, and in Canada, more than 80 000 women every year choose this method.

The first female sterilization in North America was performed in 1880 by S. S. Lungren of Toledo, Ohio. It was done at the time of a repeat caesarean for contracted pelvis. He reported it the following year in the *American Journal of Obstetrics and Diseases of Women and Children* [1]. He had first intended to remove the ovaries but, in consideration of the danger of haemorrhage: 'I tied the fallopian tubes instead with a strong silk ligature about one inch from their uterine attachment' (Figure 15.1).

Almost all the tubal sterilizations performed by various techniques during the next few decades were done at the time of caesarean section or during the postpartum period. Until about 40 years ago, most practicing obstetricians and gynaecologists were reluctant to perform a laparotomy solely for tubal ligation. Furthermore they believe that if tubal occlusion was not achieved within 24 h of delivery, morbidity would be increased drastically. We now realize that the operation may be carried out at any time. The incisions became smaller with the advent of minilaparotomy, but the techniques of tubal occlusion remained the same. The greatest step was made when laparoscopy became available and new instruments were developed to achieve tubal occlusion. Hysteroscopy is struggling to prove itself capable of achieving that goal, even adding a touch of reversibility. Would a non-surgical approach be so attractive as to replace all those techniques and increase even more the share of sterilization in

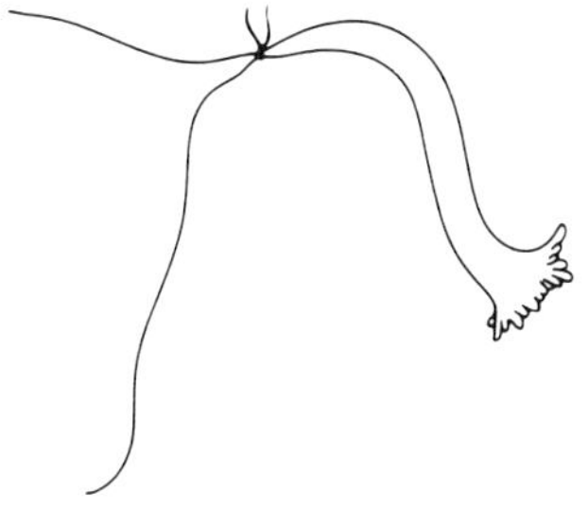

Figure 15.1. In 1880, Lungren tied the fallopian tubes with a strong silk ligature about 1 in. from their uterine attachments.

the contraceptive world? To answer this question, the author will review the most popular procedures which have been developed to achieve female sterilization; then he will introduce the transcervical technique by describing his own experience; he will conclude with a discussion which should place everything in its proper perspective.

The tubes may be approached by conventional laparotomy, minilaparotomy, colpotomy, laparoscopy, culdoscopy, hysteroscopy, and via the natural passages of the vagina and the cervical canal.

Conventional laparotomy

The following techniques are presented in the chronological order of their appearance in the medical literature, and only those that have a lasting impression are discussed.

In 1919, Madlener, a German surgeon, published a paper reporting the sterilization of 80 patients [2]. In that series, three women died of postoperative complications. He insisted that the base of the loop of the tube be crushed before ligation with non-absorbable suture material (Figure 15.2). The failure rate turned out to be 13 per 1000, resulting in waning enthusiasm for this procedure. Irving in 1924 described a method which he used exclusively for sterilization coincidental with caesarean section [3]. By burying the proximal stump within the myometrium and the distal portion between the leaves of the broad ligament, he was able to keep the ends of the severed tube away from each other, thereby producing a faultless sterilization (Figure 15.3).

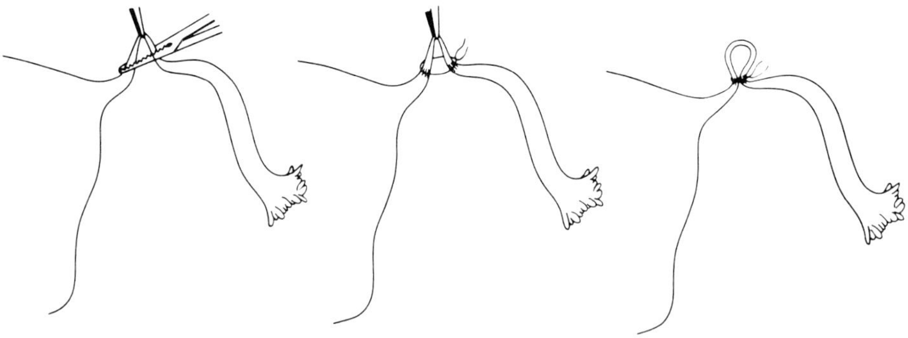

Figure 15.2. Madlener suggested in 1919 that the base of the loop of tube be crushed before ligation with non-absorbable suture material

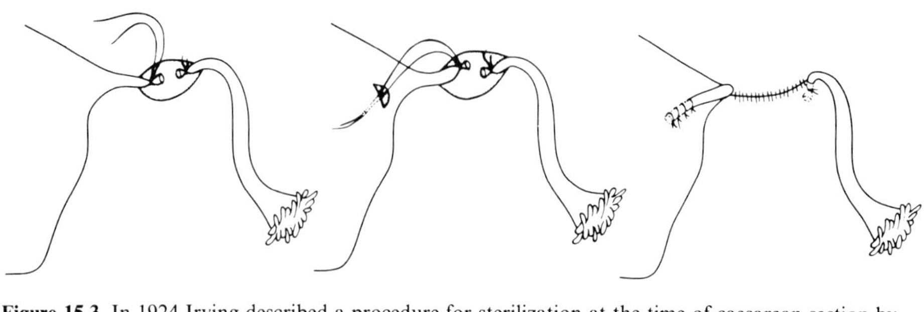

Figure 15.3. In 1924 Irving described a procedure for sterilization at the time of caesarean section by burying both stumps

Pomeroy never published a description of his technique, which is probably the most frequently used of all tubal ligation methods. In 1930, his associates Bishop and Nelms [4] reported 60 sterilizations following his principles: (1) do not crush the tube in order to avoid tubal fistula formation, and (2) do not use non-absorbable suture material, so that as soon as the suture dissolves, the proximal and distal segments separate, making recanalization unlikely (Figure 15.4).

In 1934, Aldridge described a technique which is noteworthy since it was designed to be a reversible sterilization method [5]. The peritoneum of the broad ligament is opened, creating a small bursa in which the ampulla is buried and secured in place by a few interrupted sutures between the peritoneum and tubal serosa (Figure 15.5). His paper reported only one case done and successfully reversed 5 years later. In the Canadian Jurisprudence, we have one case which reversed itself!

Other authors, mostly German, have suggested the occlusion of the fimbrial ends by displacing them into the inguinal canals, the vagina, the anterior abdominal wall, the uterovesical space, the musculature of the anterior or posterior uterine wall, etc. In 1935, Kroener proposed to occlude the tubes by distal salpingectomy or fimbriectomy [6]: the tube is doubly ligated at the ampulla and the fimbria excised (Figure 15.6). This technique is quite simple when the distal portion of the tube is free, but for some unknown reason it has never been too popular in spite of its very low failure rate.

Total salpingectomy is sometimes indicated if the tubes are diseased.

Partial salpingectomy is referred to as a 'modified Pomeroy': a mid-segment of tube

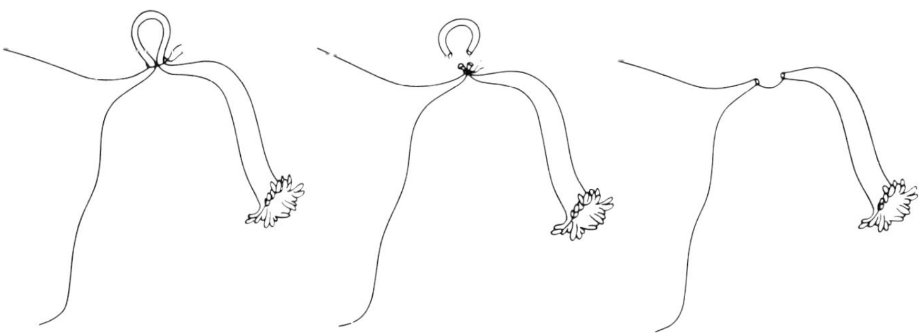

Figure 15.4 Pomeroy's techniques was published in 1930. He did not crush the tube, tied it with an absorbable suture, and excised the loop of tube

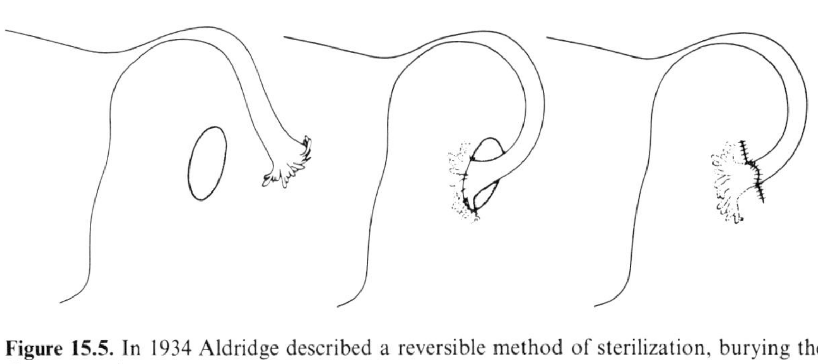

Figure 15.5. In 1934 Aldridge described a reversible method of sterilization, burying the ampulla within the retroperitoneum

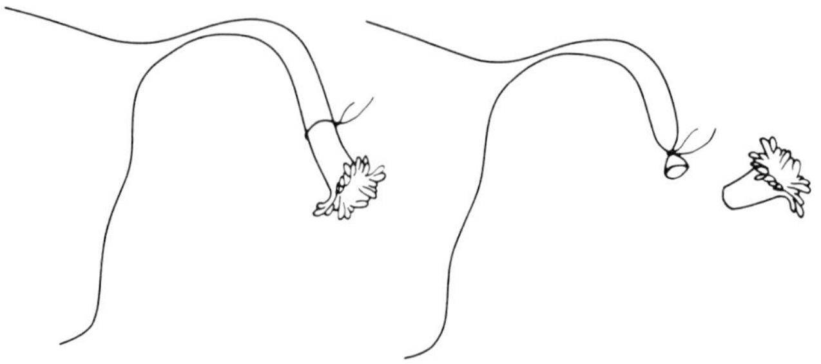

Figure 15.6. Kroener in 1935 proposed occluding the tubes by distal salpingectomy or fimbriectomy

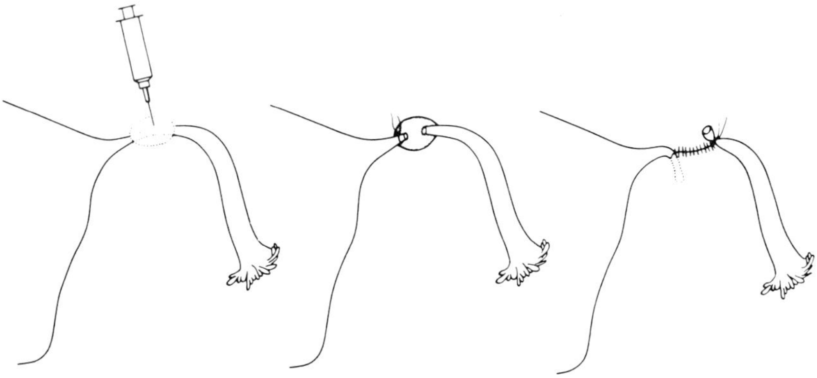

Figure 15.7. In 1945 Uchida buried the ligated proximal portion of the tube beneath the serosa and tied the distal ends outside

is removed and both cut ends are ligated separately with non-absorbable suture material. Cornual resection is when the intramural portion of the tube is removed and large mattress sutures are placed in the myometrium to achieve haemostasis.

From 1945, Uchida personally performed more than 25 000 sterilizations without a failure [7]. In his technique a saline–adrenaline solution is injected into the subserosa, separating the serosa from the muscular layer. When this oedematous bleb is opened the tube itself is easily discernible. It is then severed and the proximal portion ligated and buried beneath the serosa. The distal end is ligated together with the open fringe of the serosa (Figure 15.7). Cook presented a technique in his book *Essentials of Gynecology* in 1943 [8]. He suggested burying the proximal end of the ligated tube in the round ligament.

The most recent innovation in the field seems to have been reported by Wood [9], who uses a microsurgical technique to ligate, divide, and bury the medial stump in the mesosalpinx. He claims that by not excising any tissue, this technique should lend itself to tubal reconstruction. On the matter of reversal, it should be mentioned that all the techniques involving wrapping either the ovaries or the fimbria in synthetic materials (including condoms) to achieve temporary sterility will of course necessitate a second laparotomy for reversal.

With a large incision, complete exploration of the intra-abdominal contents is possible and any of the previously described sterilization methods may be employed, together with attention to any pathology which could have warranted the laparotomy. Conventional laparotomy does not appear to be justifiable for the sole purpose of fallopian-tube occlusion.

Minilaparotomy

Minilaparotomy under local anaesthesia in the hands of experienced surgeons is probably the safest method of female sterilization. It is also the cheapest and the most adaptable for developing countries. It can be done easily as an interval postabortum or postpartum procedure. The contraindications are few and include obesity sufficient to prevent palpation of the uterine fundus through the lower abdominal wall, and fixed uterine retroversion. Many techniques of tubal occlusion are available, the most popular being the Pomeroy (see Figure 15.4) [4].

Colpotomy

Theoretically, the vaginal route seems ideal for safe and rapid tubal sterilization, avoiding an abdominal incision. In practice though, this is far from true. It appears that the price of avoiding a small abdominal scar may be too high when the complications associated with vaginal tubal sterilization are evaluated (the possibility of cellulitis or pelvic abscess, haemorrhage, proctotomy, and cystotomy). Coital activity should be delayed until the vaginal incision has healed. This constraint may not always be complied with, and the restriction is not necessary when the abdominal route is employed. What is the advantage to a woman of undergoing tubal ligation by the vaginal approach, if deep dyspareunia precluding sexual enjoyment is a sequela?

Shepard concluded after her excellent and extensive review: ‘At the moment, the serious nature of complications encountered after vaginal tubal sterilization would appear to prohibit whole-hearted endorsement of this procedure as a quick, effective means of performing female sterilization.’ [10]

Endoscopic methods

Laparoscopy

Laparoscopic sterilization has become quite popular during the past decade. This procedure has the advantage of providing superb visualization not only of the entire pelvic cavity, but also of much of the intra-abdominal contents. There are very few, if any, situations when laparoscopy is impossible to perform. It is a sophisticated procedure, necessitating highly technical and expensive instrumentation.

Since the introduction of laparoscopic tubal sterilization, women have had access to a safe, effective and dependable method of tubal sterilization. In well-trained hands it may be performed under local anaesthesia, and in such cases the procedure is virtually comparable to vasectomy in ease of performance, safety, and efficacy. Thus the choice is now available to a couple as to which of the two will elect to be sterilized.

At the same time, although we stress the innocuous nature of laparoscopic sterilization, we also stress the seriousness of the decision to undergo sterilization, since it should be considered, for all intents and purposes, an irreversible procedure.

Electrocoagulation

Unipolar electrocoagulation

Though gynaecological laparoscopy was flourishing in Europe in the 1960s (only the gastroenterologists were using the technique in North America at that time), it was Anderson, an American, who in 1937 proposed laparoscopic electrocoagulation of the fallopian tubes in order to achieve female sterilization [11]. However, Palmer of France is credited with describing the modern technique of laparoscopic tubal electrocoagulation in 1962 [12]. The first instrument employed was the 'Palmer Biopsy Forceps', since it already had electrosurgical capabilities. Powerful, grounded, high-voltage generators producing unipolar electrical current were employed. Under such circumstances the electrical energy is concentrated at the site at which the fallopian tube is grasped by the jaws of the forceps. When current is injected, it must travel through the patient's body, whence it exits and is collected by a ground plate or return electrode in order to complete the electrical circuit. The original technique involved electrocoagulation of the tubal isthmus, followed by tubal transsection and recoagulation of the cut edges [13].

Some authors have subsequently indicated that coagulation alone without tubal transsection is equally as effective, provided the surgeon is experienced and confident that the coagulation is complete [14]. Others recommend that a specimen of the tube be excised for pathological confirmation. This step appears to have evolved as much for medicolegal as for scientific reasons [15]. Unfortunately, all too frequently the charred tube excised is quite unrecognizable, effectively defeating the primary purpose of the biopsy.

All the laparoscopic procedures so far described have employed the 'two-puncture technique', i.e. a viewing laparoscope introduced at the umbilicus and an operating instrument introduced via a second, suprapubic puncture in the midline. In 1972, Wheeless adapted this method to the operating laparoscope, thus obviating the necessity for a second puncture [16]. The 'one-puncture technique' appears to be particularly suitable for use with local anaesthesia, and requires fewer instruments and less surgical assistance.

Whether one or two punctures are employed, and regardless of the coagulation technique, (coagulation only, coagulation combined with tubal transsection or resection), the unipolar electrical system turned out to be associated with some inherent dangers. As early as 1973, Thompson and Wheeless reported eleven cases of bowel burns secondary to accidental electrical injury during tubal electrocoagulation [17]. Other reports followed, further emphasizing the fact that a potentially dangerous situation existed with the use of unipolar current. Since there was generally no rational explanation for such accidents, it was difficult if not impossible to avoid them. We now know that some of these cases were simply secondary to faulty technique, but most were related to the inherent danger associated with high-voltage, grounded generators. Some of these units, when set in the coagulation mode, were capable of producing thousands of volts, and hundreds of amps of current. As the tubal tissue was being dehydrated, the tissue resistance increased, and the generator produced more current in an attempt to overcome this resistance. Today more sophisticated generators are available, generally of solid-state construction, producing low-voltage, high-frequency current and which are not grounded but rather isolated from ground [18]. These have turned out to be much safer, but unfortunately, bowel burns still occur [19]. It is therefore the opinion of the author that unipolar electrocoagulation should be totally abolished. and that all electrocoagulation be performed using the bipolar electrical principle.

Bipolar electrocoagulation

In 1973, following reports of these accidents in the medical literature, Rioux devised the bipolar technique for tubal electrocoagulation [20,21]. This method differs from the conventional unipolar system in that the operating forceps carries both the active and the return electrode. By completely isolating the two jaws of the forceps from one another, high-frequency current can be passed through one jaw and retrieved and returned to the generator via the other. The current thus passes selectively through the tissue grasped between the jaws of the forceps. Although high-frequency current is employed, it is required to travel only a short distance, i.e. the thickness of the tube grasped within the jaws (1–2 mm). The bipolar procedure appears to be safer than the unipolar system, since the dangers of sparking are eliminated. Inadvertent electrosurgical injury to the bowel with bipolar forceps can, therefore, only occur if the bowel is grasped directly with the forceps. Such a complication is obviously a result of surgical error as opposed to instrument failure. A further advantage of bipolar electrocoagulation is that the resulting burn is discreet and localized, selectively destroying only the tube in the grasp of the forceps' jaw, leaving the mesosalpinx unaffected (Figure 15.8).

At this point, a word of caution is essential: bipolar instruments should only be employed with compatible electrosurgical units as recommended by the manufacturers, or with a generator possessing both limited output and isolated circuitry.

The previously described tubal electrocoagulation techniques possess a failure rate of approximately 2 per 1000 cases. The complication rate for laparoscopy is directly proportional to the experience of the operator and attention to the proposed safety guidelines. Electrosurgical complications have become considerably less frequent since the advent of the bipolar technique, as well as with the use of low-voltage, high-frequency generators. Furthermore, education and familiarization of physicians and operating-room personnel with electrosurgical instruments has resulted in fewer complications.

Thermocoagulation

The technique of thermocoagulation originated in Germany. The instrument literally

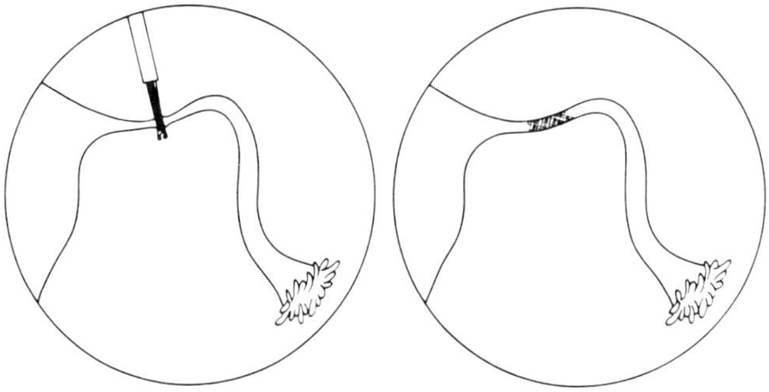

Figure 15.8. In 1973 Rioux devised the first bipolar instrument for laparoscopic tubal electrocoagulation

'cooks' the fallopian tube by means of a small element heated by an electric current. The advantage of this technique is that the current is markedly reduced from the exit potential of the standard electrical wall outlet, and is therefore much safer. The apparatus employed for this thermocoagulation procedure requires no more than 4–5 volts in order to produce the desired effect. With some of the sophisticated and automated thermocoagulation generators, the desired temperature and duration of current application may be preselected. Other generators provide an audible signal which varies according to the temperature of the heating element, indicating whether the instrument is in the heating or cooling cycle. Thermocoagulation now appears to be less dangerous than diathermy; however, full data regarding the efficacy of the technique are not as yet available.

Electrocautery

Another approach which employs the heating principle to produce coagulation as well as transsection of the tube, has been devised by the Waters Instrument Company. This apparatus possesses a small, metallic hook which is heated by electric current, produced by a battery. The tube is grasped with the hook and pulled into an insulated outer sheath. The tube is coagulated and transsected, with haemostasis being achieved by cauterization. Tissue destruction with this technique is minimal, but because sectioned ends of the tube remain in close proximity, recanalization may theoretically occur more easily than with some of the other techniques described. Unfortunately, data for evaluating the true failure rate of this method are not available.

Mechanical techniques

Clips

Two non-electrical (mechanical) laparoscopic tubal occlusive techniques have become quite popular in the past few years. The spring-loaded clip was developed by Hulka. Aware of the high failure rate associated with the use of the tantalum clip, (up to 27% according to Wheeless), yet still fascinated by the simplicity of the concept, Hulka spent years developing a clip of Lexan plastic [22]. When applied to the fallopian tube by a single-puncture technique, using a specifically designed instrument, the clip is maintained in the closed position by a stainless-steel spring, gold-plated to diminish peritoneal reaction. The basic principle involved in this technique is that the plastic jaws with interlocking teeth leave no space. The maximal pressure upon the tube is applied over a period of time, thus lessening the acute crushing effect which could result in fistula formation. This plastic clip, as opposed to the tantalum clip, leaves no room for recanalization.

The original clip applicator as described above, was adapted to the operating laparoscope. Later Lieberman *et al.* [23] favouring the two-puncture technique, devised the Samaritan clip applicator, and more recently Hulka himself has developed a second puncture applicator which is even easier to use. Follow-up figures of patients sterilized using the double-puncture clip technique show a failure rate of 20 per 1000. Our personal experience appears to be much more acceptable, being in the range of 1 per 1000 cases. The author feels strongly that improvement in the instrumentation and strict quality control of the fabrication of the clip itself will be responsible for lowering and maintaining the failure rate at a level similar to that of the electrosurgical approach, i.e. 2 per 1000 cases.

Two other clips, one devised by Bleier [24] and the other by Filshie [25], are now available. That devised by Bleier is the simpler; it has only one part made of one material – plastic. It has longitudinal striae which produced a crushing effect, and it is shorter than the Hulka clip. The locking device is purely mechanical, and must include a portion of the mesosalpinx to be effective. Unfortunately, in our hands the clip was not effective enough and we have stopped using it. It appears that the design of the clip itself is faulty, leaving room, even in the closed position, for the persistence of a channel.

The Filshie clip is, in our opinion the best one available at present. It is made of titanium which is lined with silicone rubber. The locking device is also mechanical through the mesosalpinx and, when fully closed, it leaves no space at all, thus achieving complete occlusion. It is the easiest clip to place adequately, because of the grasping effect provided by the curve on the upper jaw. Also, because of its length, it can be placed on almost any type and shape of tube, including postpartum tubes. This clip may be applied laparoscopically using a double-puncture technique [26] or a single-puncture technique, with either local or general anaesthesia. There are three single-puncture applicators available to go down operating channels of 6 mm, 7.4 mm (Storz Universal Laparoscope) or 8 mm diameter. For interval sterilization the failure rate is approximately 2 per 1000. For postpartum sterilization the figure is higher. The failure rate can be reduced if particular attention is paid to ensuring that the clip is over the whole isthmic part of the tube at the time of the sterilization. In our hands it has been highly effective (we have had no pregnancy to date (Figure 15.9)).

Falope ring

The Falope ring devised by Yoon is ingeniously simple [27]. A loop of tube is drawn into the central hollow cylinder of the ring applicator forceps, which itself can be inserted by either single- or double-puncture technique. The loaded Silastic band is then forced down over the loop of tube by the forward action of an outer cylinder, resulting in a release of the band from the applicator, and thus tubal occlusion. The portion of the tube encircled by the ring gradually becomes sclerosed (Figure 15.10).

The failure rate quoted for the ring is 6 per 1000 cases. These results are not surprising when it is acknowledged that the procedure is, in fact, a modification of the Madlener technique, with the difference that the tube is not crushed mechanically. When the tubes are slender, and lie free, i.e. are not involved in an adhesive process, they are easily drawn up within the inner cylinder. On the other hand, when a thick or

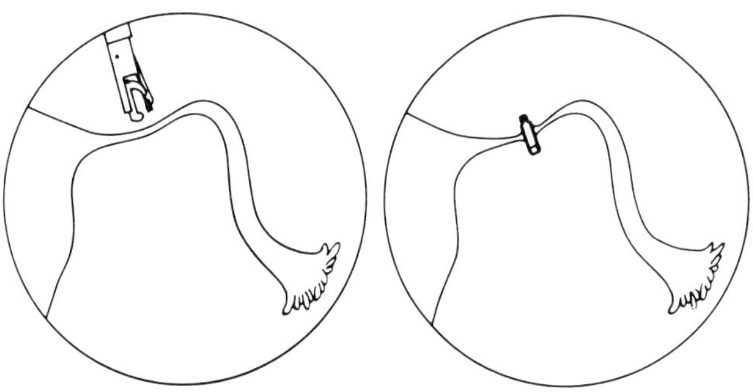

Figure 15.9. In 1972 clips were perfected by Hulka and others. Shown here is the Filshie clip

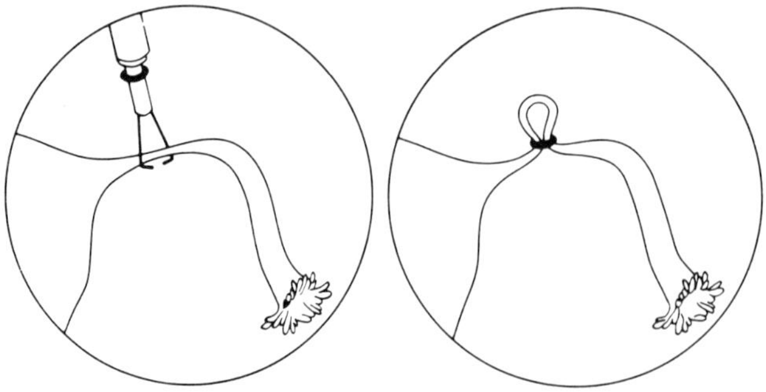

Figure 15.10. The Falope ring was devised by Yoon in 1974. It is ingeniously simple and in use the world over

oedematous tube is encountered, a slow, 'milking up' of the tube by means of a to-and-fro motion of the grasping portion of the applicator is necessary in order to draw the tube into the cylinder. In so doing, the serosa may be damaged or the tube totally transsected; this allows for an increased risk of fistula formation as with the Madlener technique.

Open laparoscopy

One cannot close a chapter on laparoscopy without mentioning open laparoscopy, devised by Hasson [28]. This technique makes laparoscopy safer by eliminating the danger associated with the insufflating needle and the blind introduction of a sharp trocar. Once the cannula is introduced all the advantages of laparoscopy are available.

Culdoscopy

Culdoscopy was described 40 years ago. It was originally a purely diagnostic procedure. Later, operative capabilities were added and it became possible to achieve tubal obstruction using many of the techniques described for laparoscopy. However the technique is obsolescent, since it is no longer being taught. Moreover, very few programmes of female sterilization are based upon its use. The reasons seems to be that culdoscopy has the disadvantages of laparoscopy (delicate and expensive instrumentation) but has none of the advantages.

Hysteroscopy

This apparently simple procedure, like laparoscopy, uses sophisticated equipment and appeals to the enthusiastic endoscopist. However, it is a tricky procedure, fraught with pitfalls and demanding a great deal of patience on the part of the surgeon; the latter is a quality sometimes lacking.

Hysteroscopic tubal occlusion will become more and more popular as instruments are simplified and reversibility of techniques improve [29]. Indeed, with the smaller instruments, hysteroscopy is becoming an office procedure which can be performed in minutes under local anaesthesia.

Three approaches are being investigated (a) the use of electrical current to coagulate the tube from inside, (b) the use of chemical agents which cause a sclerosis of the endosalpinx, and (c) the use of a plug (already shaped or formed in place) to obstruct the tubal lumen; the latter procedure embodies a certain degree of reversibility.

The use of electrical current

As with laparoscopy, electricity can be used to electrocoagulate (diathermy) or to thermocoagulate (using heat).

Electrocoagulation, whether unipolar or bipolar, is achieved by introducing an electrode with a conductive tip via the tubal ostium into the proximal portion of the tube. Identification of the ostia, however, may be difficult; in fact in only 80% of cases can these openings be identified with absolute certainty. Theoretically a flexible hysteroscope, which is still in the experimental stages of development, might provide increased facility in identifying the tubal ostia. Furthermore, since these small openings become increasingly more difficult to identify as the thickness of the endometrium increases, the early proliferative phase of the cycle is preferable for staging the procedure.

Once the electrode is introduced into the intramural portion of the tube, the electric current is applied, and permanent occlusion should result from electrocoagulation of the endosalpinx and proximal layer of muscularis. Unfortunately this is not always the case. The reported failure rate at this time is far too high (15–30%). Moreover, because the procedure becomes a blind one once the tip of the probe is introduced into the ostium, electrical injury to overlying intraperitoneal structures such as bowel may occur, and has in fact been reported. This technique has not yet been approved by the US Food and Drugs Administration.

Thermocoagulation is achieved by heating the probe itself using low-voltage current. As with the laparoscopic thermal coagulation technique, the tissue surrounding the probe is 'cooked'. No data are yet available regarding failure rates with this procedure.

The use of chemical agents

Chemical agents causing a sclerosis of the endosalpinx can be instilled into the tubes, either under hysteroscopic control, or blindly, by means of specialized injecting apparatus.

Many substances have been tried and we will name only those that have actually been used on the human with some kind of success [30].

Strong caustic agents:
- silver nitrate
- zinc chloride
- formaldehyde
- ethanol–formalin

Strong base: phenol or phenol mucilage
Sclerosing agent: sodium morrhuate
Granuloma-producing agent: talc
Cytotoxic agent: quinacrine
Tissue adhesive: methylcyanoacrylate.

Various modes of delivery of these substances exist: (a) direct tubal instillation under hysteroscopic control by catheterizing the tubal ostia, (b) blind catheterization of the ostia under fluoroscopic control using a 'test dose' of radiopaque material, (c) totally blind injection using a very sophisticated instrument: the Femcept device, and (d) loading the agent into the long arm of a T-shaped IUD and letting it diffuse slowly into the fallopian tubes. The Femcept device with methylcyanoacrylate, and an IUD (e.g. Copper T) loaded with quinacrine seem to be the most promising approaches.

Methylcyanoacrylate (MCA) is a tissue adhesive. Once it is introduced into the lumen of the tube it releases acetocyanic acid and formaldehyde, which produce necrosis of the endosalpinx. Gradually, over a period of 6 weeks, an inflammatory infiltrate replaces the tubal epithelium. This in turn is replaced by young fibroblasts which are gradually converted into dense scar tissue. The Femcept device is a very sophisticated instrument. It has a cannula 4 mm in diameter, which is inserted into the uterine cavity. Near the distal end are two opposing fluid exit ports below which is a balloon made of soft rubber, reinforced by Dacron mesh to prevent herniation through the cervix, all of which conform to the uterine cavity. The device has a handle with a plunger, and a recess to introduce the ampule of MCA. Once the cannula is inserted at the proper depth into the uterine cavity the plunger is actuated, and as the fluid is pushed into the cavity the balloon is inflated, sealing the lower part of the uterine cavity and at the same time propelling the fluid into the tubes where the scarring process is initiated. The closure rate is between 88% and 94%.

Quinacrine is a cytotoxic agent. Different delivery systems are under consideration, e.g. repeated transcervical instillation of a quinacrine hydrochloride solution, intrauterine insertion of a quinacrine hydrochloride solution, intrauterine insertion of quinacrine tablets, and more recently the use of a T-shaped IUD as the vector for quinacrine, enabling it to diffuse slowly into the tubes.

The use of plugs

Three pre-shaped plugs have reached human clinical trials.

Uterotubal junction blocking devices

The uterotubal junction blocking devices have been developed by Hosseinian [31]. They are cone-shaped plugs measuring 1 mm at the tip and increasing to about 2 mm at the base, with a length which varies from 7 mm (small) to 9 mm (large). The plugs themselves are made of silicone or polyethylene to which two metallic components are attached: (a) four anchoring spines made of elgiloy serve to fix and keep the device in place by penetrating the adjacent myometrium; and (b) the assembly screw, made of stainless steel, which attaches the anchoring spines to the plug and provides a grasping base for the device carrier, which is so designed to carry a device through the hysteroscope and implant it in, as well as remove it from, the uterus.

P-block

The P-block is a hydrogel tubal blocking device being developed by Brundin [32]. The latest model, the Mark 7 P-block has a 4 mm long and 1.2 mm wide hydrogel body fixed on a nylon 6 skeleton, which also has 2 mm wide nylon 'wings' to prevent expulsion from the tube before hydralization, which requires about 30 min. On

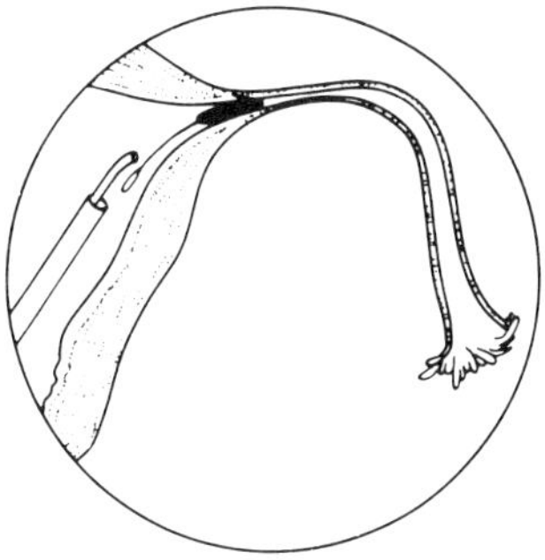

Figure 15.11. The Hamou intratubal device has been clinically tested from 1982

cannulation of the intramural part of the tube, the P-block is held in position by a flexible plunger, while the surrounding catheter (outer diameter, 2.05 mm) is removed. In many women the ostia and the intramural segment of the tubes are smaller and the device cannot be inserted. A smaller model, the Mark 8 is now being developed and should be more universally applied.

Hamou intratubal device

The Hamou intratubal device [33] is made of nylon and is the simplest one. The diameter is small (it is less than 1 mm including the anchoring system) so that it will fit most ostia. There is an intrauterine loop for retrieval. The device does not attempt to fill the lumen of the tube, but acts more or less as an intratubal device (Figure 15.11).

Another approach is to tailor the plug to the tube: these are the 'formed-in-place' silicone plugs devised by Erb and Reed [34]. It involves a flow of catalysed liquid silicone polymer into the fallopian tube through a silicone rubber obturator tip positioned at the tubal ostium. The 'formed-in-place' plug becomes bonded to the tip. The resulting flexible structure is larger in the diameter at both ends than it is in the isthmus, and thus it remains in place to effect tubal occlusion.

Theoretically, these last four techniques using plugs could be reversible, as opposed to the destructiveness of those using electricity or chemical agents. This theoretical advantage has not been proved yet, and should be used with great care when counselling a woman about her decision.

Reversal of sterilization

Philosophy

In North America and Western Europe at least, requests for reversal of sterilization procedures are increasingly frequent. What is the reason for this evolving phenomenon? Discussions and controversy have arisen on the subject of sterilization reversal. Behind several requests lurk the commonest motivating factors, which are called the 'three Ds': divorce, death, and disaster. Other factors suggested include changes in life-style and changes in economic status allowing for larger families.

What should the reaction of physicians be when faced with these facts of life? Should candidates for sterilization be specially screened? Is it possible to identify those candidates most likely to change their decisions? This is a task impossible for us to confront. However, it is clear that some cases have lacked adequate counselling of both partners. In some instances it is known that coercion has been encountered, whether overt or subtle. Physicians have often suggested or hinted that, should the situation require reversing, the procedure would be 'easy'.

The younger the patient, the greater the chance of a change of mind; this is the opinion of some authorities. Our experience has proved otherwise in many cases. Low-parity women of a younger age are among the most highly motivated to undergo sterilization procedures and to maintain their infertility permanently. In general, these include career-oriented women. Some older multiparous patients, on the other hand, have changed their minds within weeks of their original surgery and subsequently request a reversal of their sterilization procedure. As previously stated, the author suggests counselling as a major issue because of the impossible task of preselecting those patients who will most probably request future reversal [35].

When considering the subject of sterilization reversal, what should be our philosophy? Here are a few conclusions of the 4th International Conference on Voluntary Sterilization held in Seoul, Korea in 1979, where those actively implicated in voluntary sterilization movements expressed their concerns and opinions

1. There is no ideal or universal method of female sterilization.
2. No method is truly reversible.
3. At the time she is considering sterilization, a patient should never be informed of the reversal concept unless it is for the purpose of underlining the irreversibility and permanency of the procedure.
4. A physician performing the procedure should keep in mind the possible reversal of sterilization. For an equally effective method of providing permanent contraception, he should contemplate the one which could lead to possible reversal.
5. Effective procedures that do not involve the ampulla or fimbria and those that produce minimal tissue destruction with minimal interference with the vascular and nerve supply to the ovary should be considered in these cases.

Finding a technique which implies minimal interference, if at all, with the vascular and nerve supply to the ovary stems from the clinical impression that after tubal sterilization procedures, there is an increase in dysfunctional uterine bleeding and dysmenorrhoea. This increase has been underlined in a retrospective study published recently. However, to evaluate properly the relationship between tubal sterilization and the development of dysfunctional uterine bleeding and dysmenorrhoea, further prospective studies will have to be conducted [36].

Should we stop using excessively destructive methods of sterilization and direct our efforts to improving tubal reconstructive techniques? The answer is 'yes', with one single condition: that we do not compromise efficacy (in terms of a low failure rate).

Techniques

Obviously the technique to be used will be dictated by the kind of sterilization performed [37]. *Some* operations are simply irreversible, and the patient who was so advised at the time of sterilization should be retold in no uncertain terms at the first hint that she desires reversal (for example, a patient who had had an MCA injection or a bilateral salpingectomy).

Finally, other forms of sterilization are very unpredictable. For example, a unipolar diathermic coagulation can literally destroy the whole tube, leaving only a few fringes behind. A Kroener can take away the fimbria and the whole ampulla. In some other cases, however, only the fimbria are excised, leaving a complete ampulla which can bring itself nicely to an adequate salpingoneostomy. A bipolar burn or a Falope ring ligation can often be reversed by an isthmic–ampullary anastomosis; this is not as good as the isthmic-isthmic anastomosis that can be performed in most cases of clip reversal.

As mentioned, no method is 100% reversible. The clip is close to 90% reversible with microsurgical technique [38]. The other procedures are less than 50% successful, which seems quite adequate for many patients requesting reversal!

This review of the art of tubal sterilization with its perspective of reversal potential brings us to the conclusion that approximately 98% of women undergoing tubal sterilization really wish this procedure to be permanent and irreversible. From our knowledge and experience, we can offer hope to the very few women wishing a reversal with such procedures as microsurgery, *in-vitro* fertilization, and ovum transplantation. But to all intents and purposes, tubal sterilization should be considered an irreversible procedure, and it is essential for all women to be adequately counselled, so that they can fully appreciate the consequences. The procedure of choice remains that method of sterilization which maintains a high degree of efficacy with minimal tissue destruction.

Conclusion

The most recent statistics reveal the popularity of female sterilization. On a worldwide basis, more than 120 million couples rely upon this technique for contraception, and women at an increasingly younger age are choosing the method. Smaller families also provide motivation for sterilization. It would seem to be the best form of female contraception available once the desired family size is reached. A procedure of choice would appear to be hysterectomy whenever medically indicated. When concomitant intra-abdominal surgery is being carried out, the use of conventional laparotomy is justified. Ideally suited to the postpartum and mid-trimester postabortal stages, minilaparotomy may be performed in a clinic under local anaesthesia or in a hospital under general or regional anesthesia. The posterior colpotomy remains an acceptable technique in the hands of a skilled vaginal surgeon. However, without sophisticated instrumentation at hand, one has to ponder the results of increased morbidity in this procedure. Culdoscopy will not be discussed since its future seems restricted.

With the current techniques to hand, back-up abortion facilities in cases of failure must be readily available to support hysteroscopic procedures which are still experimental. One ideal method of interval female sterilization seems to be laparoscopy, and one of several electrosurgical or mechanical occlusive techniques may be used to achieve tubal occlusion.

Since no easily reversible methods are available at this time, all methods of female sterilization must be considered irreversible. It is the author's opinion that the promotion of some sterilization procedures as being reversible constitutes a form of coercion. This must be avoided.

The aim of future research should be to improve sterilization methods so that minimal tissue destruction occurs with techniques of total tubal occlusion. The ideal of course would be to find some which are universally applicable. In an attempt to single out the woman who is most likely to request reversal, sociological, anthropological, and epidemiological studies should be continued, and in these cases efforts should be made to delay the sterilization procedure.

Female sterilization has progressed considerably because of improved technology, but the road to the ideal technique still lies ahead.

References

1. LUNGREN, S. S. *American Journal of Obstetrics and Disorders of Women and Children*, **14**, 78 (1881)
2. MADLENER, M. Über Sterilisierende Operationen an den Tuben. *Zentralblatt für Gynäkologie*, **13**, 380 (1919)
3. IRVING, F. C. A new method for insuring sterility following cesarean section. *American Journal of Obstetrics and Gynecology*, **8**, 335 (1924)
4. BISHOP, E. and NELMS, W. F. A simple method of tubal sterilization. *New York State Journal of Medicine*, **30**, 214 (1930)
5. ALDRIDGE, A. H. Temporary surgical sterilization with subsequent pregnancy. *American Journal of Obstetrics and Gynecology*, **27**, 741 (1934)
6. KROENER, W. F., JR. Surgical sterilization by fimbriectomy. *American Journal of Obstetrics and Gynecology*, **104**, 247 (1969)
7. UCHIDA, H. Uchida tubal sterilization. *American Journal of Obstetrics and Gynecology*, **121**, 153 (1975)
8. COOKE, W. R. *Essentials of Gynecology*, Lippincott, Philadelphia (1943).
9. WOOD, C. Current status of sterilization. *Australian Family Physician*, **8**(5), 486–490 (1979)
10. SHEPARD, M. K. Female contraceptive sterilization. *Obstetrical and Gynecological Survey*, **29**, 739 (1974)
11. ANDERSON, E. T. Peritoneoscopy. *American Journal of Surgery*, **35**, 136 (1937)
12. PALMER, M. R. Essais de stérilisation tubaire coelioscopique par électrocoagulation isthmique. *Bulletin de la Federation des Societes de gynecologie et d'obstetrique de langue francaise*, **14**, 298 (1962)
13. STEPTOE, P. C. *Laparoscopy in Gynaecology*, E. and S. Livingstone, Edinburgh (1967)
14. YUZPE, A. A., RIOUX, J. E., LOFFER, F. D. and PENT, D. Laparoscopic tubal sterilization by the 'burn only' technique. *Obstetrics and Gynecology*, **49**, 106 (1977)
15. SODERSTROM, R. M. Legal aspects of female sterilization. In *Endoscopic Female Sterilization, A Comparison of Methods* (ed. J. M. Phillips), A. A. G. L. Downey, California (1983)
16. WHEELESS, C. R., JR. Elimination of second incision in laparoscopic sterilization. *Obstetrics and Gynecology*, **39**, 134 (1972)
17. THOMPSON, B. H. and WHEELESS, C. R. JR. Gastrointestinal complications of laparoscopic sterilization. *Obstetrics and Gynecology*, **41**, 669 (1973)
18. RIOUX, J. E. and YUZPE, A. A. Know thy generator. *Contemporary Obstetrics and Gynecology*, **6**, 52 (1975)
19. PETERSON, H. B., ORY, H. W., GREENSPAN, J. R. and TYLDER, C. W. Deaths associated with laparoscopic sterilization by unipolar electrocoagulating devices, 1978 and 1979. *American Journal of Obstetrics and Gynecology*, **139**, 141 (1981)
20. RIOUX, J. E. and CLOUTIER, D. Laparoscopic tubal sterilization: Sparking and its control. *Vie Med. Canada Franc.*, **2**, 760 (1973)
21. RIOUX, J. E. and CLOUTIER, D. A new bipolar instrument for laparoscopic tubal sterilization. *American Journal of Obstetrics and Gynecology*, **119**, 737 (1974)
22. HULKA, J. F., FISHBURNE, J. I., MERCER, J. P. *et al.* Laparoscopic sterilization with a spring-clip: A report on the first fifty cases. *American Journal of Obstetrics and Gynecology*, **116**, 715 (1973)
23. LIEBERMAN, B. A., GORDON, A. G., BOSTOCK, J. F. *et al.* Laparoscopic sterilization with spring-loaded clips: Double puncture technique. *Journal of Reproductive Medicine*, **18**, 241 (1977)
24. BLEIER, W. Hinweise und Sammelstatistik über die Tubensterilisation mit dem Kunstoff-clip. *Archiv für Gynäkologie*, 224 (1–4), 41–42 (1977)
25. FILSHIE, G. M. The Filshie Clip. In *New Trends in Female Sterilization* (eds. D. A. F. Van Lith, L. G. Keith and E. V. Van Hall), Year Book, Chicago (1983)
26. MACKENZIE, I. Z., TURNER, E., O'SULLIVAN, G. M. and GUILLEBAUD, J. Two hundred out-patient laparoscopy clip sterilizations using local anaesthesia. *British Journal of Obstetrics and Gynaecology*, **94**, 449–453 (1987)
27. YOON, I. B. and KING, T. M. A preliminary and intermediate report on a new laparoscopic tubal ring procedure. *Journal of Reproductive Medicine*, **15**, 54 (1975)

28. HASSON, J. M. Open laparoscopy. In *Laparoscopy* (ed. J. M. Phillips), Williams and Wilkins, Baltimore, p. 145 (1977)
29. SIEGLER, A. M. The rise and fall of hysteroscopic tubal sterilization. In *Endoscopic Female Sterilization, A Comparison of Methods* (ed. J. M. Phillips), A.A.G.L. Downey, California (1983)
30. RICHART, R. M. The use of chemical agents in female sterilization. In *Female Transcervical Sterilization* (eds. G. I. Zatichni, J. D. Shelton, A. Goldsmith and J. J. Sciarra), Harper and Row, Philadelphia (1983)
31. HOSSEINIAN, A. H., LUCERO, S. and KIM M. H. Hysteroscopic implantation of uterotubal junction blocking devices. In *Advances in Female Sterilization Techniques* (ed. J. J. Sciarra), Harper and Row, Philadelphia
32. BRUNDIN, J. O. Experiences with the P Block, a hydrogelic tubal blocking device. In *Hysteroscopy, Principles and Practice* (eds. A. M. Siegler and H. J. Lindemann), Lippincott, Philadelphia (1983)
33. HAMOU, J. and TAYLOR, P. J. *Panoramic, Contact, and Microcolpohysteroscopy. in Gynecologic Practice* (Current Problems in Obstetrics and Gynecology, vol 6 no. 2), Year Book, Chicago (1982)
34. ERB, R. A. and REED, T. P. Hysteroscopic oviductal blocking with formed in place silicone rubber plugs: method and apparatus. *Journal of Reproductive Medicine*, **23**, 65 (1979)
35. GOMEL, V. Profile of women requesting reversal of sterilization. *Fertility and Sterility*, **30**, 39 (1978)
36. RIOUX, J. E. Late complications of female sterilization – a review of the literature and a proposal for further research. *Journal of Reproductive Medicine*, **19**, 329 (1977)
37. GOMEL, V. Microsurgical reversal of female sterilization: a reappraisal. *Fertility and Sterility*, **33**, 587 (1980)
38. EMERY, S. and FILSHIE, G. M. Reversal of female sterilization using the Filshie clip. In *Proceedings of the Second World Congress on Endoscopic Female Sterilization* (ed. Jordan Phillips) p. 2 (1987)

Chapter 16

Vasectomy and vasectomy reversal

W. F. Hendry

Introduction

Vasectomy is by far the most reliable method of birth control [1]. This small operation can be performed under local or general anaesthetic, it takes only a few minutes, complications – though not unknown – are obvious to the patient and seldom life threatening, and the results of the procedure can be tested to make sure that it has been effective. More than 33 million couples now rely on vasectomy in the US, the UK, India and China, and it is the contraceptive method of choice in 4%–15% of couples in Thailand, South Korea, Canada, the Netherlands, and New Zealand [2]. Nevertheless, vasectomy is quite unacceptable in many societies and to some individuals, and its popularity as a method of birth control has waned a little in recent years. This has been partly as a result of the widely reported evidence of accelerated atherosclerosis observed in rhesus monkeys following vasectomy [3], even though there is no evidence of such an effect in man, and partly because of the high likelihood of litigation if fertility returns following vasectomy even when the operation was performed correctly [4]. Furthermore, it was rumoured that vasectomy was being virtually forced upon some men in rural areas of underdeveloped countries without their proper understanding, or in exchange for financial or other incentives – a practice which led to ethical concern.

Public and medical attitudes to vasectomy have changed since the halcyon days when it could be accepted simply as 'the nicest thing a man could do for a woman'. We must therefore examine critically the effects and possible complications of this procedure in order to re-evaluate its place as a method of family planning in modern society.

Traditionally vasectomy has been presented as the final event in a man's procreative life, and the irreversibility of the procedure has been constantly stressed. Little or no mention has been made of the possibility that fertility might occasionally return spontaneously, and the prospect of vasectomy reversal has generally been ignored. Indeed, most patients seen for this latter purpose express surprise to learn that the chances of success are as high as 50 per cent. Were these aspects of vasectomy more clearly understood, public acceptance of the procedure, and confidence in it, would almost certainly improve. Vasectomy reversal will therefore be considered in detail later in this chapter.

Vasectomy

Counselling

Many of the problems associated with vasectomy can be prevented by providing sensible and informative discussion with the couple concerned about the procedure beforehand. This should include a description not only of what happens when everything goes according to plan, but also a clear warning that, as with any other surgical operation, complications can and do sometimes occur. The rather 'tinselly' image sometimes projected of vasectomy as a minor procedure with negligible risk has led some men to become extremely disgruntled when, for example, they have developed a scrotal haematoma as large as a grapefruit. Litigation has followed, not because the haematoma occurred – a complication that can follow any operation – but because no warning was given that it might happen.

Failure to mention the possibility of long-term failure due to spontaneous recanalization, an event documented clearly over 15 years [5], has certainly led to a successful claim for damages, since the finality with which the vasectomy was presented and the wording of the consent form were so specific that the wife mistook her amenorrhoea for the menopause until it was too late to have the unwanted pregnancy terminated [6]. It is evident that clear warning is essential for two reasons: firstly to enable the husband to decide whether or not to have the operation, and secondly to allow the wife to take prompt steps to seek help should a pregnancy unexpectedly occur [7].

There are a number of reasons why these matters have not always been dealt with thoroughly in the past. Often the doctor who undertakes the counselling session is not the surgeon who performs the operation. The family planning specialist needs special knowledge of all types of contraception, and may be more comfortable dealing with women. Over-zealous reassurance of an anxious husband in order to induce him to have a vasectomy, perhaps after his wife has had problems with other family planning methods, may be commendable in family medicine, but it can also be frankly misleading. Popular misconceptions about the procedure can be equally misleading, and indeed some men may not wish to know too much about the operation.

Finally, the surgeon who undertakes the procedure is often junior and inexperienced, may just be doing an occasional session, and may rely on other clinical staff for the necessary counselling. It seems clear that the consent form requires considerable revision to make sure that the patient knows exactly what is involved in the procedure. Apparently, there is no longer a legal requirement for the wife to give her written consent [7], but it seems essential to ensure that she fully understands the matter.

The couple that selects vasectomy as their method of family planning tends to be relatively young, has two or fewer children, is Social Class 3 or above, and is seldom of African or Asian descent [8]. There may be anxiety or neuroticism in the wife [9]. Although the quality of marriage can improve after vasectomy, it should be recognized that in a few couples there are strains in the marriage, and they present in the hope that the procedure will save the relationship by abolishing the fear of pregnancy [10]. In other couples, the man agrees to vasectomy at a time of emotional stress, for example soon after childbirth or during financial difficulties, and such decisions hastily made by a relatively young man may be the subject of regret in later years [11].

An experienced counsellor can assess a couple requesting the procedure, and can distinguish those who have a stable relationship and have given the matter considerable thought from the 'spur of the moment' requests often made as a result of pressure in a marriage already in difficulties. Clearly, vasectomy comes as a blessing to the former couple, freeing them from worries about unwanted pregnancy and from the side-effects of the various contraceptive methods. In the latter couple however, a flat refusal is often bitterly resented and a suggestion to think things over for a month or two is often best.

Interestingly, a surgeon is sometimes pressured to perform a vasectomy as a matter of urgency, even by medical colleagues, with little or no counselling. We have always procrastinated about such requests, and clinical experience has supported this approach.

It is the objective of the counsellor to ensure that the couple understand the rudiments of male genital-tract anatomy. A sketch can be presented which distinguishes the site of sperm production in the testis from the storage reservoirs in the ampulla and vasa, and shows the vas as the tube connecting the two. The importance of the continued use of contraception is then easily appreciated until the mandatory two negative sperm counts have been produced. The possibility of spontaneous recanalization is readily understood particularly by men with a mechanical background. The prostate can be pointed out as the site of production of the 'milky' part of the semen which continues uninterrupted following the vasectomy. The possible short- and long-term complications of vasectomy are then made clear: minor local problems in 5%–10% of cases, but with only 1% or so requiring hospital treatment; a further 1% may require re-exploration for failure to achieve azoospermia, while 0.1% may fail despite producing two negativing sperm counts. It is as well to make it clear that the procedure is 99.9%, not 100% safe.

Having answered any questions that the couple may have concerning the operation, the man should be briefly examined to decide whether the procedure should be done under local or general anaesthesia. This takes only a moment or two, and is best accomplished with him standing up, so that any hernia or varicocele can be appreciated. Any significant local abnormality, or previous scrotal surgery such as orchidopexy, is an indication for general anaesthesia.

Once the counselling session and preliminary examination have been completed, arrangements for the vasectomy can be completed according to the available local facilities. A consent form should be signed and witnessed, indicating that the patient agrees to the operation and the anaesthetic and that he understands that the intention is to render him sterile, but that no warranty or guarantee is promised or inferred. The possible delegation of the operation to another surgeon should be mentioned. Reference should also be made to the small but real risk of the late return of fertility, and it should be made clear that two negative sperm counts are mandatory before the procedure can be relied upon. Finally, the limited success rate of reversal procedures should be pointed out [6]. One copy of the form should be filed in the notes and a duplicate should be handed to the patient for future reference. It seems sensible for the wife to countersign the form, although this is not now essential.

The operation

The patient should shave the scrotum and have a bath before the operation. After applying an antiseptic skin preparation (our own preference is for a solution of povidone iodine), drapes are applied around the scrotum. If local anaesthetic is used, this is introduced into the skin and the tissues of the cord with a fine needle; 2 ml of 1% lignocaine on each side is usually sufficient. A full 5 min should then elapse before proceeding with the operation, during which time the patient can be reminded of the details of the arrangements for the follow-up sperm counts.

A short linear incision is made over the vas, which is held by Allis tissue forceps. The incision is deepened until the shiny tissue of the vas itself is seen, and this is then seized with a second pair of forceps (Allis, Soonawalla, or Craft) and drawn from the wound. Approximately 1 cm of vas is excised (and sent for histological examination if this is considered advisable), and both ends are ligated with a non-absorbable ligature such as 3.0 black silk. One end, usually the distal, should be allowed to fall back into the wound, and the spermatic fascia is closed over the defect with 2.0 chromic catgut. The other end can then be released. This technique separates the ends into different tissue planes, which reduces the likelihood of recanalization [12]. Alternatively, intraluminal bipolar diathermy can be used [13]. After making sure of haemostasis, the wound is closed with interrupted sutures (chromic catgut, Dexon, or Vicryl are all satisfactory, although we prefer the last) and a spray of plastic wound protectant (such as Nobecutane) is applied.

Recently a 'no scalpel' technique has been introduced by Dr Li Shunqiang of the Peoples Republic of China [14]. He divised a technique involving 3 instruments only, one of which was a small pair of scissors. The second instrument was a pair of grasping forceps which grasped the vas together with the overlying scrotal skin. The third instruments was a pair of small pointed curved forceps. The pointed end punctured the scrotal skin and the sheath covering the vas and up to the vas. The forceps were then opened and this exposed the vas which could be seen and easily picked out of the seath. The Li technique excises a small segment of vas deferens and interposes some spermatic fascia between the two divided ends. No skin suture is employed.

A pair of Y-front pants or other firm support should be worn for a few days until the local discomfort settles. After lying down for half an hour and perhaps having a cup of tea, the patient leaves. He should be accompanied by a friend or relative if the procedure has been completed under general anaesthetic. Instructions are given in writing as to what complication may occur and what action to take (see below), and details about follow-up sperm counts are given.

Follow-up

Semen samples are examined at 10 and 12 weeks (or thereabouts) and repeated at monthly intervals until two successive samples have confirmed complete azoospermia. Other contraception can then be discontinued.

Sometimes a few dead sperms continue to appear in the ejaculate. Medicolegally this is not adequate evidence of sterility. However, provided that there are less than 10 000 completely immotile spermatozoa per ml, and a minimum of 7 months has elapsed since the vasectomy, a 'special clearance' may be given with apparent safety [15], and others have expressed the opinion that an occasional dead sperm may be ignored [16].

If considerable numbers of spermatozoa continue to appear in the ejaculate, or if any motile spermatozoa are present, the scrotum should be re-explored and the vasectomy repeated. Analysis of over 16 000 vasectomies by 19 surgeons at a single clinic in Oxford [15] has showed that the overall failure rate was 0.36%, which varied from 0.14% to 0.41% amongst surgeons who had carried out more than 1000 procedures, and was calculated to be 1.40% or more for surgeons who had performed less than 200 vasectomies. Thus experience is clearly the most important factor in assuring a successful outcome of the procedure. Of 69 failures re-explored, 52 appeared to have recanalized, while in 12 the vas appeared to be untouched, presumably because another structure in the cord had been divided. Ligation and intraluminal diathermy appeared to be equally subject to failure once individual surgeons' results were pooled. A similar failure rate of 0.6% was reported amongst 1000 vasectomies done at the Margaret Pyke Centre in London: at re-exploration, five were found to have recanalized through a fusiform granuloma, and a third vas was found in the sixth patient [17].

Late recanalization, after two negative sperm counts, occurred in six of 16 796 patients reported from Oxford [18], and in one of 1000 reported from the Margaret Pyke Centre [17]. Several legal papers have been presented relating to other cases in which pregnancy has occurred following late recanalization, despite two negative sperm counts having been observed after the vasectomy. It is obviously essential to warn the patient that this may occur in one in every 1–2000 cases. Vasectomy is, nevertheless, still the safest form of contraception, even though it is only 99.9% safe.

Complications

The detailed study of 1000 vasectomies done under local anaesthetic at the Margaret Pyke Centre in London published in 1973 [17] defined the expected complication rate. Two patients suffered vasovagal attacks during the operative procedure and required resuscitation, one for apparent cardiac arrest. Full resuscitation equipment should therefore be on hand. Minor haematomas occurred in 3.5% of cases, and required drainage in 0.7%. Twelve individuals developed minor sepsis, but only one abscess occurred which continued to discharge until a silk suture was extruded. Three cases of epididymo-orchitis were seen. Altogether, 5.6% of patients complained of minor local symptoms, including bruising, tenderness, or a mild reaction to the skin sutures. In the large Oxford Series [15], 7.7% sought medical advice for local pain, and 3.6% for bleeding. Scrotal haematoma developed in 0.9% of cases. Eighty per cent of men returned to work in 3 days, and 96% within 1 week.

Sperm granulomas occur in the epididymis in 10%–15% of patients after vasectomy, and may lead to painful, tender nodules [19]. Occasionally patients may experience severe, unremitting epididymal pain, often associated with induration. This may persist for years after vasectomy but epididymectomy is usually effective in relieving the symptoms [20].

Immunological and long-term systemic consequences

After experimental vasoligation in animals, testicular lymph and regional lymph nodes consistently contain spermatozoa [21], and spermatozoa have been found in a para-aortic lymph node 1 year after vasectomy in a man undergoing laparotomy [22]. It is therefore not surprising that circulating antisperm antibodies can be detected by sperm-agglutination tests in the serum of 60%–80% of men after vasectomy [23–25]. There is, however, no evidence of an increased incidence of other autoantibodies [25].

Antisperm antibodies can also produce circulating immune complexes. Diet-induced atherosclerosis has been shown to develop more extensively in vasectomized monkeys than in sham-operated control monkeys fed on the same diet, and was most pronounced in the abdominal aorta, coronary, carotid, and intracranial arteries [3]. This effect was attributed to immune-complex deposition damaging the vascular endothelium. Vasectomized monkeys fed on normal (cholesterol-free) monkey diet also developed more severe atherosclerosis after 9–14 years than age-matched non-vasectomized controls [26]. Subsequently, the same workers have reported that vasectomy had no significant effect on atherosclerosis in cynomolgus monkeys, irrespective of their responsiveness to dietary cholesterol [26a]. In humans, however, no excess of autoimmune, cardiovascular, or endocrine disease was found in a study of 1760 vasectomized men, followed up for a total of 4500 man-years [27]. The prevalence of prior vasectomy was the same in 55 men aged less than 50 with onset of coronary heart disease, and in a matched control group of close relatives [28].

Linet *et al.* [29] found no increase in arteriosclerotic retinopathy in 46 vasectomized men compared to control men of the same age, and there were no significant differences in the results of tests for circulating immune complexes. Petitti *et al.* [30] compared 4385 vasectomized men and 13 155 non-vasectomized men matched for age and race and found no significant differences in blood pressure, blood count, serum urea and electrolytes, or liver function tests. Walker *et al.* [31] found a significant increase in hospitalization rates only with genitourinary disease, chiefly in the first years after vasectomy, but otherwise there was no difference in new hospitalization rates amongst 6092 vasectomized men compared to controls; in a subsequent study, no increase in non-fatal myocardial infarction was demonstrated [32].

Massey *et al.* [33] matched 10 590 vasectomized men with a paired neighbourhood control for each: mean elapsed time between the vasectomy and interview or death was 7.9 years; 2318 pairs had 10 or more years of follow-up. The vasectomized men had fewer cancers, lymphomas and leukaemias, and less overt cardiovascular disease than controls; however, there was an excess of epididymo-orchitis in vasectomized men, especially in the first year after the procedure. In 8 rural communities in China, Tang *et al.* found 4596 men examined 10–25 (average 14.5) years after vasectomy to be generally healthier than 4340 control subjects, as judged by clinical examination, resting and stress ECG and fundal inspection [33a]. Only Campbell *et al.* [34] claimed to have found a possible association between vascular disease and vasectomy in man, as evidenced by some loss of distensibility of the posterior tibial arteries. Otherwise, there is no evidence whatsoever at the present time that vasectomy is associated with the development of cardiovascular or other systemic disease in man. Some of these studies have, however, uncovered evidence of a small but significant incidence of local epididymal problems after the procedure, probably as a result of sperm granulomas [19] and usually most evident in the early years after the operation. Although the remote possibility of rare or long-term systemic ill-effects of vasectomy cannot yet be completely ruled out [35], there seems to be every reason to reassure prospective vasectomy candidates on these points on the basis of currently available evidence.

Vasectomy reversal

Increasing popularity of vasectomy as a method of birth control has inevitably led to an increased demand for reversal, which probably occurs in 1–3% of the vasectomized population for a variety of reasons, including remarriage, death of children, change of heart, or altered financial circumstances. Howard [11] has studied the question 'Who asks for vasectomy reversal and why?', and found that over one-half were divorced or separated from their wives, and felt disadvantaged in courtship or remarriage by being infertile; amongst those who had remarried, many wives were said to be desperate for a pregnancy. Most requests for reversal came from men who had been under 35 at the time of vasectomy, and had often decided to have the operation done at a time of emotional crisis.

There is no fundamental reason why fertility should not be restored by reconnection of the testes after vasectomy; sperm production is well maintained in most animal species, with the possible exception of rabbits and guinea-pigs [36,37]. Certainly, normal spermatogenesis has been observed in testicular biopsies from 58 of 62 men, taken 1 month to 10 years following vasectomy [38]. However, technical difficulties with vas anastomosis, secondary changes in the epididymis, and in some cases the immunological reaction provoked by the spermatozoa, make the chances of successful restoration of fertility by vasectomy reversal only a little better than 50%.

Operative technique

Under general anaesthetic, an oblique incision is made on the lateral aspect of the scrotum, so that it can be extended up to the inguinal region to obtain more length of vas should this prove necessary. The superior end is identified first, cleaned of surrounding adhesions and mobilized enough to allow it to meet the inferior end without tension. The inferior end is then identified and cleaned. Once the mobilization is completed, an 0.5 cm linear incision is made in the inferior end of the vas just below the point of transection, and the tail of the epididymis is squeezed to express milky fluid from the vas. The superior end is similarly incised and the lumen defined with a fine nylon probe. The ends of the vasa are then brought together, using a specially designed approximator or tissue forceps.

Various techniques of anastomosis have been described. Silber [39] has developed a two-layer method of end-to-end union using an operating microscope (× 16 to × 25), ultrafine suture material (9.0 nylon), and an exquisitely careful technique. Other surgeons have less elaborate methods of vasostomy with magnifying spectacles (× 2 to × 4) and 6.0 prolene sutures. A side-to-side anastomosis is favoured by ourselves; this has the advantage of producing a wide opening between the vasa, irrespective of disproportion in their diameters (Figure 16.1). Whichever technique is used, it is essential that the stitching in the suture line should be accurate, to prevent sperm leakage into the tissues and granuloma formation which lead to scarring and secondary obstruction of the anastomosis [40,41]. Splints were favoured by some surgeons, but most are now dispensing with them as their microsurgical techniques

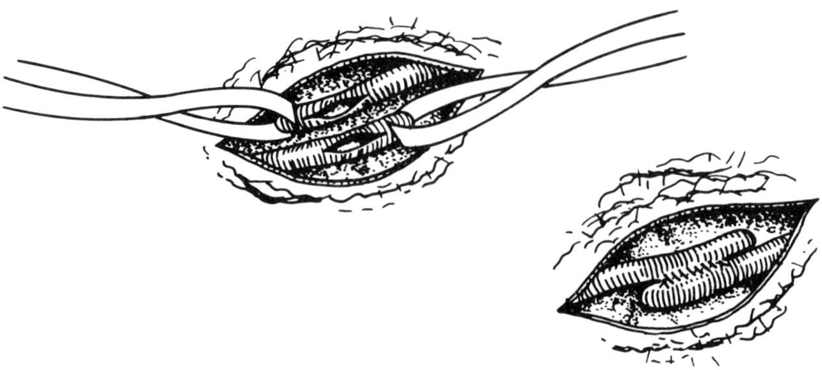

Figure 16.1. Vasostomy by overlapped side-to-side anastomosis using 6.0 prolene and no splint

improve. Comparative studies have shown an increased obstruction rate following the use of splints [42], probably caused by sperm leakage due to partial obstruction by the splint, or occurring around its point of exit.

The scrotum is closed with 3.0 catgut for the dartos muscle and subcuticular nylon or Vicryl for the skin. Follow-up sperm counts are done at 3, 6 and 12 months.

Results

The sperm count rises slowly after vasectomy reversal and usually reaches a plateau by 6 months. A collective review of 13 papers [43] showed that normal sperm counts were reported in 37%–92% (average 60%) of cases, with pregnancies in 10%–60% (mean 44%) of wives. In another collective review of 20 papers [44], 49% of 2685 cases showed return of sperm to the ejaculate, with 21% of wives of 2177 men becoming pregnant. The results of some series have been considerably better than this. For example, Silber [37] has reported a pregnancy rate of 71% in the first 42 patients followed for 15 months. Comparative studies have shown slightly superior results with a microsurgical technique [45].

Soonawalla and Lal [46] reported patency and pregnancy rates of 81.4% and 43.9% respectively in 194 cases using a macroscopic stented technique, which improved to 89% and 63.2% in 339 cases with a non-stented microscopic technique.

Several other factors have been shown to have an influence on the likelihood of success. The finding of sperm in the fluid from the testicular end of the vas indicated a favourable prognosis, whereas the absence of such sperm were associated with an increasingly poor prognosis with lengthening time since vasectomy. Overall, the likelihood of regaining a normal sperm count fell from 91% within 10 years of vasectomy to 35% after more than 10 years [39]. This may have been a reflection of the development of secondary changes in the epididymis [47]. Vasectomy increases the pressure in the testicular end of the vas which is transmitted to the epididymis. Rupture of tubules in the epididymis may produce granulomata and epididymal obstruction, and the epididymis should therefore be examined in cases with no fluid in the vas to see whether epididymovasostomy is indicated. Granuloma formation at the cut testicular end of the vas is associated with significant reduction in dilatation of the vas; better-quality vas fluid was observed in the absence of such dilatation, possibly as a result of protection against back pressure [39]. Vasectomy can also damage the nerves lying adjacent to the vas [48] and degenerative changes have been described in the alpha-adrenergic nerve supply to the testicular end of the vas and the cauda epididymis; these nerves regenerated slowly after vasovasostomy, and this may account for the slow recovery of normal ejaculate content after vasectomy reversal [49].

Antisperm antibodies develop in the serum of 60%–80% of men following vasectomy [23–25], but their effects on fertility following vasectomy reversal are poorly understood. For example, Sullivan and Howe [50] found agglutinating antibodies in the serum of no less than 48% of 29 men whose wives became pregnant, although this was significantly less than in 16 men whose wives did not, of whom 94% had such antibodies. The relation between pre- and post-vasectomy reversal antisperm antibodies and fertility was clarified considerably by Linnet *et al.* [51] who showed that antibodies were detectable in seminal fluid of only two of 29 men before bilateral vasovasostomies, but were present in ten men (34%) afterwards. Twenty of these men were trying to produce children: 11 pregnancies resulted amongst the 13 women whose men had no antibodies in seminal plasma, but only one among the

Table 16.1 Incidence of pregnancy in spouse 1 year or more after vasectomy reversal related to serum TAT titre (from Parslow *et al.* [51])

Serum TAT titre	*Total no.*	*Information available*	*Sperm count (m/ml)*			*? Pregnancy*	
			0	*<20*	*≥20*	*Trying*	*Success*
≤16	40	32	5	7	20	29	15 (52%)
32–256	40	36	1	14	21	32	17 (53%)
≥512	41	31	2	9	20	28	7 (25%)

seven whose men had such antibodies. This highly significant association established a relationship between *seminal plasma* antibodies and fertility after vasectomy reversal.

We measured antisperm antibodies in serum and seminal plasma in 130 males before and after vasectomy reversal, and the occurrence of pregnancy was analysed in those partners who were trying to produce a pregnancy. All patients were followed for at least one year. Sperm agglutinating antibodies were found in the serum of 79% of patients; seminal plasma antibodies were present in only 9.5% before reversal, and this rose to 29.5% afterwards [52]. Overall, pregnancies occurred in the partners of 44.6% of those men who were trying to produce children. Production of pregnancy was significantly less likely when the preoperative serum antisperm antibody titre was 512 or more, but no decrease in fertility was seen with titres below this (Table 16.1). Similar numbers of pregnancies were produced by patients with or without seminal plasma antibodies, in titres of up to 16. This is different from the conclusions of Linnet *et al.* [51], and from spontaneously infertile males. Further studies have shown that this distinction may be due to the antibodies being of a different class. Most of the antibody produced after vasectomy is IgG, and some may transude into the seminal plasma, whereas in spontaneously infertile males the seminal plasma antibody is probably produced locally in the genital tract as IgA; it appears that the locally produced antibody has a greater adverse effect on fertility [53].

Failed vasectomy reversal

With good surgical technique, vasectomy reversal should successfully restore a man's fertility in over 50% of cases [54]. If the operation is unsuccessful, with sperms appearing in the ejaculate only transiently or not at all, the scrotum should be re-explored. Our results in 23 such cases are summarized in Table 16.2 [55].

There appear to be four distinct causes of failure of vasectomy reversal. The most common by far, which should be anticipated in about one-half of these patients, results from stenosis or blockage of the previous vasovasostomy. It is known that spermatozoa tend to leak out of the anastomosis when vasovasostomy is performed, and these may produce local granulomas. Hagan and Coffey [41] showed that the presence of spermatozoa at the site of anastomosis led to sperm granuloma formation and that this appeared to be an important cause of failure of vasovasostomy. In 1977 Silber [39] showed that excellent results can be obtained by re-doing the vasovasostomy using an obsessively careful technique. We favour our method of vasovasostomy using an overlapped side-to-side anastomosis with continuous 60 prolene, which offers considerable advantages. Not only is a large opening obtained between the two parts of the vas, but the use of continuous prolene suture produces a

Table 16.2 Results of re-exploration of scrotum in 23 patients who remained azoospermic after vasectomy reversal (from Royle and Hendry [55])

			Follow-up sperm count (m/ml)			
Category	*Treatment*	*No.*	*0*	*<20*	*20≥*	*Pregnancies**
1 Blocked vas	Redo vas-vas	12	1	3	7	5/8 (62%)
2 Epididymal block	Ep-vas	4	1		3	2/4 (50%)
3 Antisperm antibodies (≥1024)	Surgery + prednisolone	7	1	3	3	0/7
						7/19 (37%)

(* Trying for 6 months or more)

watertight anastomosis, which discourages the leakage of spermatozoa from the anastomosis, and hence reduces the tendency towards granuloma formation. Furthermore, the use of a side-to-side technique eliminates any technical difficulties due to differences in the calibre of either end of the vas. As may be seen from the excellent results in terms of restoration of normal sperm count, and the incidence of pregnancy in wives, the success rate in this group is equivalent to that obtained with a first vasovasostomy (Table 16.2).

The second most common cause of failure of reversal is epididymal blockage, presumably from back pressure from the site of the vasectomy, leading to rupture of epididymal tubules with local sperm granuloma formation within the epididymis. Histological examination of a section of epididymis removed at the time of epididymovasostomy will often demonstrate rupture of an epididymal tubule with surrounding sperm granuloma formation; this leads to the secondary blockage in the epididymis upstream of the original site of the vasectomy. Silber has described a technique for mobilizing the epididymis and anastomosing it to the vas [56]. We have confirmed that excellent results can be obtained following epididymovasostomy in these cases, although restoration of normal sperm count generally takes rather longer than following vasovasostomy.

The problem of the patient who develops very high antisperm antibody response to his vasectomy continues to defy successful treatment. In our previous studies we showed that pregnancy was possible despite high antisperm antibody titres, but we have defined a small sub-population in whom, despite re-exploration of the scrotum and prednisolone therapy [57], restoration of fertility does not seem to be possible; this is apparently due to the immunological response to the spermatozoa. The problem continues to present a significant therapeutic challenge.

Finally, spermatogenesis may have ceased. Our analyses [55], and those of Bagshaw *et al.* [38], show by testicular biopsy studies that significant impairment of spermatogenesis following vasectomy is in fact extremely uncommon. Nevertheless, the possibility should be considered amongst this population of patients, many of whom are entering middle life at the time that this surgery is carried out.

Summary and conclusions

Vasectomy remains the safest method of birth control, and there is much to commend it in the setting of a stable family relationship. There is, however, considerable evidence that some aspects of this operation have been wrongly presented in an attempt to widen its popularity and increase public acceptance. A simple procedure it may be, but it is not totally free of complications; it sometimes has to be repeated and, rarely, it may fail even after the most stringent precautions. It is the duty of those who counsel prospective candidates, and of surgeons who undertake this procedure, to make sure that these facts are clearly understood, and that this is recorded on a signed and witnessed consent form.

Any organization which includes vasectomy in its programme of family planning should include advice and referral for vasectomy reversal, in exactly the same way that the pill may be stopped or a coil be removed. Fertility can be successfully restored by vasovasostomy in 50% of men who wish to have their vasectomies reversed, often after changes in personal circumstances beyond their immediate control.

References

1. VESSEY, M., LAWLESS, M. and YEATES, D. Efficacy of different contraceptive methods. *Lancet*, **1**, 841–842 (1982)
2. Vasectomy – safe and simple. *Population Reports*, **11**, 61–99 (1984)
3. ALEXANDER N. J. and CLARKSON, T. B. Vasectomy increases the severity of diet-induced atherosclerosis in *Macaca fascicularis*. *Science*, **201**, 538–541 (1978)
4. KOONTZ, W. W. and RUSSELL, J. B. Thoughts on the prevention of urologic liability claims. *Journal of Urology*, **118**, 695–697 (1977)
5. PUGH, R. C. B. and HANLEY, H. G. Spontaneous recanalisation of the divided vas deferens. *British Journal of Urology*, **41**, 340–347 (1969)
6. BRAHAMS, D. Damages awarded for failed vasectomy. *Lancet*, **2**, 704–705 (1984)
7. Editorial. Late failure of vasectomy. *Lancet*, **1**, 794–795 (1985)
8. HOWARD, G. Motivation for vasectomy. *Lancet*, **1**, 545 (1978)
9. HOWARD, G. Anxiety and neuroticism in couples requesting vasectomy. *British Journal of Family Planning*, **6** (3), 67–69 (1980)
10. HOWARD, G. The quality of marriage before and after vasectomy. *British Journal of Sexual Medicine*, **6**, 13–15 (1979)
11. HOWARD, G. Who asks for vasectomy reversal and why? *British Medical Journal*, **285**, 490–492 (1982)
12. ESHO, J. O. and CASS, A. S. Recanalization rate following methods of vasectomy using interposition of fascial sheath of vas deferens. *Journal of Urology*, **120**, 178–179 (1978)
13. SCHMIDT, S. S. and FREE, M. J. The bipolar needle for vasectomy. I. Experience with the first 1000 cases. *Fertility and Sterility*, **29**, 676–680 (1978)
14. HUBER, D. Advances in voluntary surgical contraception. *Outlook*, **6**, pp. 2–6 (Ed. J. Sherris) Path and Piact, Washington. (1988)
15. PHILP, T., GUILLEBAUD, J. and BUDD, D. Complications of vasectomy: Review of 16 000 patients. *British Journal of Urology*, **56**, 745–748 (1984)
16. BLANDY, J. P. Vasectomy. *British Journal of Hospital Medicine*, **21**, 520–527 (1979)
17. BARNES, M. N. *et al.* One thousand vasectomies. *British Medical Journal*, **4**, 216–221 (1973)
18. PHILP, T., GUILLEBAUD, J. and BUDD, D. Late failure of vasectomy after 2 documented analysis showing azoospermic semen. *British Medical Journal*, **289**, 77–79 (1984)
19. SCHMIDT, S. S. Spermatic granuloma: an often painful lesion. *Fertility and Sterility*, **31**, 178–181 (1979)
20. SELIKOWITZ, S. M. and SCHNED, A. R. A late post-vasectomy syndrome. *Journal of Urology*, **134**, 494–497 (1985)
21. BALL, R. Y. and SETCHELL, B. P. The passage of spermatozoa to regional lymph nodes in testicular lymph following vasectomy in rams and boars. *Journal of Reproduction and Fertility*, **68**, 145–153 (1983)
22. BALL, R. Y., NAYLOR, C. P. E. and MITCHINSON, M. J. Spermatozoa in an abdominal lymph node after vasectomy in a man. *Journal of Reproduction and Fertility*, **66**, 715–716 (1982)
23. HELLEMA, J. W. J. and RUMKE, P. Sperm autoantibodies as a consequence of vasectomy. I. Within 1 year post-operation. *Clinical and Experimental Immunology*, **31**, 18–29 (1978)

24. HELLEMA, H. W., SAMUEL, T. and RUMKE, P. Sperm antibodies as a consequence of vasectomy. II. Long-term follow-up studies. *Clinical and Experimental Immunology*, **36**, 31–36 (1979)
25. ROSE, N. R. and LUCAS, P. L. Immunological consequences of vasectomy. II. Two-year summary of prospective study. In *Vasectomy: Immunologic and Pathophysiologic Effects in Animals and Man* (eds. I. H. Lepow and R. Crozier), Academic Press, New York, pp. 533–560 (1979)
26. ALEXANDER, N. J. and ANDERSON, D. J. Vasectomy: consequences of auto immunity to sperm antigens. *Fertility and Sterility*, **32**, 253–260 (1979)
26a CLARKSON, T. B., ALEXANDER, N. J., and MORGAN, T. M. Atherosclerosis of cynomolgus monkeys hyper- and hyporesponsive to dietary cholesterol: lack of effect of vasectomy. *Arteriosclerosis*, **8**, 488–498 (1988)
27. GOLDACRE, M. J., CLARKE, J. A., HEASMAN, M. A. and VESSEY, M. P. Follow-up of vasectomy using medical record linkage. *American Journal of Epidemiology*, **108**, 176–180 (1978)
28. WALLACE, R. B., LEE, J., GERBER, W. L. *et al.* Vasectomy and coronary disease in men less than 50 years old: absence of association. *Journal of Urology*, **126**, 182–184 (1981)
29. LINNET, L., MOLLER, N. P. H., BERNTH-PETERSEN, P. *et al.* No increase in arteriosclerotic retinopathy or activity in tests for circulating immune complexes 5 years after vasectomy. *Fertility and Sterility*, **37**, 798–806 (1982)
30. PETTITI, D. B., KLEIN, R., KIPP, H. *et al.* Physiologic measures in men with and without vasectomies. *Fertility and Sterility*, **37**, 438–440 (1982)
31. WALKER, A. M., JICK, H., HUNTER, J. R. *et al.* Hospitalization rates in vasectomized men. *Journal of the American Medical Association*, **245**, 2315–2317 (1951)
32. WALKER, A. M., JICK, H., HUNTER, J. R. and MCEVOY, J. Vasectomy and non fatal myocardial infarction: continued observations indicates no elevation of risk. *Journal of Urology*, **130**, 936–937 (1983)
33. MASSEY, F. J. *et al.* Vasectomy and health: results from a large cohort study. *Journal of the American Medical Association*, **252**, 1023–1030 (1984)
33a TANG, G. H., ZHONG, Y. H. and MA, Y. M. *et al.* Vasectomy and health: cardiovascular and other diseases following vasectomy in Sichuan province, People's Republic of China. *Int. J. Epidemiol.*, **17**, 608–617 (1988)
34. CAMPBELL, W. B., SLACK, R. W. T., CLIFFORD, P. C. *et al.* Vasectomy and atherosclerosis: an association in man? *British Journal of Urology*, **55**, 430–433 (1983)
35. Leading Article. Safety of vasectomy. *Lancet*, **2**, 1057–1958 (1979)
36. FAWCETT, D. W. Interpretation of the sequelae of vasectomy. In *Vasectomy: Immunologic and Pathophysiologic Effects in Animals and Man* (ed. I. H. Lepow and R. Crozier), Academic Press, New York, pp. 3–21 (1979)
37. SILBER, S. J. Vasectomy and vasectomy reversal. *Fertility and Sterility*, **29**, 125–140 (1978)
38. BAGSHAW, H. A., MASTERS, J. R. W. and PRYOR, J. P. Factors influencing the outcome of vasectomy reversal. *British Journal of Urology*, **52**, 57–60 (1980)
39. SILBER, S. J. Microscopic vasectomy reversal. *Fertility and Sterility*, **28**, 1191–1202 (1977)
40. SCHMIDT, S. S. Anastomosis of the vas deferens: an experimental study. II. Successes and failures in experimental anastomosis. *Journal of Urology*, **81**, 203–205 (1959)
41. HAGAN, K. F. and COFFEY, D. S. The adverse effects of sperm during vasovasostomy. *Journal of Urology*, **118**, 269–273 (1977)
42. THOMAS, A. J., PONTES, J. E., BUDDHDEV, H. and PIERCE, J. M. Vasovasostomy: evaluation of four surgical techniues. *Fertility and Sterility*, **32**, 324–328 (1979)
43. HULKA, J. F. and DAVIS, J. E. Vasectomy and reversible vasocclusion. *Fertility and Sterility*, **23**, 683–696 (1972)
44. WICKLUND, R. and ALEXANDER, N. J. Vaso-vasostomy: evaluation of success. *Urology*, **13**, 532–534 (1979)
45. LEE, L. and MCLOUGHLIN, M. G. Vasovasostomy: a comparison of macroscopic and microscopic techniques at one institution. *Fertility and Sterility*, **33**, 54–55 (1980)
46. SOONAWALLA, F. B. and LAL, S. S. Microsurgery in Vasovasectomy. *Indian Journal of Urology*, **1**, 104–108 (1984)
47. SILBER, S. J. Epididymal extravasation following vasectomy as a cause for failure of vasectomy reversal. *Fertility and Sterility*, **31**, 309–315 (1979)

48. PABST, R., MARTIN, O. and LIPPERT, H. Is the low fertility rate after vasovasostomy caused by nerve resection during vasectomy. *Fertility and Sterility*, **31**, 316–320 (1979)
49. ALEXANDER, N. J., FULGHAM, D. L., TOYOOKA, D. C. *et al.* Innervation of the rabbit ductus deferens after vasectomy and vasovasostomy. *Biology of Reproduction*, **21**, 161–171 (1979)
50. SULLIVAN, M. J. and HOWE, G. E. Correlation of circulating antisperm antibodies to functional success in vasovasostomy. *Journal of Urology*, **117**, 189–191 (1977)
51. LINNET, L., HJORT, T. and FOGH-ANDERSEN, P. Association between failure to impregnate after vasovasostomy and sperm agglutinins in semen. Lancet, **1**, 117–119 (1981)
52. PARSLOW, J. M., ROYLE, M. G., KINGSCOTT, M. M. B. *et al.* The effects of sperm antibodies on fertility after vasectomy reversal. *American Journal of Reproductive Immunology*, **3**, 28–31 (1983)
53. PARSLOW, J. M., POULTON, T. A., BESSER, G. M. and HENDRY, W. F. The clinical relevance of classes of immunoglobulins on spermatozoa from infertile and vasovasostomised males. *Fertility and Sterility*, **43**, 621–627 (1985)
54. COS, L. R., VALVO, J. R., DAVIS, R. S. and COCKETT, A. T. K. Vasovasostomy: current state of the art. *Urology*, **22**, 567–575 (1983)
55. ROYLE, M. G. and HENDRY, W. F. Why does vasectomy reversal fail? *British Journal of Urology*, **57**, 780–783 (1985)
56. SILBER, S. J. Microsurgical vasoepididymostomy. In *Reproductive Infertility Microsurgery in the Male and Female* (ed. S. J. Silber), Williams and Wilkins, Baltimore, 132–146 (1984)
57. HENDRY, W. F., TREEHUBA, K., HUGHES, L. *et al.* Cyclic prednisolone therapy for male infertility associated with antibodies to spermatozoa. *Fertility and Sterility*, **45**, 249–254 (1986)

Chapter 17

Progress towards a systemic male contraceptive

S. L. Jeffcoate

Introduction

Every 'scare' occasioned by reports on possible side-effects of systemic contraception (whether oral or injectable) in the human female generates the question 'What about the male pill?'. The short answer is that progress is very slow and limited, for reasons which are detailed in the specific sections and in the general conclusions that follow. Whilst much experimental work is being done, few clinical trials are in progress and no method is anywhere near routine use. The methods divide, fundamentally, into two approaches (though some drugs, such as gossypol, may have both types of action): reduction of sperm numbers, and inhibition of sperm function. Each method needs to be assessed by five criteria (neatly summarized by the acronym, 'SCARE'): safety, cheapness, acceptability, reversibility, effectiveness.

Interference with sperm production

Methods designed to interfere with testicular spermatogenesis, and thus to reduce, preferably to zero, the numbers of sperm in the ejaculate are of three types: hormonal inhibition of hypothalamic–pituitary function, specific inhibition of pituitary FSH secretion or action, and direct testicular action.

Inhibition of hypothalamic–pituitary function

These approaches, using either steroids or LHRH analogues (or combinations), are equivalent to methods in use in women. They are aimed at inhibiting the secretion of pituitary gonadotrophin so that the testis is deprived of its stimulatory drive and spermatogenesis ceases. A major drawback is that as well as FSH secretion being inhibited, LH secretion is also reduced, with a resultant fall in testosterone secretion from the Leydig cells. Since males require testosterone for their libido and potency (as well as hair growth, muscles, etc.) androgen replacement is required, thus increasing the cost, complexity and potential hazards of the methods.

Steroids

Steroids have been the subject of a number of studies, both experimental and clinical [1,2]. Although androgens and progestogens have been tried separately, it is generally considered that combinations of the two which maximize pituitary inhibition and also replace androgen, are preferable. Perhaps the most likely to succeed is 19-nortestosterone, which combines androgen and progestogen action in a single molecule and has been found to be effective in monkeys, and in a small trial, in men [3]. Other steroids such as danazol or the antiandrogen, cyproterone acetate, either alone or in combination, have been disappointing. The major and probably fatal specific disadvantage of the steroid methods are: doubts about safety and acceptability (systemic controlled release systems avoiding the oral route could help here); cost (the amounts of steroid required to inhibit pituitary–testicular function are about 100 times greater than for pituitary–ovarian function in the female); effectiveness (see below). Reversibility is not a problem.

LHRH analogues

LHRH analogues are of two types [4]. The 'superactive' LHRH agonists are the most developed and widely used. After an initial stimulatory phase lasting 2–3 weeks, these agonists inhibit gonadotrophin secretion by blocking pituitary LHRH receptors (down-regulation). The LHRH antagonists are less well developed, but increasingly potent derivatives are becoming available. For both types the disadvantages are: cost (new methods of peptide synthesis on an industrial scale may reduce this) and the potential side-effects of continued low androgen levels which would need to be supplemented. This combination has been shown to be effective in monkeys.

As in other areas of pharmacology development of controlled-release systems (e.g. with the peptide incorporated in biodegradable implants which give zero-order release for weeks or months) will considerably improve the acceptability of these LHRH analogues. Reversibility is no problem but it seems unlikely that they will ever be widely used for male contraception.

Inhibition of FSH

Specific inhibition of FSH, which controls spermatogenesis, leaving LH secretion intact would have clear advantages over the methods inhibiting hypothalamopituitary function, since androgen replacement would be unnecessary. Unfortunately it is not possible yet, nor likely to be for the foreseeable future.

Inhibin

Inhibin is a dimeric polypeptide secreted by testicular Sertoli cells which selectively inhibits pituitary FSH secretion. It has recently been isolated and synthesized by recombinant DNA techniques. In theory it could be a rational approach to male contraception without interfering with Leydig cell function, but it is an expensive and complicated approach and progress is slow.

Immunological inhibition of FSH

Immunological inhibition of FSH has been studied in non-human primates. It involves a standard active immunization procedure, with boosters, using FSH as an antigen. In practice, other materials (adjuvants) are used to maximize antibody responses, and these cause unacceptable local skin lesions (from inflammation to ulcer formation). Although these methods are effective in inducing reversible azoospermia in monkeys without affecting Leydig cell function, antibody responses are variable from subject to subject and need to be monitored so that appropriate boosters can be given. For these reasons, it is difficult to envisage any immunological approach (whether active or by passive transfer) being used in male contraception; this conclusion applies also to anti-LHRH immunization, which has been tried in a number of species.

Direct inhibition of spermatogenesis

A number of drugs, industrial agents (e.g. pesticides), and other agents (e.g. irradiation) are known to damage seminiferous tubule function in man, reversibly or irreversibly, without affecting androgen production from the Leydig cells [5]. Only one (gossypol) is the subject of serious investigation at the present time.

Gossypol

Gossypol is perhaps the most promising of the current approaches to a systemic male contraceptive [6]. It is a toxic pigment present in high concentration in the seed and bark of the cotton plant and in oil extracted from it. Following the observed association between cooking with cotton-seed oil and male infertility in parts of China in the 1950s, clinical trials were initiated and reported in 1978 and 1981. Nearly 9000 men have taken part in these trials: gossypol was found to be over 99% effective in inducing azoospermia, or severe oligospermia. Gossypol also reduces sperm motility. Few side-effects were reported, hypokalaemia being the most important. In animals, however, there is only a narrow gap between effective and toxic doses with marked species and strain differences. There are also doubts about reversibility: as many as 10% of subjects are permanently azoospermic. Gossypol exists as two isomers which may have different effectiveness : toxicity ratios, although they are difficult to separate chemically. These and an increasing number of derivatives and analogues are being intensively prepared and studied. An effective, safe, reversible pill based on these studies seems a long way off.

Conclusions

In addition to the specific drawbacks attached to the individual methods described above, there is a major limiting problem with methods aimed at a chemical reduction or abolition of sperm numbers. Not only is there at least a 3-month delay (because of the time-scale of spermatogenesis) between initiation of therapy and an effect, but also even a major (e.g. 90%) reduction of sperm numbers will still leave some spermatozoa, and a potentially fertile man. In my view this makes approaches at interfering with sperm function more likely to be successful.

Interference with sperm function

Efforts at inhibiting the fertilizing capacity of human spermatozoa suffer from a major handicap: lack of knowledge of the factors involved in the normal process of maturation and capacitation, and in the control of this process. Two main approaches are under study: immunological and pharmacological.

Potential use of anti-sperm antibodies

About 10% of males with infertility have anti-sperm antibodies (though the prevalence varies in different centres and according to the laboratory method used). There is a bewildering variety of these antibodies: they can be of the IgG, IgA or IgM classes, and present in male or female blood plasma or in seminal plasma. They can interfere with sperm transport, fertilization of the ovum, or even implantation. Treatment which reduces the antibodies is reported to be successful in inducing fertility, although it should be said that this is a field of some controversy.

These clinical observations have been used as a starting point for the possible development of immunological methods whereby sperm are immobilized or otherwise rendered infertile by artificially induced antibodies. Basic research is aimed at 'mapping' the considerable number of antigenic sites on the sperm head using monoclonal antibodies *in vitro*. These studies are likely to yield important information on sperm structure and function, but whether they will lead to a viable means of male contraception is less certain. Major objections to active immunization in man have already been mentioned, and in the case of anti-sperm antibodies it seems likely to be most effective (and may *only* be effective) if it is the female partner who harbours the antibodies.

Pharmacological approaches

In the absence of clear and detailed knowledge of the process of sperm capacitation and the factors regulating fertilization, most of the approaches have arisen serendipitously.

6-chloro, 6-deoxy sugars

These have been tested in a number of species, especially rodents, because of the dependence of sperm metabolism in hexose sugars in seminal plasma. Some, for example 6-chloro, 6-deoxyglucose, are highly effective at inhibiting the activity of epididymal spermatozoa. Unfortunately they are also markedly neurotoxic, particularly in primates, but their study may contribute to the development of a future male contraceptive by knowledge gained from their use as research tools.

Sulphasalazine and propranolol

These two drugs are widely used clinically (for ulcerative colitis and to induce beta-adrenoceptor blockade, respectively); they have been found, coincidentally, to cause infertility in a number of male patients by reducing sperm motility. These effects are reversible, and whilst the drugs themselves are not necessarily suitable for contraception, once again they could provide the starting point for other initiatives.

Conclusions

It can be seen that progress towards a safe, cheap, acceptable, reversible and effective male contraceptive is slow. In general, methods aimed at interfering with sperm function are more likely to succeed than those interfering with spermatogenesis itself. Unfortunately, since the process of capacitation takes place in the female genital tract after ejaculation, it is likely that it will be women who have to take the male pill! This may not be so crazy, because even in Western societies contraception is perceived to be a female concern, and many women express the view that they would rather control their own destiny than rely on a man to take a pill.

Another reason for slow progress is a lack of basic knowledge of male reproduction and fertility, compared to that of the female, at a time when there are constraints on research funding both in the public sector and in the pharmaceutical industry. Even if a promising lead is found the time-scale is a long one before a product is widely used, because of the stringent toxicological studies and licensing procedures compared with 25 years ago when the female pill was first widely available. The prospects are, therefore, gloomy.

References

1. NIESHLAG, E., WICKINGS, E. J. and BREUER, H. Chemical methods for male fertility control. *Contraception*, **23**, 1–10 (1981)
2. PRYOR, J. P. The role of steroids as male contraceptives. In *Progress Towards a Male Contraceptive* (ed. S. L. Jeffcoate), J. Wiley, Chichester. pp. 135–142 (1982)
3. SHÜRMEYER, T., KNUTH, U. A., BELKEIN, L. and NEISCHLAG, E. Reversible azoospermia induced by the anabolic steroid, 19-nortestosterone. *Lancet*, **1**, 417–420 (1984)
4. SANDOW, J. Inhibition of pituitary and testicular function by LHRH analogues. In: *Progress Towards a Male Contraceptive* (ed. S. L. Jeffcoate), J. Wiley, Chichester, pp. 19–39 (1982)
5. JEFFCOATE, S. L. (ed.) *Progress Towards a Male Contraceptive*. J. Wiley, Chichester (1982)
6. Editorial. Gossypol prospects. *Lancet*, **1**, 1108–1109 (1984)

Index